The Confederate
Yellow Fever
Conspiracy

The Confederate Yellow Fever Conspiracy

*The Germ Warfare Plot of
Luke Pryor Blackburn, 1864–1865*

H. LEON GREENE

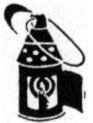

McFarland & Company, Inc., Publishers
Jefferson, North Carolina

LIBRARY OF CONGRESS CATALOGUING-IN-PUBLICATION DATA

Names: Greene, H. Leon, 1944– author.
Title: The Confederate yellow fever conspiracy : the germ warfare plot of Luke Pryor Blackburn, 1864–1865 / H. Leon Greene.
Description: Jefferson, North Carolina : McFarland & Company, Inc., Publishers, 2019. | Includes bibliographical references and index.
Identifiers: LCCN 2019001062 | ISBN 9781476668901 (softcover : acid free paper) ∞
Subjects: LCSH: Yellow fever—Northern States—History—19th century. | Blackburn, Luke Pryor, 1816–1887.
Classification: LCC RA644.Y4 G74 2019 | DDC 614.5/41—dc23
LC record available at https://lccn.loc.gov/2019001062

BRITISH LIBRARY CATALOGUING DATA ARE AVAILABLE

ISBN (print) 978-1-4766-6890-1
ISBN (ebook) 978-1-4766-3100-4

© 2019 H. Leon Greene. All rights reserved

No part of this book may be reproduced or transmitted in any form or by any means, electronic or mechanical, including photocopying or recording, or by any information storage and retrieval system, without permission in writing from the publisher.

Front cover: photograph of the steamship *Alpha* (City of Vancouver Archives, CVA 137-106, photographer Stephen Joseph Thompson); *inset* photograph of Dr. Luke Blackburn (National Library of Medicine)

Printed in the United States of America

McFarland & Company, Inc., Publishers
 Box 611, Jefferson, North Carolina 28640
 www.mcfarlandpub.com

Acknowledgments

I wish to thank the many people who assisted in the production of this book. Andrew M. Baylay at the Bermuda Archives in Hamilton, Bermuda, tirelessly searched for the documents relevant to the Bermuda aspect of the story. His staff, including Karla N. Ingemann, Mandellas A. Lightbourne, and Elizabeth Walters, likewise were continuously gracious to my seemingly endless requests. Ellen Jane Hollis at the Bermuda National Library similarly interrupted her busy schedule for my unannounced visits, suggesting ancient books and documents that proved valuable to the story. Margaret Lloyd of the Bermuda National Trust dropped what she was doing for days as she helped me research the background of the Hamilton Hotel and Slater's Boarding House. Doug Doughty at the Bermuda Yacht Club helped me to understand the geography of Hamilton, Bermuda, in the 1860s. Peter Frith at the Bermuda National Trust, in charge of the Globe Hotel Museum of Confederate History, encouraged me and provided valuable insights into the activity of St. Georges in the 1860s. David Wingate educated me about the history of Nonsuch Island in Bermuda and its role as a Quarantine Station. Keith Forbes manages a phenomenal Web site for Bermudian history (http://www.bermuda-online.org/history.htm) that helped me separate the forest from the trees. Dawn Eurich and Romie Minor at the Detroit Public Library graciously made Halmer Hull Emmons' papers available for my review. Staffs at the National Archives in Washington, D.C., especially John P. Deeben, and College Park, Maryland, were knowledgeable and helpful in tracking down obscure documents for me. Jim Holmberg and his assistants Aaron Rosenblum, Heather Stone, Jana Meyer, and Jennie Cole at the Filson Historical Society in Louisville, Kentucky, assisted me in the perusal of the Blackburn Family Papers and the Churchill Family Papers. Matthew Harris and Deborah Dunn at the Margaret I. King Library at the University of Kentucky in Lexington, Kentucky, provided me copies of the microfilm collection of the Blackburn Family Papers. Marianne Cawley, Molly French, and Nicholas Butler at the South Carolina Room of the Charleston County Public Library, Mary Jo

Fairchild at the South Carolina Historical Society, and Wade H. Dorsey at the South Carolina Department of Archives and History in Columbia, South Carolina, helped me track the lives of the characters in the story after the Civil War. Harlan Greene at the Jewish Heritage Collection, College of Charleston, Special Collections Department, Addlestone Library, suggested clues to pursue other Hyams family members in Charleston. Thanks to Rebecca Quinton, librarian, historian, and genealogist of the Hopkinsville (Kentucky) Library for her help locating the appropriate tax records in Christian County; to Lynn Stillwell, the Helena, Arkansas, circuit court clerk, for allowing me to search through the ancient record books under her guardianship; to Pat Ward of the Phillips County Public Library for searching through old documents and maps from the Civil War era; to Shane Williams of the Helena Historical Society Museum for sharing his extensive knowledge of the region in the 1860s; to Bill Branch, the exhibit curator of the Delta Cultural Center in Helena, Arkansas, for interrupting his busy day and spending a few hours with me telling about the history of the Delta; to Ron Kelley, historian and museum program assistant at the Delta Cultural Center in Helena, Arkansas, for searching for data about Godfrey Hyams in their archives, and to the descendants of the Hyams family (Sonny and Goldie Newcomb and Martha Gleerup) in Trenton, Kentucky, for opening their home and hearts to my many questions about their ancestors. Thanks, also, to Fay Fenske, in charge of interlibrary loans at the Bellingham (Washington) Public Library, for locating obscure books and documents for me.

Thanks to the many people who helped me to find photos, diagrams, and illustrations for this story: Annie Macanulty at the New Westminster Public Library in New Westminster, British Columbia, Canada; Jeannie Hounslow at the City of Vancouver Archives, Vancouver, British Columbia, Canada; Brock Switzer at the Mariners' Museum, Newport News, VA; David Asprey at the Caledonian Maritime Research Trust, River Clyde, Glasgow, Scotland; B.J. Gooch at the Transylvania University Library, Lexington, KY; Cheri Daniels at the Kentucky Historical Society, Frankfort; and Heather McNabb at the McCord Museum, Montreal, Quebec, Canada.

Thanks to John Carter and John Walstad, friends and local Civil War enthusiasts, who read an early version of the manuscript and provided valuable suggestions for the organization of this work. Finally, thanks to the two anonymous reviewers chosen by McFarland to critique this book. Their suggestions greatly improved the flow and coherence of the manuscript.

I am grateful for the help of all these true historians and archivists who assisted and humored me, the amateur historian in their midst. To a person they performed their duties with enthusiasm and even delight, making one want to join their ranks. As that amateur historian, I accept responsibility for any and all inaccuracies in the text.

Table of Contents

Acknowledgments   v
Preface   1
Introduction   4

1. Luke Pryor Blackburn, Lover of the South and Its Culture   7
2. The Scourge of Yellow Fever   19
3. The Canadian Confederacy   23
4. Maritime Shipping and the Union Blockade of Confederate Ports   28
5. Civil War Medicine and Dr. Blackburn   38
6. Dr. Blackburn's Early Confederate Service   46
7. Godfrey Joseph Hyams, Co-Conspirator   53
8. Nefarious Schemes and Diabolical Plans   68
9. Plans for the Importation of Pestilence: The First Shipment of Articles Contaminated with Yellow Fever   86
10. The Second Shipment of Articles Contaminated with Yellow Fever   119
11. Trials in Canada   142
12. Trials in the United States   153
13. Jefferson Davis: His Involvement in the Plots and the Consequences   170
14. The Fate of the Co-Conspirators   185

15. Godfrey Joseph Hyams: The Aftermath ... 195
16. Dr. Luke Pryor Blackburn: Ghoul or Governor? Is This the Same Man? ... 205

Chapter Notes ... 221
Bibliography ... 242
Index ... 245

Preface

The Civil War is the darkest blot on American history. For four years the conflict split the nation with fighting that extinguished the lives of over 600,000 men and women and maimed countless hundreds of thousands of others. War tore families asunder when some fought for the South while others outfitted themselves in Northern uniforms. Combatants used all manner of warfare, and malevolent soldiers even devised new methods of killing.

This story exposes in detail the South's attempts to devastate the North with a technique we would now call germ, or biologic, warfare. It was the Civil War's version of a weapon of mass destruction. Such an approach was not unique to the South. Both sides experimented with unconventional warfare—burning cities, poisoning the water supply, introducing disease, kidnapping high government officials, and killing the heads of state. These newer forms of destruction were not only unconventional, but many also were considered immoral even before governments established rules of warfare. "Gentlemanly" fighting had previously required troops to stand face to face, shooting columns of men in broad daylight. Even what we today call guerrilla warfare was considered to be out of bounds. Both sides rejected terrorism as a legitimate form of fighting. But germ warfare was exactly that—terrorism. It could decimate the enemy's population, killing thousands or even millions while instilling panic in the survivors. This method was simple and cheap. But even germ warfare is not new, as military strategists and serious misanthropes used it in the 1700s and early 1800s. Such a plot surfaced in 1864 and 1865 during the Civil War, but the story has never been told in detail.

Many authors have written briefly about the saga of Dr. Luke Pryor Blackburn and his attempt to bring down the North, but often the story is told with skeptical words. Some authors seem to have been unsure if those events reported from 1864 and 1865 really happened. A superficial examination of the evidence suggests that the tale may be exactly that—a fantasy created by the political opponents of an upright Southern gentleman. However, evidence still exists more than 150 years after the alleged event. I've unearthed letters, documents, diaries, court records, newspaper reports, ledgers, and testimony that have never been examined in detail. Archives in Detroit; Lexington, Virginia; Louisville; Charleston, South Carolina; St. Louis; Boston; Cincinnati; Washington, D.C.; College Park, Maryland; Helena, Arkansas; Hopkinsville, Kentucky; Newport News, Virginia; Hamilton, Bermuda; Vancouver and New Westminster, British Columbia; and Montreal, Quebec, and Toronto, Ontario, have yielded new insights into the workings of this alleged plot. Even photos from this era shed light on the details of a misguided attempt to destroy the North. This event occurred. It was real. But who was actually involved? How did it really happen?

This book will introduce the reader to two very different men who implausibly worked together. They had backgrounds as different from each other as day and night. Dr. Luke Blackburn lived high in social circles, was a wealthy landowner, physician, Kentucky aristocrat, and championship horse breeder. Godfrey Joseph Hyams, on the other hand, came from lowly beginnings in a poverty-stricken region of England, worked as a shoemaker, often owed much, and rarely owned even a mule. While this book is not a complete biography of either man, the reader must understand the backgrounds of both men to fathom the most historically significant events in the lives of the two and to grasp the dynamics of their interaction. Did they actually collude to import pestilence to the North? If so, how could members of the two ends of the social spectrum work together? Were their motivations the same? How did their partnership influence their ultimate fates? Were others involved in this scheme? Did high-level Confederate operatives, even President Jefferson Davis, approve of the plan? This story is not just a biography of the two major participants, it is also an account of the contributions of other Confederates working from Canada.

The cause of the South faltered in 1864. Battles were not going well, and the North was gaining advantage over the South. Confederates needed some novel approaches to warfare. Badly outnumbered, the South was even having difficulty procuring food, weapons, ammunition, basic supplies, transportation, and medicine. These deficiencies dictated new strategies. Techniques previously considered to be immoral were reconsidered. Dr. Blackburn, an ardent lover of the South, had some ideas to improve the Confederate fortunes.

Did either Luke Blackburn or Godfrey Hyams participate in this plan to import disease to the North? Did either stand trial? Was anyone ever convicted for this scheme? Did they serve time in prison, or were they fined? What happened to the other co-conspirators? This book explores the many unanswered questions surrounding Blackburn's and Hyam's roles in this diabolical plot.

A Note on Spelling and Punctuation

Many conventions for spelling and punctuation, as well as sentence structure, were different in the 1860s compared to now. In general, I chose not to note each variation from today's standards because the reading of documents more than 150 years old would have become much too tedious. Only if the meaning of a passage was obscure or if the interpretation hinged on the exact presence or absence of a comma, for example, did I append "[sic]."

Documents from the 1860s frequently had what appeared to be rather random capitalization and punctuation throughout sentences. Furthermore, dashes were often used in the place of periods. In all quotations, I maintained the original punctuation and variations and anomalies of upper case and lower case handwriting, however unusual they seemed to be.

This book is entirely history; it is not historical fiction. As such, all quotations are taken from documents from the period, and references to the documents of origin are noted. In no case did I attribute a quotation that was not extant in documents, newspapers or archival materials. Information that is common knowledge or that was derived from multiple similar common sources was not necessarily referenced.

Finally, newspaper accounts provided many of the sources for this work. While these origins for data can be unreliable, events from the 1800s often have no other points of reference. Furthermore, newspapers then (more commonly than today) gave detailed verbatim reports of conversations, meetings, trial testimony, and the like. Where possible, I used sources other than newspapers; however, I was often forced to rely upon newspapers for specific quotations when no other sources were available. I used the following sources for quotations and citations from newspapers of the era:

Ancestry, www.ancestry.com.
Bermuda Royal Gazette, http://cdm15212.contentdm.oclc.org/cdm/landingpage/collection/BermudaNP02.
Chronicling America, http://chroniclingamerica.loc.gov/newspaper.
Fold3, www.fold3.com.
Google News, https://news.google.com/newspapers?hl=en.
Newsbank/GenealogyBank, www.genealogybank.com.
Newspaper Archive, www.newspaperarchive.com.
Newspapers, www.newspapers.com.

Introduction

The governor's race of 1879 in the Commonwealth of Kentucky was entering its final stages. The Democratic candidate, Dr. Luke Pryor Blackburn, who had been overwhelmingly nominated as the party's flagbearer in May 1879, seemed to be pulling ahead of his Republican competitor, Walter Evans. The campaign had been hard-fought, and Dr. Blackburn was leading because he had a not-so-secret weapon—he was a local hero. For decades he had been one of the world's experts on infectious diseases, especially yellow fever. Countless times he had volunteered to go to communities in Kentucky hard hit by an epidemic, and he always seemed to be able to stop the march of death through these remote hamlets. Moreover, he had similarly responded to epidemics in other states, and even internationally. Most recently he had been dubbed the "Hero of Hickman" for his tireless efforts to treat those afflicted with yellow fever in Hickman, Kentucky. How could any candidate compete against a compassionate local hero? Never mind that Blackburn had almost no political experience. His foray into politics decades earlier had given him a lackluster record in the legislative arena, but his fellow Kentuckians were not concerned. Dr. Blackburn wanted to be governor, and his reward for being a heroic and compassionate physician should be to win the election.

However, just before the balloting, the 19th century Kentucky equivalent of what we now call the "October Surprise" appeared, except that it was July. An October Surprise is the late revelation of some piece of data designed to alter the course of an election. Ofttimes it's the hint of a scandal implicating one of the candidates. It is released so close to the election that the accused has little to no time to respond to the accusations. Such was the case in Kentucky in 1879.

Some newspapers began to question a remarkable name coincidence. It would seem that the press had excoriated another person also named Dr. Luke Blackburn for allegedly trying to import yellow fever to the North from Bermuda in 1864 and 1865. Kentucky had been a border state, but even those voters who had identified with the Southern cause felt that the diabolical namesake Dr. Blackburn was a fiend, a devil. He had run his scheme from Canada, and apparently he had remained in Canada after the Civil War. Such outrageous behavior was uniformly condemned at the end of the Civil War—both by the North and by the South—but these episodes had occurred nearly 15 years earlier. The question, however, arose: "Could our candidate for governor Dr. Blackburn be the same as the fiend Dr. Blackburn?"

Newspaper reporters and common citizens alike began to ask the question as the gubernatorial campaign was drawing to a close: "Are the two Dr. Luke Blackburns the same?" The *Cincinnati Gazette* took the lead in investigative reporting. Beginning in late May 1879 the *Gazette* relentlessly pursued leads, talked with witnesses, and tried to extract statements from the candidate Dr. Blackburn. A story had surfaced in 1869 that claimed the candidate Dr. Blackburn had confessed to the yellow fever plot a few years after the Civil War ended. The newspaper would later report that Blackburn had disclosed the story to "some gentlemen who listened to it from the Doctor's own lips in 1869."[1] In this 1869 account, actually a confession if it were true, Blackburn asserted that he had originally tried to find yellow fever patients in New Orleans and Charleston but had been unsuccessful. From Canada, Blackburn learned of the yellow fever epidemic in Bermuda, and he arranged passage there allegedly to help the ailing citizens of Bermuda with his extensive knowledge of the disease and how to treat and prevent it. He then tried to ship yellow fever to the North. Blackburn had "expressed deep regret at its failure." But were these two Dr. Blackburns the same man?

The Blackburn of 1879, the one running for the office of governor of Kentucky, seemed evasive before the election. He said the questions were so outlandish that they didn't even deserve a reply. Newspapers around the country reported the story, mostly for its shock value. Kentucky papers seemed to be less concerned, and their coverage of the story was more limited. The veracity of the story itself was questioned, let alone the identity of the perpetrator. Could it have been possible that anyone, much less a physician (and a beloved physician, at that), would have participated in such a plot? Who but the devil incarnate would try to kill hundreds of thousands of innocent civilians to advance the cause of the South? Who? Was this Dr. Blackburn—the "Hero of Hickman," the Democratic candidate for governor—the same man as the fiendish Dr. Blackburn? Would the truth be known by Election Day on August 4, 1879?

1

Luke Pryor Blackburn, Lover of the South and Its Culture

Dr. Luke Pryor Blackburn was a healer. A doctor. One whom you could trust with your very life. Or could you? How did he go wrong? Or did he? A Kentucky native, Luke Blackburn lived most of his life in Kentucky, served with dignity as the governor of Kentucky from 1879 to 1883, and died in Kentucky, where his legacy as a medical doctor, public health officer, governor, philanthropist, and prison reformer would stand unblemished were it not for his alleged activities during the Civil War.

Many honorable men did dishonorable acts during that conflict, as do other men and women under duress. Often it is quite difficult to condemn another person for such actions. The greater good frequently seems to dictate what happens during a war; on the other hand, it is also said that the end never justifies the means. While desperate conditions may seem to demand desperate measures, such a course may not be the wisest. Nevertheless, the failing fortunes of the South in the Civil War ("The War of the Rebellion," as the Northerners called it, and "The War of Northern Aggression," as the Southerners viewed it) seemed to demand desperate measures. Guerrilla tactics, terrorism, and use of disease as warfare were definitely available options. Would the dissemination of disease be considered to be a well-intentioned attempt to shorten a war that was already taking hundreds of thousands of lives, mostly those of soldiers? Or should this tactic be rejected for its barbarity? Use of disease as a weapon would bring disease and death to hundreds of thousands of persons, many of them civilians. Was someone willing to act in this manner a hideous fiend or simply a devoted lover of the South?

• • •

Luke Pryor Blackburn was born on June 16, 1816, at Spring Station, Woodford County, Kentucky. His father, Edward M. Blackburn, worked as a lawyer, farmer, and horse breeder. His mother was Lavinia Bell Blackburn. Other ancestors included lawyers, doctors, politicians/statesmen, missionaries, and pastors/theologians. The family had an honorable past with a worthy heritage. The immediate family comprised twelve living children (nine boys, three girls); two other boys died before the age of two. Luke Pryor had been the fourth born in the family. The entire clan enjoyed a life of relative wealth and upper-class status. By 1850 Luke's father, Edward, had many servants: 10 "free white," 31 "free colored," and 21 "colored slaves."[1] Luke Blackburn himself in Natchez owned 18 slaves by 1850.[2]

At age 16 Luke began studying medicine under the tutelage of his uncle, Dr. Churchill Blackburn. Luke's interest in medicine was intense, even as he studied the local illnesses, including cases of cholera rampant in Kentucky in 1833. Of course, physicians then knew little about the mechanisms of disease, and many theories attributed illnesses to causes mentioned only in folklore and witchcraft today. Experts blamed "miasmas," or vapors, as the carriers of illnesses, and this theory would certainly account for the way many infectious diseases propagated rapidly across the landscape. These gases originated from locations where rotting matter lay. Early-era epidemiologists thought that decomposition of otherwise innocuous animal and vegetable material was responsible for the production of illnesses. Doctors blamed the wrong causes, and the medical establishment clung to an inappropriate treatment mantra. It called for the doctor to "bleed, blister, vomit, cup, and purge." Remove blood; apply treatments that cause the skin to blister; induce vomiting; place vacuum cups on the skin to "draw out" dangerous poisons; and cause diarrhea. Sanitation in Kentucky (and elsewhere in the world) during this era existed only in its crudest form. Diseases traveled rapidly, and epidemics disseminated widely. Even the concept that bacteria caused infection was barely emerging. The germ theory of disease didn't appear until Louis Pasteur discovered it in the 1860s and 1870s. Pasteur introduced the concept of pasteurization in 1865, but he didn't develop it fully until 1876. He argued in 1874 that microbes caused infection, but he didn't isolate staphylococcal and streptococcal bacteria until 1879, and he connected some diseases with microbes only in 1880. Robert Koch did his pioneering work on the bacterial theory in the late 1870s. He did not publish his classic paper on the etiology of infectious diseases until 1879. Joseph Lister published his theory of antisepsis with carbolic acid (phenol) in 1867, but doctors accepted it only years later. Then—as now—the medical community embraced new discoveries slowly, but it took far longer in the 19th century to convey new theories even after their detection. So Blackburn labored under the mantles of both lack of information and serious misinformation as he studied the illnesses of his fellow Kentuckians.

Theories about the propagation of yellow fever specifically included "fomites," an early term that would later be ascribed to "germs"—bacteria or viruses as we know them today, or those "miasmas," gases that wafted through communities infecting those who were exposed. No one at that time knew that a virus caused yellow fever. No one even knew what a virus was. In 1865 "germ" meant "a point of growth" or "that from which any thing springs." The word "virus" was similarly vague; it meant "contagious or poisonous matter" or "the spirit, aim, or drift of any thing injurious."[3]

Epidemics spread rapidly. Yellow fever could be devastating, killing up to half of its victims. Emergence of an epidemic of yellow fever was always accompanied by widespread panic. Residents deserted entire towns as a wave of yellow fever approached an area. No effective treatment existed for this disease. With an incubation period of 3–6 days, it begins with a fever and headaches, then generalized aching (especially the neck, back, and legs), eye pain and extreme sensitivity to the light (photophobia), jaundice (yellow color imparted to the skin and eyes by breakdown products of hemoglobin in the blood), nausea, vomiting, disorientation, delirium, and seizures. Sometimes a brief remission of symptoms seems to indicate the illness has run its course, but a secondary onslaught heralds liver involvement. Bloody stools and bleeding into the skin and gums often come next. This diffuse bleeding includes upper gastrointestinal hemorrhage that leads to the characteristic "black vomit," the result of blood oozing from the stomach and being degraded by gastric acid—so-called "coffee-grounds vomitus." Then coma often heralds impending death. A victim can progress from completely healthy to death in 48–72 hours. It was an illness that instilled terror for its severity, rapidity, and lethality. A Southern malefactor would eventually devise a plot to use yellow fever as a weapon to destroy the North.

Cholera was another illness that caused panic. To be accurate, not all epidemics that were called cholera in the 1830s when Blackburn was learning medicine were actually cholera as we know it. The diagnosis "cholera" was a general description for acute and serious gastrointestinal illnesses characterized by fever, diarrhea, and prostration. Doctors had no bacterial cultures, antibody tests, or other diagnostic aids we take for granted today. Nevertheless, cholera struck Paris (Woodford County), Kentucky, where Luke Blackburn was studying and doing his apprenticeship, in the summer of 1833. It acquainted him with the basics of epidemiology, and it certainly gave him an appreciation for the chaos that infectious diseases can cause. Could Luke Blackburn already have been envisioning what biologic warfare might be able to do? Little did anyone know that approximately 20 years later someone would use experience with disease-induced chaos to attempt to bring down the North during the Civil War. Yellow fever and smallpox would be the diseases, and a man would be the agent delivering this form of warfare.

Smallpox was also greatly feared by all. Recognized today as a viral disease (though, of course, this fact was not known during Civil War times), smallpox begins as a fever, followed by the characteristic skin rash. It has an incubation period of about 12–14 days, with a range from 7 to 17 days. Fever is followed by muscle aches (especially backache), weakness, headache, nausea, and vomiting. These last for about 2–4 days, after which the early rash begins. Mortality of the major type of smallpox approached 30 percent. It was a fearsome disease that similarly spread panic in the general population. Furthermore, it was another candidate for germ warfare. (Even though physicians could administer a crude smallpox vaccine during the Civil War era, large segments of the population remained unvaccinated.)

Blackburn served his medical apprenticeship with his uncle for two years, then he enrolled in his formal medical education at Transylvania University in Lexington, Kentucky, studying there from 1833 to 1835. Transylvania University had been founded in 1798, with its medical department established in 1799. It was a very prestigious institution at the time, on a par with Harvard and Yale. MD degrees were granted until 1881, when the medical school closed. Graduation requirements were rather flexible, and some were actually quite vague. The candidate had to be at least 21 years old, of "good moral character," must have studied under a "competent preceptor," and had to attend two full courses of medical lectures, at least one of which was at Transylvania University. Lecture series began the first Monday of November and ended the first week in March. Four years of medical practice counted as equivalent to one of the series of lectures. Most candidates chose this route, attending one series of courses and then practicing for four years, usually under the tutelage of another physician, before actually receiving the MD degree. The candidate had to pass two sets of exams, one before the medical faculty and one before the president and trustees of the university. In addition, a candidate had to do a medical dissertation on a subject of his own choosing, though it had to be approved in advance by the faculty.[4] Blackburn chose cholera—the second disease in the dreaded triumvirate of yellow fever, cholera, and smallpox—as his dissertation subject.

In his thesis, entitled "Cholera Maligna," Blackburn waxed poetically about the disease Cholera Maligna and its causes (Figures 1A and 1B).[5] He submitted his thesis on February 20, 1835, with his address listed as Woodford County, Kentucky (Versailles, Kentucky, was the county seat, and Blackburn would soon settle there). Submitted in elegant handwriting, the thesis was a scant eighteen pages long. A consummate politician and poet even then, Blackburn dedicated his thesis to Dr. Charles Caldwell, professor of the Institutes of Clinical Practice at Transylvania University. Dr. Caldwell was at least partially responsible for reviewing and grading the thesis, and Blackburn knew who held his future. Caldwell was an egotistical professor; the sheer length of his own autobiography (454 pages) gives us some indication of how important he might have thought himself to be.[6] (Caldwell himself was also an expert on yellow fever.) Blackburn said that his thesis was "a feeble evidence of that high estimation which I entertain for you [Dr. Caldwell], not only as a lecturer but as a man, whose genius and intellect are such as to call forth the aspiration of every ardent and energetic youth to the prosecution of that important profession which you do ably support. May your happiness and prosperity never be marred, by the frown of jealousy or the hand of malevolence; but may you glide smoothly down this current of time with an expanse of genius and an increase of knowledge until time shall emerge in the ocean of eternity."[7]

One only needs to read a small portion of Blackburn's thesis to understand the paucity of medical knowledge at that time. He wrote of those "miasmas," "agencies," "predisposing and exciting" causes, and "specific and common" causes, without actually identifying any of them. Emphasizing the distinction between animal and plant food sources, Blackburn claimed that animal-derived foods were better for one's health. Railing against the "habits of intemperance," he argued for a life of moderation. He spoke against "all acid drinks, particularly cider, thin sour wines, bad water, ice water, beer and porter" as causes of cholera. The admonition against ice water would be repeated in 1850, as President Zachary Taylor was erroneously said to have died from a form of cholera that emanated from ingestion of a combination of milk, cherries, and ice water. Blackburn also mentioned the "moral exciting causes of cholera maligna … [as being] grief, fear, and despair." He claimed lack of space and time for omitting the treatment of cholera in his thesis, simply reminding the reader that calomel (mercurous chloride, commonly used as a purgative) was useful "in larger or smaller doses."[8]

Almost prophetically, Blackburn wrote of the need to "disarm this monster [cholera] of its terrors": "Epidemics are not at all dependant [sic] for their propagation on contagion, they are readily transmissible in other modes." He noted that epidemics are not limited geographically in their spread, but "the yellow fever … prevailed in Europe and America simultaneously."[9] Could these statements presage his use of "this monster" (an epidemic) to try to wreak his own terrors, devising his own method of propagation to distribute an illness across multiple geographic regions?

Blackburn graduated with his MD degree in March 1835 (not even 20 years old yet). He immediately began seeing patients in both Lexington and Versailles. As a generous and honorable man of medicine he saw both paying patients and the ones who couldn't afford a doctor. Another cholera epidemic reared its ugly head in the summer of 1835. Blackburn was immediately overwhelmed by the needs of the sick, especially in Versailles, his hometown. There he practiced the most noble of professions, approaching patients with dignity and grace. When the epidemic abated, he remained in Versailles, in

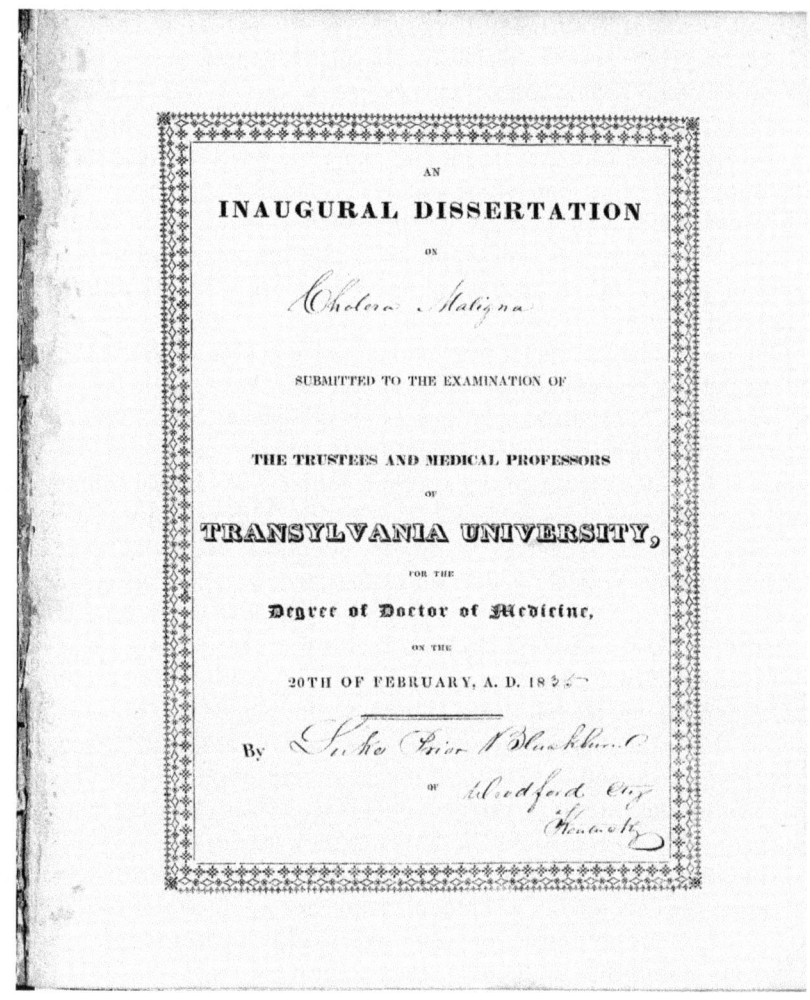

Figure 1A. Luke Pryor Blackburn's doctoral thesis, "An Inaugural Dissertation on Cholera Maligna." Blackburn was interested in infectious diseases from the beginning of his medical career (Kentucky Digital Library. Accessed at: http://kdl.kyvl.org/catalog/xt7ttd9n427b_1?).

part because there he was closer to some of his family (Versailles in Woodford County was only 33 miles from Paris in Bourbon County, both French namesakes but in opposite directions from Lexington). Also, many other physicians in the area had either died from cholera or had deserted their towns, so Blackburn had an immediate following and his practice grew rapidly. As his practice yielded him a very good income, he began to branch out and invest in many business ventures in Kentucky, including hemp rope and bagging. Dr.

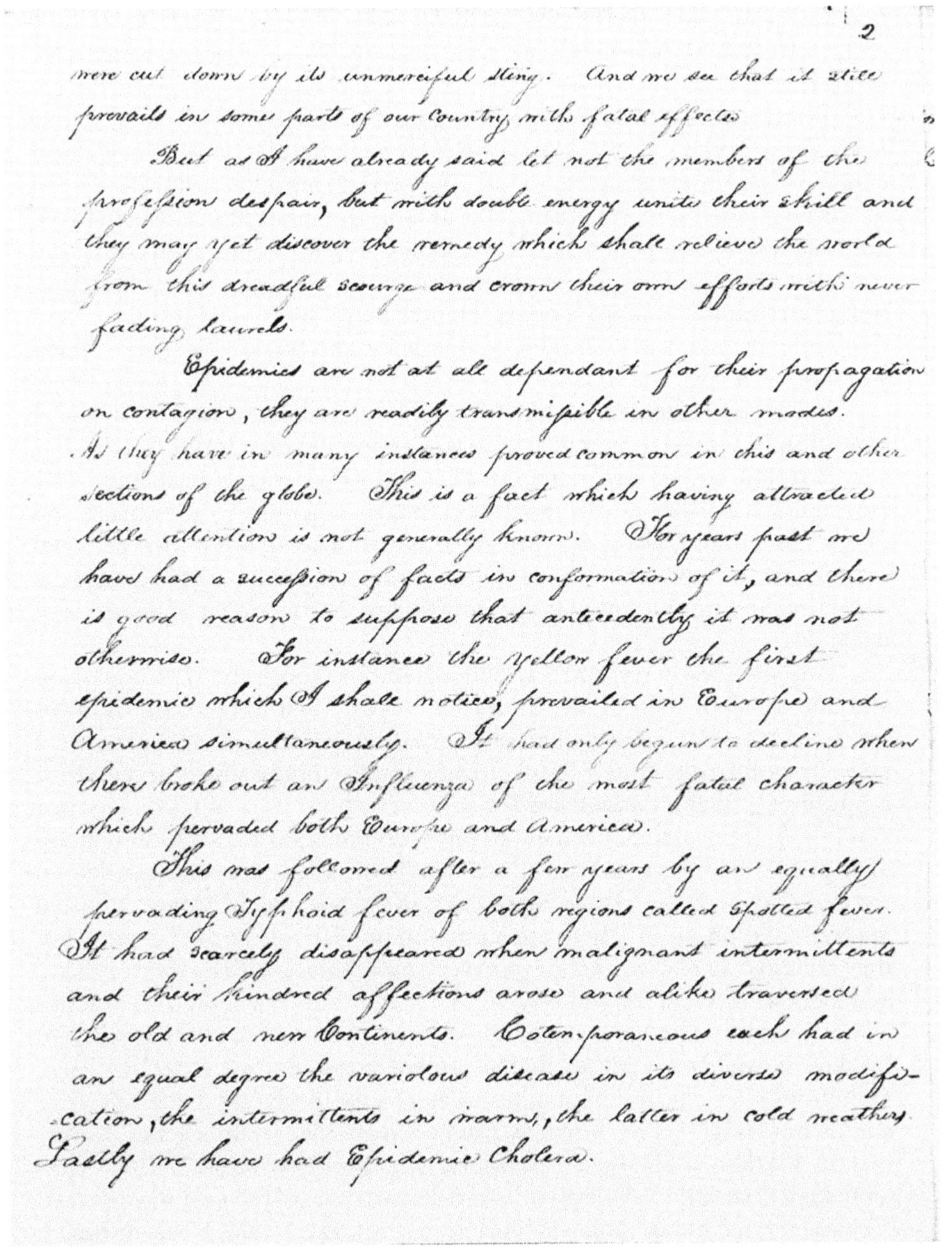

were cut down by its unmerciful sting. And we see that it still prevails in some parts of our Country with fatal effects.

But as I have already said let not the members of the profession despair, but with double energy unite their skill and they may yet discover the remedy which shall relieve the world from this dreadful scourge and crown their own efforts with never fading laurels.

Epidemics are not at all dependant for their propagation on contagion, they are readily transmissible in other modes. As they have in many instances proved common in this and other sections of the globe. This is a fact which having attracted little attention is not generally known. For years past we have had a succession of facts in confirmation of it, and there is good reason to suppose that antecedently it was not otherwise. For instance the yellow fever the first epidemic which I shall notice, prevailed in Europe and America simultaneously. It had only begun to decline when there broke out an Influenza of the most fatal character which pervaded both Europe and America.

This was followed after a few years by an equally pervading Typhoid fever of both regions called Spotted fever. It had scarcely disappeared when malignant intermittents and their kindred affections arose and alike traversed the old and new Continents. Cotemporaneous each had in an equal degree the variolous disease in its diverse modification, the intermittents in warm, the latter in cold weather. Lastly we have had Epidemic Cholera.

Figure 1B. In his doctoral thesis he already acknowledges that disease can be transmitted by other than natural causes: "Epidemics are not at all dependant [sic] for their propagation on contagion, they are readily transmissible in other modes" (Kentucky Digital Library. Accessed at: http://kdl.kyvl.org/catalog/xt7ttd9n427b_4?).

Blackburn married Ella Gist Boswell on November 24, 1835.[10] Their only child, Cary Bell Blackburn, was born on April 29, 1837. He became a physician as well.

Blackburn's interests remained centered on infectious diseases, yellow fever in particular. Dr. Blackburn the elder soon became the acknowledged expert in the United States in the treatment and control of yellow fever. But he initially didn't fare well financially, and his nonmedical investments generally failed. He remained in the Versailles area for about eight years and entered politics in 1843 as a Whig elected to the Kentucky House of Representatives from Woodford County. He left politics after a single term, and the family moved first to Frankfort, Kentucky, and then to Natchez, Mississippi, in 1846.

In Natchez, Blackburn entered Southern high society, where his financial condition improved dramatically. He was appointed director of the Natchez City Hospital, and he also maintained his private practice of medicine.[11] City Hospital was a rather dismal institution that treated mostly the indigent and slaves. Under Dr. Blackburn's direction, and with some of his own personal investment, it improved considerably. Further, also at his own expense, he began expanding the hospital specifically for the treatment of sailors and mariners.

Patients greatly respected and loved Dr. Blackburn for his compassion and attention. In 1846 he declared to his family that his income from his practice alone, not counting his hospital salary, would be $3,000 per year, a princely sum for the time.[12] In his private practice in town he charged $2 for a house call. If the patient needed a prescription, most doctors charged another $1. If the patient lived out of town, doctors charged an additional fee of $1 per mile of travel for the house call. They billed repeat visits, even on the same day, at the same rate. For patients in the hospital, Blackburn adjusted his fee based on race: "There are a good many patients at the hospital, but they are most all blacks, and they are very profitable, a dollar a day for them, and a dollar & a half for whites...."[13] By 1853 Blackburn's combined practice would yield him $10,000 per year. He was now well-to-do.[14] In that year, Dr. Blackburn would even declare that he wanted to tour Europe, especially Paris, to improve his medical skills, but his wife objected, declaring that his practice and income might suffer from any prolonged absence from Natchez. Nevertheless, Blackburn obtained a passport, issued on May 9, 1857, which contained his description since photos weren't yet a part of the passport process. It characterized him as follows: "Forehead–oval, Eyes–light, Nose–ordinary, Mouth–rather large, Chin–oval, Hair–brown, Complexion–florid, Face–full."[15]

Luke and Ella Blackburn were kind to neighbors and patients alike. Though they owned slaves (18 in 1850 in Natchez, Mississippi, and 74 in Mississippi Township, Desha County, Arkansas, in 1860, "co-owned" by his brother Churchill H. Blackburn),[16] they considered their slaves to be friends. Ella wrote profusely to relatives back in Kentucky, and she frequently ended her letters with admonitions to remember her to the slaves there, while sending the good wishes of her Mississippi slaves to kin in her home state. A typical letter's conclusion might say, "Tell the servants howdy for me—Nat [a servant in Mississippi] is busy now, setting out shrubbery and making a garden, at our new house, we are all well, + doing much."[17] There was also, "Remember us kindly to all the servants—all of ours send you their respects—they were very much disappointed that you did not come down."[18] The Blackburns attended the Presbyterian church in Natchez, making influential friends through this connection, yet Ella, in particular, always dreamed of returning to Kentucky.[19] Blackburn's friendships included Jefferson Davis, who had also attended Transylvania University.

Blackburn was elected health officer for Natchez, Mississippi, in 1848, and as such he was finally able to implement some of the techniques he believed would help to stem the spread of epidemics. He instituted quarantines, and he isolated those men who had contagious diseases, most often yellow fever, cholera, and smallpox. The techniques he used to prevent the spread of illnesses also unsuspectingly controlled the mosquitoes that actually transmitted yellow fever, and these methods improved unsanitary conditions that had promoted the spread of cholera. As Blackburn biographer Nancy Baird summarizes, eliminating standing water, cleaning dirty trenches, covering cisterns, cleaning the area around wells, and improving the cleanliness of latrines all contributed to the improvement of general health and reduced the spread of epidemics.[20]

Dr. Blackburn responded to the yellow fever epidemic in New Orleans in 1848, and there he successfully instituted a quarantine that quelled the spread of the disease. He required that ships with ill sailors be quarantined for two weeks to allow any emerging cases to become evident. Here again his techniques gained the upper hand, and the scourge of the "yellow jack," as yellow fever was often called, came under control. Blackburn extended his personal influence on the control and treatment of yellow fever when he responded to that epidemic. His fame increased, and it would soon lead him to both international travel and a chance to help the Confederacy.

In 1845 the United States Congress had expanded the Marine Hospital Service (the precursor to the Public Health Service Hospital system today, also known as the "Marine Hospitals"), one of which was ultimately built in Natchez along the Mississippi River. Blackburn was appointed chief of service of this hospital, which was built between 1849 and 1852 and opened in 1852. He resigned the directorship of the Natchez City Hospital. His wife, Ella, still dreamed of returning to Kentucky, but Blackburn was too busy seeing his patients both in his office (which was located in his home) and at the Marine Hospital to consider moving back to his home state. Blackburn continued his charitable medical care to the poor and to blacks, expanding his reputation as a truly compassionate physician.

Another yellow fever epidemic hit Natchez during 1853–1855; rapidly about 10 percent of the population died from the disease. Blackburn quickly established and enforced a strict quarantine that may have saved hundreds of lives that would have otherwise been lost. Ella Blackburn had experienced a mild case of yellow fever earlier in life, so she had natural immunity, though of course no one then understood how she had acquired the resistance to the disease. Blackburn himself hadn't experienced a clinical episode of yellow fever, but it is highly likely, given his vast exposure to the disease, that he had also lived through a mild case and had immunity himself.

Doctors possessed few effective treatments for most illnesses of that era, although they tried many remedies upon hearing reports and rumors that something might be successful. Medical treatment of yellow fever at the time was no different. It included administration of fluids, quinine (good for malaria but not for yellow fever), and calomel. Doctors administered calomel (mercurous chloride) primarily as a purgative, though they also gave it in low doses, a treatment called an "alterative," or a cure-all for many diseases. "Alterative" during the Civil War era meant "a medicine which gradually induces a change in the habit or constitution, and restores healthy functions without sensible evacuations."[21] Doctors also prescribed antimony, rhubarb, ice, turpentine, castor oil, potassium citrate, and whatever seemed to reduce the fever. In reality, everyone knew that not much worked. Blistering and cupping treatments were also common. Cupping used techniques of placing hot glass cups on the patient's skin, the rim of the glass creating suction as the glass cooled. Some physicians even used physical suction machines that formed blisters on the skin. Blistering could be caused by the cupping glass or sometimes was caused by chemical agents placed on the skin to cause blisters. Doctors believed that these techniques somehow withdrew detrimental liquids from the patient's body. Opium, laudanum (a mixture of alcohol and opium), and other painkillers were used lavishly, though these agents also had powerful effects against coughing and diarrhea. Efforts to prevent the spread of the illness usually involved producing some type of noxious smoke to kill the "miasmas," those airborne agents believed to produce the disease.

• • •

Although Blackburn relinquished the post of health officer in October 1853 he continued to lobby for ever-more–strict quarantine measures. He emphasized the need for intercepting ships upon their arrival in United States waters at the mouth of rivers leading inland rather than farther upriver.

In March 1855 Ella began to reveal in her letters to Lavinia Blackburn that her health was worsening. Her handwriting changed perceptibly during these months. Usually small, dainty, and well formed, her penmanship became larger and rather sloppy. Ella wrote, in March 1855, "My health has been bad all winter. It has been a great effort for me to write even to Cary [their son], + at times I could not hold a pen, for I have been suffering with neuralgia, for some months, and when it attacks my right hand I can't use it."[22] On September 30, 1855, she penned, "My hands pained me, so much, that I was not able to use them, not even wash my face, I had overtaxed them, in writing too much. They are a little better, to day."[23] And in December 1855 she said, "My health is improving, but I am dreadfully nervous, cannot stand any noise or excitement[.] [T]he swelling has gone out of my hands but they are as weak, almost as an infant but this I know, I am most decidedly better."[24] Perhaps even her mind was beginning to fail, as one of her last letters was dated "Thursday morning, 19th of Feb, Natchez, 1858." The 17th of February 1858 was a Wednesday, and the 1858 date would have been 15 months after her death on November 11, 1856. She wistfully reported, "I wish that we had a comfortable home, in Kentucky, so that we could be near those that we love so dearly, and I am determined as soon as Dr. [Blackburn] is able to buy a farm there, to persuade him to go, for life is short, in this world, and we ought to try and be happy whilst in it...." She was unhappy and realized that her remaining life might be short.[25]

Blackburn went to Philadelphia in September 1856 to take their 18-year-old son, Cary, to begin his medical training as an apprentice to Dr. Samuel D. Gross, an eminent physician, surgeon, and teacher. While Dr. Blackburn and Cary were there, yellow fever broke out at Fort Washington near Long Island, New York, and Dr. Blackburn responded to help treat patients infected by the epidemic. His help there seemed to be pivotal, the yellow fever quickly coming under control. When he returned home to Natchez, Ella was sick with an undiagnosed fever. She had suffered for a long time from "dropsy," a term used then most commonly for congestive heart failure. She also had some form of a chronic unspecified nervous condition, causing her hand pain ("neuralgia," in her words) and swelling, especially in the right hand, making it impossible for her to write letters, an activity in which she previously had been prolific. She died on November 11, 1856.[26]

Dr. Blackburn was devastated and could not stop grieving. Friends encouraged him to leave Natchez for a while. He had talked about wanting to tour hospitals in Europe, and he finally embarked on such a trip in spring 1857 and visited hospitals in England, Scotland, Italy, France, and Germany. While there he met Julia Maria Preston Pope Churchill,[27] a 27-year-old fellow Kentuckian who was touring Paris with her sister and niece. Blackburn, 40 years old when they met, would ultimately marry this young woman, on

November 17, 1857, in Kentucky. First living in Natchez, they moved to New Orleans in January 1858. They would live in New Orleans only briefly, but while they were there Blackburn's son established a medical practice with his father. Luke and Julia would have only one child, a girl they named Abby, who died in infancy in June 1860.[28]

2

The Scourge of Yellow Fever

Yellow fever today is considered to be a disease of the tropics, a scourge of southern Atlantic islands, the Caribbean, and points south. Yellow fever in the 21st century is a disease unknown in the United States, and the mere mention of it elicits quizzical looks from nonmedical persons. However, in the 1800s it was feared throughout the coastal regions, though more in the South than in the North, and particularly during the warmer seasons. Soon after an initial case of yellow fever appeared, thousands of additional victims would emerge in the immediate area. Physicians noted that this contagion often was introduced to a region when a ship from tropical climates (usually the Caribbean and points south) arrived in a local port with sick crew members. Contaminated ships ultimately were required to hoist the "yellow jack," a yellow flag signifying that someone on board was ill, perhaps with yellow fever. Thus, the disease was dubbed "yellow jack." (It was also nicknamed "bronze John," "black vomit," the "saffron scourge," and "gaol fever"—because the epidemic often appeared in the confines of prisons.)

In the 1800s the disease was rampant throughout the United States as well as in the tropics. Extending far up the East Coast, this illness—now identified as a viral disease—ran in cycles, often coincident with warm weather. Outbreaks of yellow fever were common from Key West on the Gulf Coast as far north as even the upper mid-Atlantic states. New York was first hit in 1702. Philadelphia experienced one of its worst major epidemics in 1793. Out of a population of over 40,000 there were 4,040 who died of the disease, and another 12,000 fled the city to avoid the wrath of that illness.[1] Yellow fever decimated other cities and states, one of the worst epidemics occurring in 1798. That year, over 200 people died in Boston, hardly a tropical environment. In New York the 1798 epidemic claimed 2,086, and in Philadelphia 3,500 succumbed to the "yellow jack" (Figure 2).[2] Baltimore was hit in 1819; Middletown, Connecticut in 1820; and Key West in 1824. However, the southern climes were the most vulnerable—Charleston, Wilmington, Pensacola, Savannah, New Orleans, Mobile. During the Civil War era, yellow fever was rampant along the coastal regions. In 1862 Wilmington, North Carolina, saw many flee the city, and of the 3,000 remaining behind 1,200 died of yellow fever.[3] It was a disease that inspired "shock and awe," instilling panic in all who saw it coming.

Yellow fever played a role during the course of the Civil War in many cities, New Orleans—the Crescent City—being one of them. The year 1861 was unusual, as not a single fatal case of yellow fever occurred in New Orleans. Perhaps the absence of the disease aided Union troops in capturing the city in April 1862. Newspapers of the day reported the widespread condemnation of the notion of purposely spreading yellow fever—or any disease, even if the target population was the army of the North. But, in fact, some residents of New Orleans desired—even prayed for—the scourge to come to the Federal occupying troops who had taken the city. The Crescent City had seen its share of epidemics, and its citizens knew that foreigners or visitors always fared worse than natives of the city. While residents of New Orleans didn't completely understand the principle of immunity that could be conferred by contracting a mild or subclinical case of the disease, they knew that yellow fever first killed the visitor or stranger to the city. Long-term residents were often spared. Therefore, it was sometimes called "the stranger's illness." Yellow fever visited the city reliably in waves every few years. In 1853, 1854, 1855, and 1858 the total killed by yellow fever in New Orleans numbered about 18,000.[4]

A yellow fever epidemic usually lasted for about three months, and residents of New Orleans thought that the arrival of such pestilence might give the Confederates a chance to retake the Crescent City, or at least that it would punish the Yankees for invading it. So local residents prayed that yellow fever would come quickly to kill the Yankees. The outcome would be the same if someone purposely brought the illness to New Orleans by some physical means, but praying seemed to be more socially and morally acceptable.

General Benjamin F. Butler, the Union officer in charge of the occupying troops in New Orleans and therefore responsible for their health, succeeded in keeping yellow fever at bay. His quarantine kept any ships suspected of harboring the disease at anchor and away from New Orleans for 40 days. He also believed that yellow fever was caused by the combination of animal and vegetable filth, mixed with the "seeds" of the disease, whatever these might be, so he labored to rid the city of both forms of refuse. By so doing, his quarantine likely stopped the introduction of the "seeds" (the virus, it would later be discovered) into the city, and cleaning the streets of refuse perhaps removed some of the breeding grounds necessary for the multiplication of the mosquito *Aedes aegypti*, the tiny assassin actually responsible for trans-

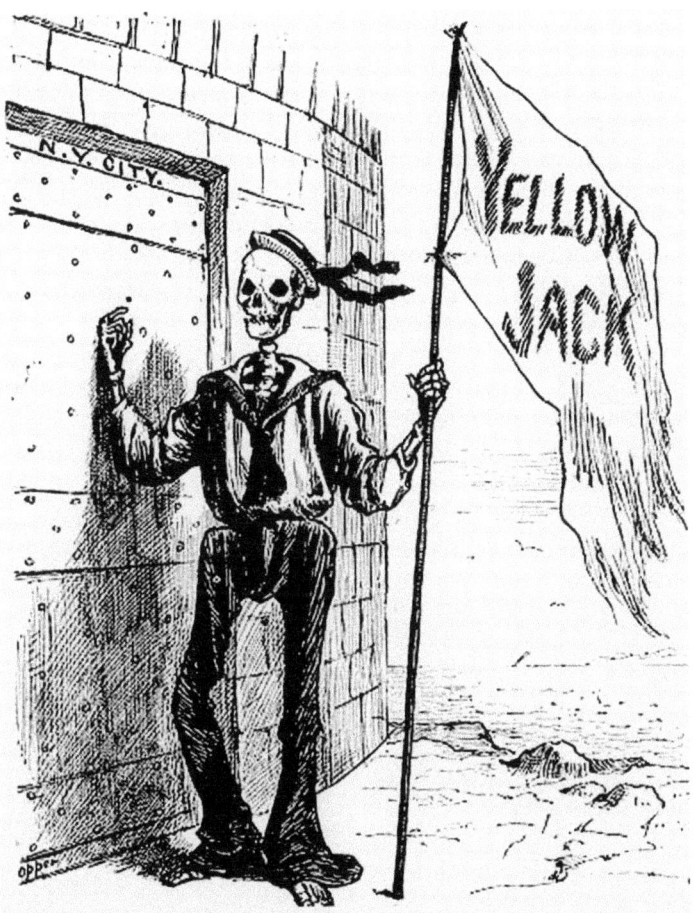

Figure 2. The Yellow Jack. Yellow fever, also called "yellow jack," "bronze John," and "black vomit," was feared throughout the United States in the mid-19th century. It was not limited to tropical environments, and could appear in locales as far north as Philadelphia, New York, and Boston. This cartoon from 1878 depicts the scourge of yellow fever, represented by an Italian sailor dressed as Death, knocking on the door of New York City. The caption of the drawing in 1878 read, "SHALL WE LET HIM IN? Mr. Mayor and gentlemen of the Board of Aldermen, the answer rests with you" (*Frank Leslie's Illustrated Newspaper*, September 21, 1878, Vol. XLVII, No. 1199, p. 48).

mitting the disease. Mankind had to wait until 1901 for Walter Reed to discover the mode of transmission of yellow fever, but Butler's techniques were inadvertently successful. They were an ideal combination of quarantine and sanitation. The prayers of the populace—at least for the moment—were thwarted. In May and June of 1862 residents of New Orleans anticipated—

yes, continued to pray for, and expect—yellow fever striking the Union troops. In an early form of mental terrorism or psychological warfare, two citizens of New Orleans sympathetic to the Southern cause walked around the city with measuring tapes and notebooks, approaching any Union soldier they might see. When asked what they were doing, they said they were working for a company that had been contracted to make 10,000 coffins for the Union troops who were going to die of yellow fever and they wanted to be sure they built the proper sizes to accommodate the Northern men.[5]

Butler's efforts to control the disease were amply rewarded. In 1863 only two deaths from yellow fever occurred in New Orleans, six in 1864, and one in 1865. When New Orleans civil authorities later acquired the task of enforcing quarantine and sanitation from the Union military in 1866, the iron fist of the Union military occupiers was released, and the civilians subsequently in control relaxed the methods. Cholera claimed 1,200 victims, while the "saffron scourge" killed 185 in 1866. In 1867 yellow fever rebounded in strength to claim over 3,000 victims. So the prayers of some New Orleanians were finally answered but too late to affect the course of the Civil War.

3

The Canadian Confederacy

To understand the role Dr. Blackburn and his associates played in the Civil War one must appreciate the relationship between Canada and the combatants in the Civil War—the North and the South. Officially Canada was a neutral party in the United States' Civil War. Canada was the "United Province of Canada" from 1841 to 1867, a part of the British Empire. The British declarations of neutrality were to be observed both in Canada and the other parts of Great Britain. Likewise, the islands and countries surrounding the United States theoretically remained neutral in the conflict. Cuba, Bermuda, and the Bahamas officially aligned with neither side, though all three soon served as unofficial bases of operation for Confederate blockade-runners. As with any war, proponents for both sides could be found everywhere. However, the preponderance of Canadian sentiment and activity favored the South by a margin of 5:1.[1] Reasons for this polarization were complex and multifactorial: economic, religious, political, and historical. Newspapers both reported and created much of this division with almost a 3:1 ratio of Southern-leaning publications.[2] Therefore, it didn't take long for Confederate Rebel sympathizers to migrate north of the United States-Canadian border. Rebels knew that Canada would be a safe haven, and Canada had strategic geographic advantages to those trying to support the Southern cause. Canada was a perfect location for sporadic raids across the border into the North, where Union forces had some of their forts and encampments and where many Confederate prisoners were incarcerated (Figure 3).

Canada had been divided into Lower Canada and Upper Canada (the two together were often called "British North America"), later to become Canada East and Canada West respectively. Lower Canada (Canada East) included Montreal, Quebec, and Ottawa; Upper Canada (Canada West) contained Toronto and Ontario. These areas were all British colonies. Nova Scotia, Newfoundland, New Brunswick, and Prince Edward Island were also British colonies separately governed at the time of the Civil War (Hudson's Bay Company ran Rupert's Land). Legal separation existed among the prov-

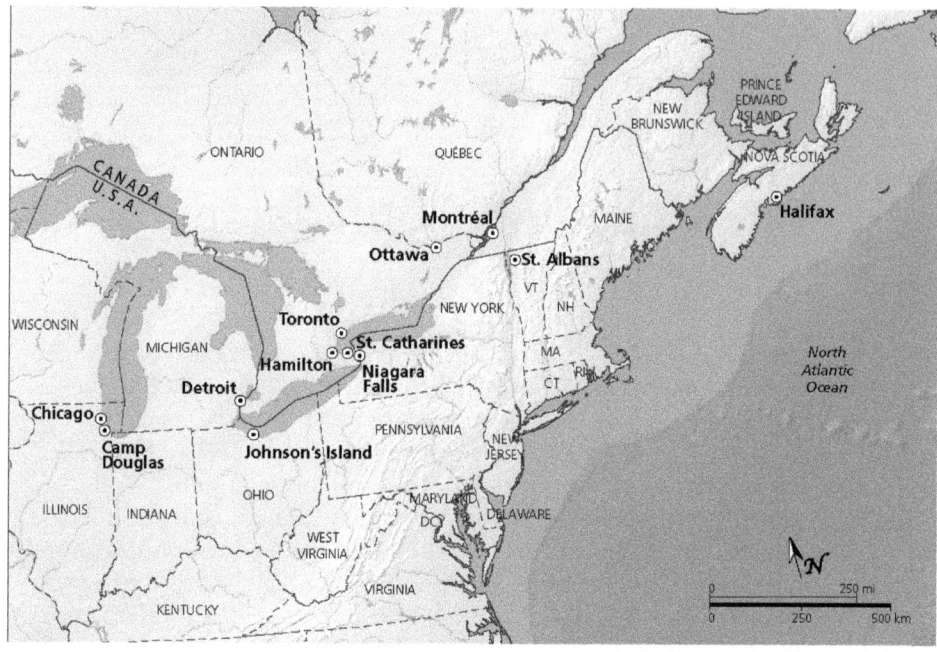

Figure 3. The Canadian Confederacy. The Canadian Confederacy functioned primarily out of Toronto and Montreal. Blockade-runners used Halifax as a port to make connections to the South, but Nova Scotia technically wasn't yet a part of Canada. Confederates staged raids and concocted schemes to harrass the North from Canadian border towns, with attacks on Fort Douglas in Chicago; Johnson's Island near Sandusky, Ohio; St. Albans, Vermont; and even into Boston and New York City (Kulshan Cartographics, Bellingham, Washington).

inces. Courts adjudicated disputes locally. That is to say, if a criminal broke a law in Nova Scotia, for example, the case could not be tried in Canada East or Canada West, even though all were British provinces. These jurisdictional issues would become very important to the court cases that would arise as a result of the Civil War—and any future case against Dr. Blackburn, in particular.

The centers of Confederate activity in Canada were Montreal, Toronto, the Canadian side of Niagara Falls, and—to a lesser extent—Nova Scotia. In Montreal, Confederates most often frequented a hotel named St. Lawrence Hall (Figure 4). Southerners referred to both St. Lawrence Hall and Montreal as "Little Richmond." "The Hall," as locals called it, was located in the center of Montreal, near the Notre Dame Cathedral, the Champ de Mars Square, and popular restaurants, theaters, and meeting places. This lavish five-story building had ballrooms, newsstands, dining rooms, a post office, a telegraph station, and a library and reading room.

3. The Canadian Confederacy

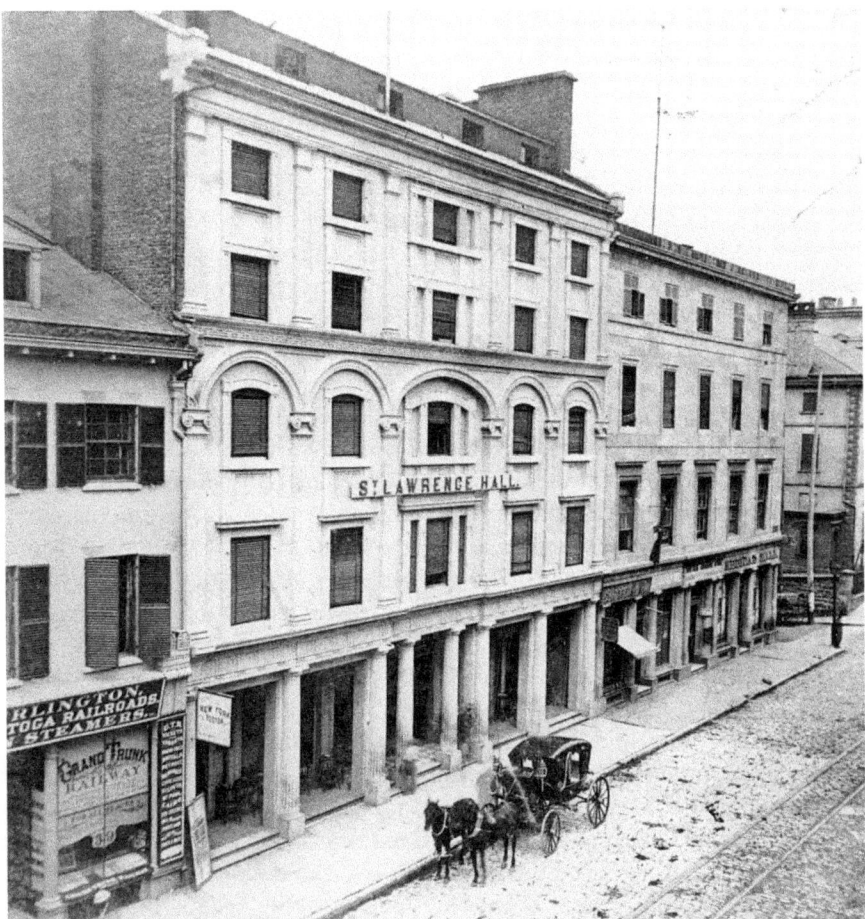

Figure 4. St. Lawrence Hall in Montreal was the central meeting place for the Confederates in Canada. Lavish by any standards, it served the elite of the Canadian Confederacy (McCord Museum, Montreal; photograph by James George Parks, c. 1865–1870, purchased from Edward McCann, © MP-1975.36.5.1).

The actor John Wilkes Booth met with other Confederates at St. Lawrence Hall on at least two occasions—October 18–27, 1864, and January 1865. On October 18, 1864, a ciphered letter reported that "their friends would be set to work as he had directed."[3] This letter may have been related to Booth's plan to develop a plot to kidnap Lincoln. Some historians dispute whether kidnapping was ever a serious option in the plan; clearly Booth's intent on the night of April 14, 1865, was not kidnapping. Booth was reported to have said the following in Montreal in October 1864: "For Abe's contract is near up and whether re-elected or not, he will get his goose cooked."[4] All this time, the Confederate Secret Service was gathering men and momentum to undermine the Union war effort. John Wilkes Booth, John Surratt, and Lewis Powell (alias Lewis Payne or Lewis Paine) met in Montreal at least twice to discuss actions they could use to stop Lincoln and his forces. On October 18, 1864, Booth met with other conspirators in Room 150 at St. Lawrence Hall. The attendees included Jacob Thompson, Clement Clay, Beverly Tucker, George Sanders, Dr. Montrose A. Pallen, Dr. Luke Blackburn, a Mr. Lee from Richmond (one of Robert E. Lee's relatives, likely Edwin Gray Lee), James D. Westcott of Florida, and probably others. The exact dealings completed there are unknown, but Booth might have refined his plans at these meetings to put a stop to Lincoln. Whether he had a "Plan B" at the time that included assassination is unknown. Nevertheless, in spite of these well-documented meetings, no *direct proof* exists that Booth and the other Confederates plotted Lincoln's kidnapping or murder there. Booth then went back to the states, appearing onstage in New York in November 1864. On November 29, 1864, Jefferson Davis received a communication from Waldeman Alston, a recently escaped Confederate prisoner, regarding the need "to rid my Country of some of her deadliest enemies, by striking at the very hearts [sic] blood of those who seek to enchain her in slavery,"[5] presumably referring to actions directed against high government officials.

Dr. Luke Blackburn would travel extensively through Canada, frequently residing in Montreal, Toronto, and Halifax. Montreal was the largest city in Canada at the time, and it had many amenities, making it a desirable place for the Confederate agents to sequester themselves. For Southern gentlemen and ladies it had everything they needed for a lavish existence, at least by the standards of the 1860s. Confederates in Canada—at least the upper-level Confederate commissioners and their friends—lived an elegant lifestyle. Confederate funding seemed endless, and its higher-ranking agents lived well and traveled freely. Confederates loved and demanded fancy hotels. Southerners loved mint juleps, brandy, and fine cigars. The St. Lawrence was purportedly the only hotel in the entire country that served all of these fineries. Blackburn would experience all of its offerings.

Other meeting places in Montreal were the Ottawa Hotel, and—for lower-class accommodations—the Donegana Hotel.[6] The Donegana had passed through many iterations. First it was a home, then a political residence, then a school, then a hotel. It burned in 1849 but was rebuilt. First an elegant accommodation, it lowered its standards a bit in the 1860s. Located at the corner of Notre-Dame Street and Bonsecours Market in Montreal, it sported 150 rooms, and in 1866 it advertised "Hot and Cold Bath Rooms," three meals and a tea, and billiard tables. The Donegana remained open through the winter for the first time in 1861 to cater to Confederates as a men-only establishment, housing many escaped and penniless Confederate soldiers. Union

Secretary of State William H. Seward found that the management of the Donegana was unsympathetic to Union requests for rooms, and he was unable to house his agents there. An article in the *New York Times* in 1863 lamented the sentiment of Canadians toward the Union and decried their hoteliers' hospitality: "I found but one hotel in Montreal where a Union man could stop and sojourn, without being insulted daily and hourly at the table and in the parlors. That is the Ottawa Hotel, kept by S. Browning, an American gentleman. The Donegana and St. Lawrence are as full of secesh [Confederate secessionists] as an egg is full of meat. Sympathy or good-will toward us here in the North is a thing of the past in Canada. The war interrupts their trade, and they are constantly wishing it was closed."[7] Blackburn's wealth dictated that his residence would be the St. Lawrence when he visited Montreal and the Queen's Hotel when in Toronto.

The Saverly House was a Confederate haunt in Halifax. Hesslein's was the hotel of choice in St. John, and the Clifton House was the center of activity in Niagara. The American Hotel at the corner of Front Street East and Yonge Street served in Toronto as the Confederate headquarters, and the Queen's Hotel, on Front Street West at York Street, near the train station, was also popular with Southerners. But St. Lawrence Hall at King and Centre streets in Montreal was the epicenter of Confederate activity for the entire country. The registers for these hotels comprised a virtual encyclopedia of Southern agitators residing in Canada. Agents and counteragents followed each other endlessly, and such connections were part of the reason the Confederate plans to sabotage sites in the North would be so singularly unsuccessful. Nothing was secret, and everyone was being followed. Nevertheless, St. Lawrence Hall remained popular to the Confederates, with even President Jefferson Davis fleeing there after his release from prison in 1867.

4

Maritime Shipping and the Union Blockade of Confederate Ports

Abraham Lincoln recognized the importance of shipping by boat for the economy and survival of the South, and he instituted the naval blockade from Virginia to Texas on April 19, 1861, only days after the start of hostilities of the Civil War. This blockade was meant to strangle the South, and it was called the "Anaconda Plan" (Figures 5 and 6). During early 1861, the Union had only about 50 vessels to pursue this isolation of Southern ports from supplies originating in Britain and Europe.[1] They needed to control about 3,500 miles of coastline from Maryland to the Gulf of Mexico border between Texas and Mexico, but soon the Union navy would expand to sufficient numbers such that the blockade was effective.[2] As the blockade tightened, the runners used smaller and smaller ships, vessels that were more maneuverable, faster, and having more shallow drafts to be able to enter ports that weren't as deep. These smaller ships were often less stable and certainly couldn't carry large quantities of coal, making intermediate stops such as those provided

Opposite top: Figure 5. The Confederate blockade-runner *Robert E. Lee*. Blockade-runners were usually coal-fired and steam-powered, with auxiliary sails. They were fast, sleek, and ran low in the water. They succeeded initially during the Civil War because they could outrun the Union blockading ships. This photograph was taken in 1864 after the Confederate ship *Robert E. Lee* had been captured and rechristened the Union USS *Fort Donelson*. *Opposite bottom:* Figure 6. Famous depiction of the naval isolation of Confederate ports—"Scott's Great Snake," or "The Anaconda Plan." Drawn by J. B. Elliott in 1861 (note that his spelling left a bit to be desired: "Kanzas" "Nutrality," "Pensylvania," and "Dam" instead of "Damn"). General Winfield Scott proposed to strangle the South by blockading Southern ports, preventing transfer of goods and supplies to the Southern war effort. Abraham Lincoln approved this plan on April 19, 1861, just days after the Civil War began (Library of Congress).

SCOTT'S GREAT SNAKE.
IOWA
ILLINOIS
INDIANA
OHIO
NEW YORK
PENSYLVANIA
MISSOURI
KANZAS
KENTUCKY
VIRGINIA
INDIAN TERRITORY
ARKANSAS
TENNESSEE
NORTH CAROLINA
GEORGIA
SOUTH CAROLINA
MISSISSIPPI
ALABAMA
TEXAS
LOUISIANA
FLORIDA

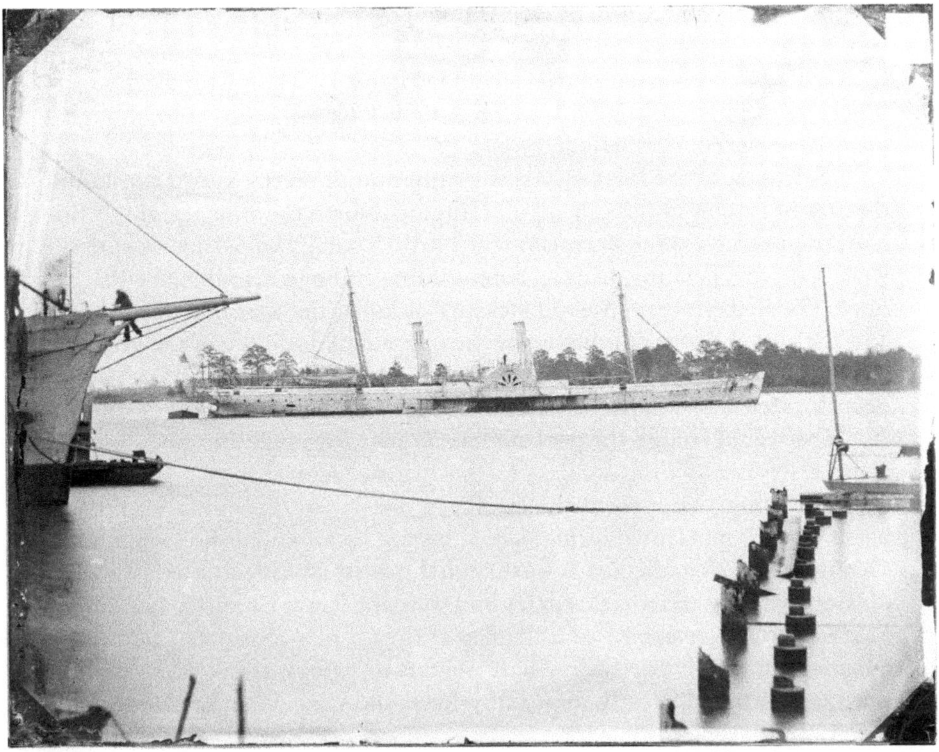

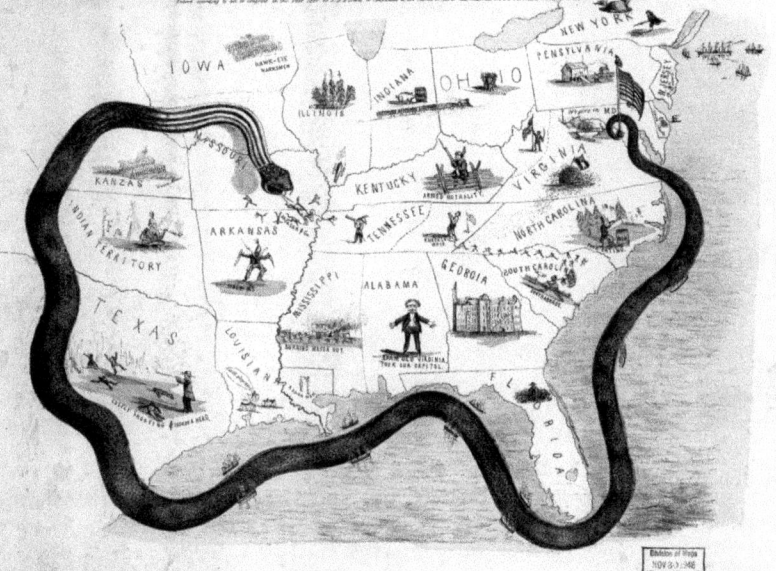

by Bermuda and Nassau more valuable (Figure 7). The vast majority of the blockade-runners officially flew the British flag; few were bold enough to hoist the Confederate banner.

Bermuda of the late 1850s was a rather quiet, sleepy island community that sat 674 miles to the east of Wilmington, North Carolina. Having a population of about 11,000, Bermuda was a British colony whose major activities were shipping, farming, fishing, boatbuilding and repair, and the British military. The British Royal Naval Dockyard stood at the west end of the island, and the east end was dominated by the commercial activity of the port of St. Georges (Figures 8A and 8B).[3] (While Bermuda's government center had been located in Hamilton since 1815, most Confederate blockade-running shipping went through the port at St. Georges.) Although Bermuda was officially a British holding, subject to the British Neutrality Act, Bermudians overwhelmingly supported the Southern cause, and Bermuda would soon become an important intermediate shipping location for the Confederacy. (Testimony to that allegiance was the fact that upon Lincoln's assassination, the only flags lowered in respect for him were the flag at Union Consul Charles Maxwell Allen's residence and the flag at the French consulate.) Bermudian allegiance was only partly drawn by politics or natural affinity. The island of Bermuda profited greatly financially from the Civil War. Some blockade-

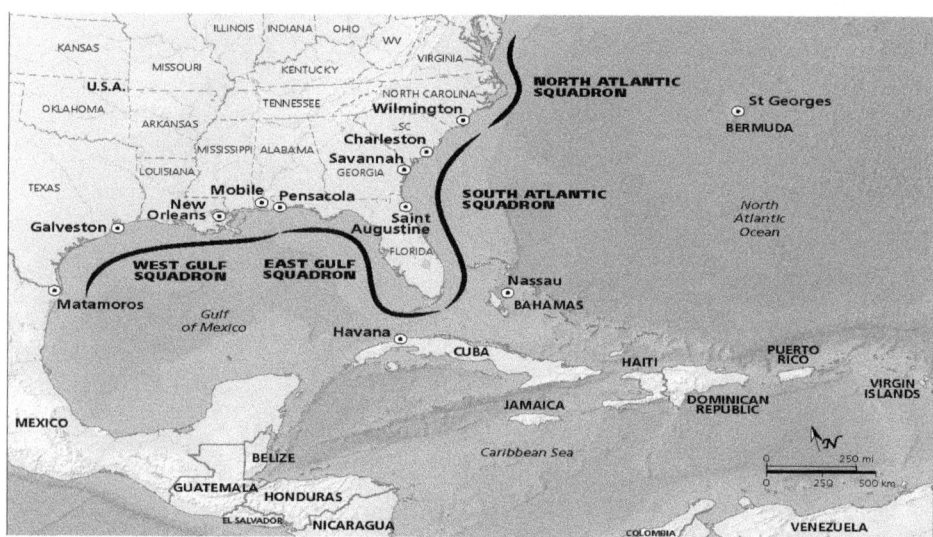

Figure 7. Union Blockading Squadrons under the "Anaconda Plan." Union naval forces were divided into four regions: the North Atlantic, the South Atlantic, the East Gulf, and the West Gulf. Over the course of the Civil War, Northern blockade of the Southern ports became more effective (Kulshan Cartographics, Bellingham, Washington).

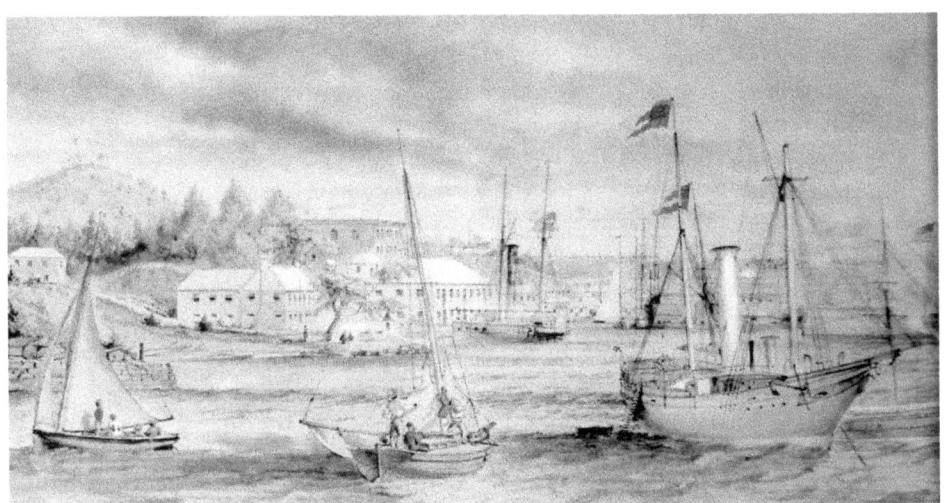

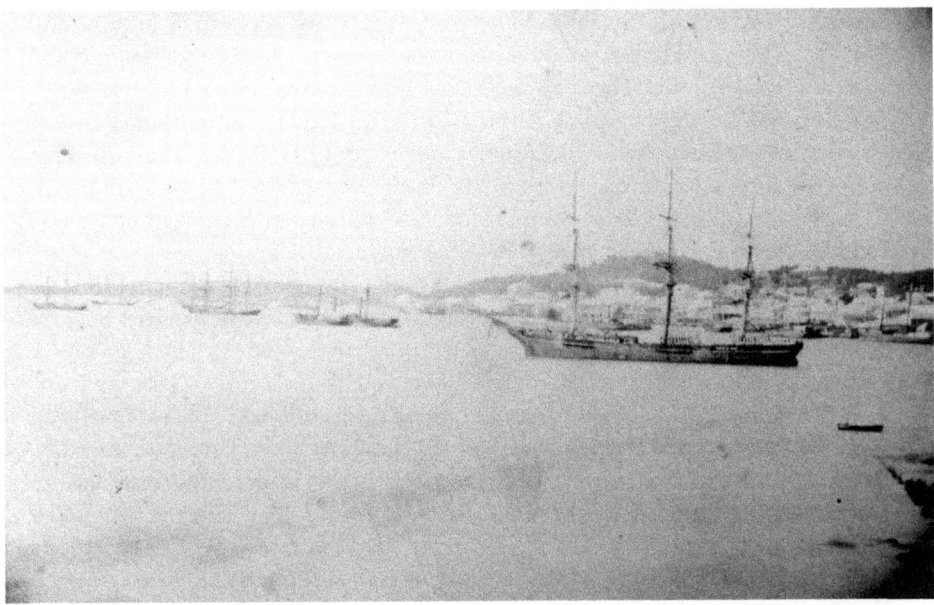

Top: Figure 8A. St. Georges Harbor, painted by Edward K. James in c. 1864. Bermuda was a transfer point for goods and supplies for the South, the major Bermudian port cities being Hamilton and St. Georges. Confederate blockade-runners centered their activity at St. Georges, where larger ships from Europe would unload their freight and place it on smaller, sleeker, faster vessels that would deliver supplies to the South, most commonly through the ports of Wilmington, North Carolina, Charleston, South Carolina, and Savannah, Georgia (St. Georges Historical Society, https://en.wikipedia.org/wiki/File:St._George%27s_Harbour_circa_1864.jpg). *Bottom:* Figure 8B. St. Georges Harbor, Bermuda, 1869. Even after economic stimulus of blockade-running during the Civil War disappeared, the harbor at St. Georges was quite active (Bermuda Archives, Photographic Collection, Image #2547).

running ships were strictly commercial; some were owned and coordinated by the Confederate government. Dr. Blackburn would experience life in Bermuda with its support of the Southern cause.

Chief exports from the South to Britain and Europe were cotton ("white gold") and tobacco. On the return trip from Britain and Europe, large sailing ships contained munitions and other supplies needed by the Confederacy. As the war progressed, smaller, sleeker, and faster ships replaced the larger vessels plying the route between Bermuda and the South. These newer blockade-runners needed coal to fire their engines, and they were theoretically less prone to capture or destruction by the Union blockading squadrons. So the stop in Bermuda allowed the goods intended for the Confederacy to be transferred from the larger ships from Europe to the smaller vessels bound directly for the South through Confederate ports, usually Wilmington, North Carolina, but also to Savannah, Mobile, Galveston, and Charleston. Alternate transfer ports for blockade-runners were located in Nassau, Bahamas, and Havana, Cuba, and less often in Matamoros, Mexico. Frequent passenger and mail service also plied the seas between Halifax, Nova Scotia, and Bermuda, and between Bermuda and St. Thomas, Virgin Islands. Government officials in Halifax were satisfied to let their citizens profit from the trade growing from the Confederate use of its port. Union Secretary of State William H. Seward was fully aware of the Confederate activity in Halifax, but he was unable to halt it through diplomatic channels.

Initially isolated by both distance and provincial thought processes, Bermudians soon began to understand that the unrest in the American states would have a profound impact on Bermudian fortunes. The Civil War changed the face of this island community and made it one of intense Confederate commercial activity. One Bermuda resident said, "There is nothing to talk of here but war.... Active preparations are being made, I may say, throughout the Island."[4] By the time the war was well underway, Confederate-bound vessels clogged Bermudian ports. Union consul Charles M. Allen reported in October 1863 on St. Georges: "The harbor is so full of vessels there is scarcely a chance for one to anchor—all secessionist."[5] Allen decried the domination of Bermudian shipping by Confederates but said, "I have learned to keep quiet and [enter] into no arguments.... Every hole and corner is filled with Southernors [sic]."[6]

Ships' captains embarked on their hazardous duties for handsome salaries. The British pound was the currency used in Bermuda. Exchange rates varied as the Civil War progressed, with Confederate currency falling in value toward the end of the war, as it appeared that Confederate dollars might become worthless. But in general a U.S. dollar was worth about 0.2 British Pound Sterling (£) in 1860 and 0.13 £ in early 1865.[7] Wages might be paid either in British pounds or in U.S. dollars or often in gold.

4. Maritime Shipping and the Union Blockade

A captain would likely earn about £1–2 (about $8–16) per day, with a bonus of £25 (about $200) for a successful trip. An entire round-trip could last 20–40 days, so £100 (about $800) was the average pay to travel from Bermuda to, for example, Wilmington, North Carolina. Later in the war, captains of private vessels doing blockade-running could earn up to $500 in U.S. gold per round-trip. Captains of Confederate-owned ships received about $200, and a bonus of another $200 was added if the trip was successful. (Some captains of particularly dangerous and lucrative runs were reported to have made up to $5,000 per run.) In addition, however, some captains were allowed to bring personal merchandise along on the trip to sell, and this activity could dramatically increase the captain's wages. Good captains were also paid a retainer between runs, and this supplement could run up to 10 shillings (about $2.50) per day.[8] The crew would number 35–60 men. Firemen on private vessels would make the equivalent of $100–150 per round-trip; common sailors on private ships drew $50 ($80–150 later in the Civil War, though crews of Confederate-owned vessels made considerably less). This wage was high compared to sailors doing shipping other than Confederate blockade-running. Later in the Civil War a blockade-runner could earn more in three trips than a regular commercial sailor earned in an entire year. Most crew members were able to secure their next job after about two weeks in port, but this gap lended itself to troublemaking, as bars and brothels were abundant.[9]

Dock laborers in Bermuda before the Civil War made about 3 shillings 6 pence per day; by early in the war they made 5 shillings; and by 1863—mid-war—they were able to command 8 shillings per day.[10] By comparison, a common laborer in Bermuda in 1863 earned about 6–8 shillings per day during the same time period; by 1864 the wage had risen to 12 shillings per day. These wages would become important when considering the prices attached to the storage and transport of items to be used for germ warfare against the North. Furthermore, agents of the South would be offered exorbitant sums of money in comparison to a laborer's yearly wage for their part in the scheme to destroy the North by importing yellow fever.

Cotton sold for $500 per bale as the war reached its midpoint. Demand was high. England had 1,800 cotton mills in the 1860s that produced 1.5 billion yards of manufactured cotton goods during these years. Many purchases for the South were funded by the sale of cotton, a prime source for exchange (tobacco was the number two crop sold to Europe from the South). Bales of cotton weighed 400–500 pounds; a small steamer could hold 500 bales, and cotton that was sold for 6 cents per pound in Wilmington fetched as much as 56 cents per pound in Britain by the end of the war.[11] This "white gold"[12] was one of the major commodities that supported the purchase of contraband goods in Europe for the Confederacy. Prices for other goods in great demand soared, too. Flour sold for $300 per barrel; coffee sold for $12 per pound.

Other indices of income and cost of living in the 1860s are reflected in the yearly salaries of other jobs and professions. The governor of Bermuda made £500/year (about $4,000); the police magistrate of Hamilton, Bermuda, £120/year (about $960); a librarian, £50/year (about $400). Salaries were low; prices were high.[13]

All the while, Bermudians enjoyed the good life. Increased commercial activity caused a boom in the economy, and one report described conditions on Bermuda as a "Life of high gaiety."[14] While the cost of living was high (more than 125 percent of that in New York City), Bermudians generally prospered.[15] Salaries of clerks were about $500–1000 per year; Major Smith Stansbury, the commanding officer of the Bermuda Confederate Ordnance Department of the Confederate States Army, wrote that a good clerk needed even a much higher salary. The Confederacy wanted to pay $700–800 per year, an amount that Stansbury called "utterly inadequate." Stansbury argued that they should be paid at least $1,200–1,500.[16] George P. Black, a Confederate clerk, ultimately made $1,000 per year; Gustave Alexander,[17] another clerk who came to Bermuda at about the same time as Black, made the same salary.[18]

While the port at St. Georges, Bermuda, provided water 21 feet deep, some of the American ports were shallower. Bermuda had an abundance of wharves, storage buildings, and warehouses, as well as a cadre of dockworkers. By early 1862, blockade-running was the dominant industry for St. Georges. Bermuda was more distant from the Southern shores than Nassau, Bahamas, but there was no lack of need for both sites to supply the Confederacy. Private vessels were more common in Nassau, while the Confederate Ordnance Bureau (under the direction of Major Josiah Gorgas) used Bermuda for its main base of operations. Thus, consumer goods usually passed through Nassau, while guns and ammunition were ordinarily sent to the South from Europe through Bermuda. The British had about 1,000 troops stationed on Bermuda, and at the outset of the war, 25 British ships patrolled between Bermuda and Halifax. Within one year, the troop numbers had grown by an additional 445—to 1,445—and the British navy had 42 ships. However, the British navy rarely interfered with the contraband traffic of the blockade-runners.

Coal was the major energy source for the steamships, wood being too expensive. All of the coal had to come from elsewhere, as none was mined in Bermuda. Large storage facilities near the St. Georges docks kept huge quantities of coal, but coal shortages were common. This meant that blockade-running ships often were stranded in the Bermudian port. Amazingly, the ships used by blockade-runners were considered to be disposable items. When being pursued by Union navy ships near Southern ports, Confederate captains would often purposely run them aground and burn them rather than let them become prizes for the Union navy. The smaller steamships cost £10,000–30,000 (about $80,000–240,000), while their cargo was worth approximately £50,000 (about $400,000). The price of 500 bales of cotton in Britain at the beginning of the Civil War was about £21,000 (about $168,000).[19] By mid-war it was $250,000.

Both Union and Confederate forces had key personnel at the Bermudian port of St. Georges. Consul Frederick B. Wells first represented the Union. He was followed by Consul Charles Maxwell Allen, who was assigned to Bermuda in August 1861, although Allen didn't arrive in Bermuda until November. Allen's wife Susan and their five children later joined him. He served there until his death in 1889. Allen's Union counterpart in Halifax, Nova Scotia, one of the ports most frequented by Confederate sympathizers, was Consul Mortimer M. Jackson. Major Josiah Gorgas first served the Confederate interests in Bermuda. He was initially responsible for the shipping of ordnance for the Confederacy through the island. However, by early 1862 the job had grown so large and the volume of weapons and supplies passing through the Bermudian port so great that Gorgas first sent Major Norman S. Walker to Europe with $2 million dollars in cotton bonds to purchase more blockade-running ships. Then Gorgas appointed Walker to help with the coordination of supplies passing through Bermuda. Walker arrived in Bermuda in February 1863. In contrast to the rude treatment the Bermudians afforded Consul Allen, Walker and his family were welcomed warmly into Bermudian society. John Tory Bourne was the Bermudian Confederate commercial agent who most frequently dealt with Major Walker.

Consul Allen diligently reported the activities of the blockade-runners, often with exasperation at the British government since Bermuda was supposed to be a neutral port (some referred to it as the "Offshore Confederacy"). Allen was adept at discovering and reporting activities designed to help the Confederacy, though resources to combat such activity were meager or nonexistent. Blockade-runners from Bermuda—sometimes as many as three or four a day—departed unchallenged from Bermuda.[20] On a few occasions Union ships policed the areas approaching the entrances to Bermuda's harbors, but they judiciously avoided major conflicts on the seas near the island. While Queen Victoria had issued proclamations that forbade transport of guns or weapons from Britain to the North or the South, these proclamations were ignored by almost everyone. The queen made her Proclamation of Neutrality on May 13, 1861, saying that she "strictly charged and commanded all her subjects to observe a strict neutrality during the hostilities [between the Union and the Confederacy] ... and to abstain from violating or contravening either the laws and statutes of the realm in this behalf, or the law of nations in relation thereto." She forbade her subjects from entering the military service of either side, from serving upon any vessels of transport for either side, from "fitting out, arming, or equipping" either side, and specifically from engaging in blockade-running.[21] Englishmen routinely disobeyed these rules. The majority of British citizens and businessmen, as well as many in the British navy, remained pro–Confederacy throughout the war.

Consul Allen worked almost alone during the Civil War era and with inadequate funds. Visitors frequently prevailed upon him and his wife to help them out of logistical, personal, and legal difficulties, with Allen often making even his home and personal provisions available to the lost or stranded sailor. Bermudians initially despised Allen, although after the war he became more accepted and even well liked by local residents. Early in his duties, on December 30, 1861, Allen wrote, "The present state of things makes it very unpleasant for me here just now as there is a very bitter feeling against everything and everybody belonging to the United States [the North] and many here seem to go upon the supposition that I am responsible for the whole difficulty."[22] Later he would say, "It is wonderful to see how ready they are to believe anything that favors the South and ready to disbelieve anything that favors the North."[23] However, by the end of his tenure as consul in 1889, nearly a quarter of a century after the Civil War, he was one of the most beloved political figures on the island.

The *Bermuda Gazette* daily reported activities of the North and the South to citizens of Bermuda, and this newspaper was decidedly pro–Confederacy, molding and directing the sentiments of its readers to reflect that. It frequently told of the "atrocities" committed by the Union troops, and it glorified Jefferson Davis and his speeches while denouncing Abraham Lincoln for the stands he took.

Blockade-running was a dangerous endeavor. Many ships were captured and many were sunk. At the start of the war nine blockade-running trips succeeded for each one that was captured or sunk.[24] By 1863 the ratio was 4:1; by 1864, 1.7:1; by 1865, 1:1. Mail and passenger ships from and to Halifax, however, were virtually never harassed, sunk, or captured.[25] At the start of the war, Bermuda and the Bahamas vied for dominance in trade, but after 1862 Bermuda ascended in importance. Yellow fever in the summer generally hit the Bahamas worse than in Bermuda, and the Union's Southern Atlantic Blocking Squadron concentrated its efforts on the Bahamas, to the relief of Bermudian shipping.[26] Sailors spent wildly when they had shore leave. St. Georges had one area of particularly ill repute called Shinbone Alley, located at the base of the road to Barrack Hill. Edward Cork Swan, a man with connections to Dr. Luke Blackburn and who would soon become prominent in the Bermuda yellow fever plot, lived here. Bars proliferated in the neighborhood, as did prostitution.[27]

The increased shipping activity and traffic had a negative side. Yellow fever and smallpox were frequently imported from other islands. Bermudian

4. Maritime Shipping and the Union Blockade

health officials established quarantine stations and procedures for arriving sailors who appeared to be sick. Nevertheless, epidemics frequently threatened Bermudian society. Bermuda is a group of about 181 islands, most of them tiny, and even the main island is only about 22 miles long and 2 miles wide. Any communicable disease arriving on one part of the main island could be easily transmitted to the rest of the island or to any of the smaller surrounding islands.

5

Civil War Medicine and Dr. Blackburn

Dr. Luke Blackburn moved back to Kentucky from New Orleans in 1860. There he established a medical practice in Louisville, but he would soon become an agent of the Confederacy in the Civil War, though he did not join the Confederate Medical Corps. One must ask why a physician like Dr. Luke Blackburn chose not to join the corps. He was well trained; he was an expert in infectious diseases; he could have risen high in the corps' medical hierarchy and been influential for the Southern cause. Furthermore, he might have even gained fame in this position. The South relied upon volunteers until the First Conscription Act in April 1862, which limited the draft between the ages of 18 and 35. Later draft acts expanded the age range from 18–45 (September 1862) and from 17–50 (February 1864).[1] Blackburn was 44 when the war broke out in April 1861. But was age the only reason he declined to offer his services to the Medical Corps?

Doctors of Blackburn's era had not yet seen what we consider today to be the major medical discoveries. The germ theory of disease hadn't been promulgated; antibiotics were unknown; antisepsis was an undiscovered concept; vaccines were nearly nonexistent; cleanliness was an afterthought, if that.[2] Also, surgery was crude. Most doctors of the day were not experienced in it. Many had never seen a bullet wound, and most had never performed an amputation. Such surgical knowledge and experience would be needed for battlefield medicine during the Civil War.[3]

The Confederate Medical Branch, which Dr. Blackburn might have been tempted to join, was organized similar to the Union Medical Corps.[4] Personnel were classified into three groups: surgeons (their rank was similar to a major in the cavalry), assistant surgeons (the rank of captain), and contract or acting assistant surgeons (the rank and pay equal to a second lieutenant; many of these would become surgeons or assistant surgeons as the war continued). Usually the battalion level had an assistant surgeon, and occasionally a company had an assistant surgeon. Having both a surgeon and assistant surgeon was the staffing level usually reserved for a regiment.

Hospitals were only a short distance from the front lines. The concept of ambulance services originated during the Civil War with Dr. Jonathan Letterman in the Union army.[5] Either an infirmary detail or an ambulance crew brought the wounded to the field hospital for care. Ambulances were wooden carts, some of which could hold four patients. By 1862 each Union regiment had two wagons, one of which was used as an ambulance and one to ferry supplies. By August 1863 each Union regiment had three wagons.[6] Advances in skills and techniques for the Confederate Medical Branch often came from captured Union hospitals, and Confederate patient transport systems followed the Union's leading.

Assistant surgeons did mostly first aid, while the surgeons were responsible for definitive care. First aid consisted of stopping major bleeding (tourniquet, ligature, or compressive bandages), temporarily setting broken limbs, and administering oral fluids, stimulants, and painkillers. Most major wounds were handled at the field hospital. Patients were then transferred by horse and buggy, makeshift ambulance, or train to more distant regional hospitals. Doctors had a staff of enlisted, noncommissioned assistants, starting with the hospital steward, whose education and skills were quite varied. Some had begun medical training (medical school was usually two years, followed by some type of apprenticeship); some had experience in a pharmacy. Hospital stewards had additional help from the enlisted men to perform nursing duties and to care for the wounded soldiers.

The Medical Corps lived and ate with the infantry soldiers in open fields under harsh conditions. Food rations were often one-half to one-quarter of what was ideally needed and prescribed, and soldiers and doctors alike often existed under semi-starvation conditions. Exhaustion and prostration were constant companions. Even during battle, the "field hospitals" (transformed houses, churches, barns, or even the open fields) were located close to the fighting, one-half to one mile to the rear of the front line. The first hospitals were open-air, but small tents (holding about six patients) soon became the norm. They, too, were within range of stray bullets or cannonballs. Dr. Blackburn may not have relished such an existence.

Some reports, including a statement made by President Jefferson Davis while he was in confinement at Fortress Monroe after the Civil War,[7] suggested that the surgeons and assistant surgeons in the Confederate army were poorly qualified, even "quacks." In fact, the level of medical skill was very limited on both sides of the Civil War, but more because of the general lack of medical knowledge rather than specific deficiencies in the Confederate physicians. The doctors were, in fact, generally well screened, and a medical board examined each doctor entering the medical service, as well as those who were already a part of the army. Indeed, the level of medical care by today's standards was woefully inadequate, but similar medicine and surgery were practiced on both civilians and military throughout the states at the time, in both the North and the South.

The Medical Corps of the Union was small at the beginning of the Civil War. Estimates suggest that only 115 doctors initially served the entire Union army when hostilities erupted. As the conflict began, 27 doctors resigned from the ranks of the North. Three of them returned to private practice, and 24 enlisted in the Confederate army because they were from the South and their sympathies rested with the Rebels. These 24 actually became the core of the fledgling Confederate Medical Corps.[8] They brought with them their training from the Union, as well as their techniques, their instruments, their concept of organization of hospitals, and even the paperwork and forms that they had used when they were working for the North. So the organization of the Confederate medical system was virtually identical to its Northern counterpart. It was within this Confederate Medical Corps that Dr. Blackburn could have made his mark had he so chosen.

Doctors had a unique approach to the conflict. Feeling that they had been caught in the fray, rather than being responsible for the fighting, and believing that their duty was to relieve suffering, rather than inflict wounds, they often found themselves treating the victims of the opposing side of the war. At the beginning of the Civil War, when the enemy captured a doctor he was incarcerated like any other prisoner of war. However, soon these doctors began treating members of the prison population, and thereafter their captors allowed them to function as doctors not only within their own prisoner camps but permitted them to treat troops of the other side, as well. Confederate doctors treated Union troops, and vice versa.

One Confederate physician, Dr. Paul Christian Yates, wrote a short biography of his service in the Civil War.[9] On one occasion, he went to a Federal hospital to see if he could render assistance to any wounded Union soldiers there. Two Union doctors were present who were doing nothing for the patients. They had given up hope because they had been told that they would likely die the next day because the Confederate Rebels were going to kill all of the Union troops in battle, even those they captured. The rumor had been circulated that the Rebels were working under a "black flag," which meant that the Confederates were to take no prisoners. Dr. Yates declared this rumor to be false and proceeded to treat the Union soldiers. One soldier in particular was suffering greatly, having been "shot through the elbow joint, which was full of maggots and very painful":

> I [Dr. Yates] said [to the Union doctors present], "Take that arm off immediately, or you will have blood poison[ing]."
> Then, he [the patient] said [to Dr. Yates], "Please do it for me."

I have never amputated. I said, "Get ready."
We put him on the table and put chloroform to his nose.
He [the patient] says, "I tell you what I wish."
The [other Union] doctor shook him and said, "Hush."
I said, "Let him tell it. What do you wish?"
He said he wished he had all the Rebels except Jeff Davis in a big cauldron, and a big fire under that. He would boil them down to a pint, and pour that down old [Jefferson] Davis' throat.
I said, "Was that all?"
He said, no, he wishes he had all the Gun-Powder in a heap, and all the Rebels Army [on] it; he would torch it off, and blow them all to hell.
By this time he was under chloroform. I cut the arm off near the shoulder, fixed it nicely, and brought him out from under the chloroform, and he felt much better.
I said, "Young man, what do you wish now?"
He said he wished he was home with his mother.
I said, "That is a very different wish to what you did make [a few minutes ago]."
He asked what it was.
On being told, he looked at me and said, "You have done for me what my own doctor would not do. I will take it back as far as you are concerned." But be damned if he would ever take it back as far as the rest of the Rebels were concerned.
They [the other wounded Union soldiers] all looked upon me as a friend, and expressed many regrets when I had to leave them, which was after all of the worst cases had been attended to.[10]

By May 1862 doctors captured were immediately released to return to their own troops. Therefore, in general, the neutral status of the medical profession was honored. Dr. Blackburn might have been able to function—even flourish—in this system.

Confederate medical personnel at the peak of the conflict were estimated to comprise 834 surgeons and 1,668 assistant surgeons, for a total of 2,502.[11] The Union's complement of doctors was about four times that many. One must remember, however, that the size of the respective populations of the North and the South were quite different. The population of the North was about 22 million, in the South about 9 million. Eligible men of fighting age were about 4.6 million in the North and 1.1 million in the South. The Union army totaled 2,128,948 soldiers who fought during the entire war.[12] The Confederate army numbered 1,082,119. At any one time, the largest fighting force the Union army had was 1,000,516, the Confederate army being 304,015. On average, the Union strength was 614,000, the Confederate 213,000.[13] The army of the North thus was three to four times as large as that of the South at any given time. By the end of the war more nurses had become available to assist in the medical and surgical duties. About 20,000 nurses served in the Civil War, a combined number from both the North and the South. However, Dr. Blackburn didn't join these forces. He apparently had other plans.

• • •

Major infectious diseases during the Civil War era included typhoid, dysentery, malaria, yellow fever, tetanus, measles, smallpox, chickenpox, mumps, whooping cough, and various types of pneumonia. Virtually every soldier on both sides experienced at least one diarrheal illness during his service. Disease far outweighed battlefield injury or death in removing a soldier from his duty. Two of three deaths were caused by illness, as opposed to an injury sustained in battle. Diarrhea and dysentery alone claimed more victims than wounds. Typhoid, dysentery, and pneumonia were the three major killers in all of the camps.

Camp sanitation and hygiene were the responsibility of the Medical Corps. However, little attention was paid to these aspects of the soldier's health because physicians knew little about the relationship between cleanliness and health, and little manpower was available to pursue these goals. Medicines were in short supply, both for the Confederate army and for the population of the South in general. Few Southern medicine-producing laboratories existed. Nearly the entire supply of drugs was dependent upon smuggling, blockade-running, or the capture of medicines from Northern hospitals as spoils of battle. The South was agricultural; the North was industrial. Production in the South consisted of cotton, wheat, sugar cane, rice, fruits, and livestock.

Both Southern Army and Southern civilian doctors had to resort to nonstandard herbal remedies for many, if not most, needs.[14] Teas and potions made with roots, barks, and branches supplanted conventional medicines. Occasionally, whiskey, brandy, and quinine were the only available medicines, and even these were frightfully expensive. Quinine sometimes sold for $100 per ounce; in today's dollars, quinine was $2,000 per ounce. Rations of common medicines in Confederate army hospitals were woefully inadequate—192 pints of medicinal alcohol were supposed to be enough for 1,000 soldiers for one year (though additional quantities might be obtained through the quartermaster's general allotment), 16 ounces of iodine likewise. Red oak, snake root, mayapple, peachtree leaves, slippery elm, mandrake tea, and a myriad of other homemade and herbal medicines became commonplace. Even old herbal remedies had to be abandoned for substitutes when the original herb was exhausted: ipecac was replaced by Carolina hipps; digitalis became bugleweed. When opium supplies were exhausted, doctors used motherwort. Calomel disappeared, and dandelion became its substitute. The pharmacopeia became a veritable gardener's stock.

Not only was the supply of medicines for the Confederate doctors difficult because of the lack of manufacturing sites for them in the South, but also the priority for transporting goods put the hospitals at a disadvantage. First priorities were the provisions for the troops needed at the battlefront: ammunition was crucial and went first; food and rations came next. Only after these items were transported did the medical supplies make their way to the front lines. Often, even if medicines were available, they didn't arrive at the front lines in a timely fashion. The Union naval blockade of ports was indeed quite effective in limiting the medical supplies needed by the South. Dr. Blackburn may have considered these limitations as part of the reason why he chose not to join the Medical Corps.

Contrasted to the supply of other medicines, chloroform and ether were widely available and used almost invariably for soldiers with serious wounds or those needing amputation. Chloroform anesthesia had been discovered by James Young Simpson in 1847, ether in the 1840s (some say by Crawford Williamson Long in 1842, others say by William T.G. Morton in 1846). The anesthetic properties of these two substances revolutionized surgery. Civil War doctors knew the value of good anesthesia, and most operations utilized one or both of these substances. Anesthesia was given in over 80,000 surgeries performed on the troops in the Civil War.[15] A sampling of over 8,900 cases revealed that chloroform was used in 76.2 percent of them, ether in 14.7 percent, and a combination of both in 9.1 percent. Administration was relatively simple and often a minimally trained assistant performed the anesthesia. The liquid chloroform (or ether) was applied to a porous cone placed over the patient's mouth and nose. It evaporated and was inhaled by the wounded soldier; as soon as he was rendered senseless, the surgeon began his work. Toxic reactions were rare, and many of the deaths attributed to the anesthetic were, in fact, the result of the severity of the wound or the operation. Since most operations were amputations, and most could be performed in 10–15 minutes, the duration of the anesthesia was brief. As today, the risk of the operation (and of the anesthesia) was related to the duration of the surgery; most patients survived the immediate operation itself. Subsequent deaths were often the result of infectious complications. Death ascribed to the anesthetic occurred in 0.54 percent of cases using chloroform, in 0.30 percent of cases with ether, and in 0.24 percent with the combination of chloroform and ether. Since preoperative evaluation for heart and lung disease wasn't performed, many patients who died might have had preexisting conditions that led to the anesthetic catastrophe.

Initially, doctors were expected to bring their own equipment and surgical instruments. By 1862 most doctors had four army-supplied kits at their disposal—one for major surgery, one for minor surgery, a field case, and a pocket kit. Major operations were undertaken at the field hospital near the battlefield. Amputation was the most common operation performed (hence, the name "sawbones" given to the battlefield physicians). Good surgeons could perform an amputation in 10 minutes. Speed was the essence of skillful practice. A quick operation meant that the soldier needed less precious anesthesia—chloroform, ether, or a mixture of the two. Dr. Blackburn had neither these skills nor battlefield experience.

Amputations were more lethal the closer the incision was to the soldier's trunk. That is to say, amputation of a foot was less likely to cause death than amputation at the knee. A hand amputation was safer than the removal at the elbow. Overall, about 25–28 percent of amputees died during the operation. Hip amputations were fatal 83 percent of the time; removal of an entire upper arm resulted in death 24 percent of the time. About 75 percent of all war wounds were to the arms or legs. The Union alone saw 30,000 amputations. Abdominal, head, and chest wounds were almost always fatal. Doctors often triaged these patients to wait until other soldiers with more salvageable wounds were attended, worsening the self-fulfilling prophecy that head, abdominal, and chest wounds would be fatal. But Dr. Blackburn was not trained as a surgeon.

Unfortunately for the victim of the bullet, doctors *expected* the wound to become infected. It was a normal part of the process; if pus didn't appear, something was wrong with the "normal" healing of the wound. This situation reigned because doctors didn't understand anything about the need for cleanliness. Instruments—if cleaned at all—were simply rinsed and passed from one amputation to another. Sponges were used from one patient to the next after only a quick rinse. Doctors proudly wore their bloodstained and pus-besmirched clothes from patient to patient. Clean dressings were almost non-existent, and surgery sites were covered with clothing or strips of torn cloth from the battlefield. (Joseph Lister began the era of antiseptic surgery only in 1865, at the close of the war.) When infection spread to the bloodstream ("blood poisoning" or "pyemia"), fully 90 percent of its victims died. Tetanus was another accompanying disease of war wounds, with a mortality rate of 87 percent. Bone infection (osteomyelitis) after an amputation was common. Overall, the mortality from an immediate amputation, regardless of location, was 25–28 percent; amputations performed later, after the wound was infected, had a death rate of 52 percent.[16]

Weaponry also changed about the time of the Civil War. The Minié ball (soldiers called it the "minnie") was developed in the late 1830s–1840s to provide greater accuracy and longer range (it could travel 200–250 yards in a reasonably straight line, while older bullets were limited to 50 yards, at best).[17] Ironically, the Minié was adopted for the U.S. Army in 1855 by then-Secretary of War Jefferson Davis, who was soon to become the president of the Confederacy. Although called a "ball," it was actually conical in shape and was still loaded through the rifle barrel. The soft lead of the projectile penetrated flesh more effectively than older rifle bullets, tending to destroy more tissue and shatter bone along its course, causing wounds beyond repair and forcing amputation.

Statistics for mortality and morbidity during the Civil War were not kept with precision, but estimates are available. A total of about 624,000 soldiers died. Union soldiers killed in action or mortally wounded numbered 110,100; 224,580 died of disease; 24,881 died of other causes. The total deaths numbered 359,561. Confederate soldiers killed in action or mortally wounded numbered 94,000; 164,000 died of disease; 31,000 died of other causes. Deaths totaled 289,000. Union wounded were 275,175; Confederate 194,026. About one-quarter of all soldiers died (Union 23 percent, Confederate 24 percent). If a soldier was taken prisoner of war, his chance of dying in captivity if he was a Union soldier was 15.5 percent; if he was a Confederate prisoner it was 12 percent.[18]

These facts again demand that question: Why did Dr. Blackburn not volunteer to become a member of the Confederate Medical Corps? Though he may have been too old to be a regular Confederate medical officer at the outset of the Civil War, perhaps it wasn't age alone that drove his decision. The answer likely is that routine doctoring was not the type of practice Blackburn saw as his first choice to aid the Confederacy. He was experienced as a medical doctor, not as a surgeon. As an expert in infectious diseases he could have been useful, but he chose other options. He was devoted to the Confederate cause and could not remain inactive. He served as a nonmedical agent for both Kentucky and Mississippi at the inception of the Civil War, and he would expand his activity later during the conflict. These would be his contributions to the Confederate effort.

6

Dr. Blackburn's Early Confederate Service

In 1861 and 1862 Dr. Blackburn worked to obtain arms for the Southern cause. His first duty was as an assistant to the governor of Kentucky, Beriah Magoffin. Magoffin initially tried to remain neutral in the secession frenzy, balancing the Union and Confederate sympathies of the residents of Kentucky. In part, he may have simply wanted to await the possession of sufficient arms to support hostilities. Kentucky had a state guard, with 61 companies, but it lacked weapons and ordnance.[1] Magoffin received requests from both the North (Secretary of War Simon Cameron) and the South (Secretary of War L.P. Walker) to provide troops for the war and refused both requests. He believed states had the right to secede from the Union, but initially he wouldn't commit to the support of either side. Further demonstrating his desire for strict neutrality,[2] he sought weapons for Kentucky troops from both the North and the South. He justified this approach by asserting Kentucky's neutrality and specifying that the weapons were strictly to be used for defense, not for either Southern-supporting or Northern-supporting offense.

Magoffin dispatched Blackburn to New Orleans to procure arms with a promise of $50,000 for the task (money was obtained from loans drawn on Kentucky banks) and sent Simon Bolivar Buckner on a similar mission to the North (Buckner was unsuccessful). Kentucky banks had loaned the money for weapons only on the condition that Kentucky remain neutral in the war. Blackburn suggested that Kentucky needed "2,000 muskets, 600 kegs of gunpowder, and two pieces of ordinance [sic]."[3] It's unclear from what advice Blackburn made this request, since Blackburn as a physician would have had little knowledge of the military needs of the Kentucky State Guard.

Blackburn went to New Orleans for arms but also allegedly as a spokesperson for Kentucky. It's difficult to understand whether Blackburn was speaking for Magoffin or for himself. Newspapers announced that he

6. Early Confederate Service

would speak about Kentucky's need for arms and ammunition at Lafayette Square, the center of public debate in New Orleans.[4] He boldly proclaimed Kentucky to be firmly on the side of the Confederacy, in opposition to public declarations of neutrality from Governor Magoffin. It could have been an example of having a "well-placed source" announce a policy to see how the news would be received back in the home state. On April 24, 1861, Blackburn wrote to LeRoy Pope Walker, the first Confederate of secretary of war: "I have come here accredited from the Governor of Kentucky for arms. Mississippi has none to spare. We have plenty of men and money. We have no heavy ordnance, and only 10,000 muskets. Kentucky is all right, but powerless for the want of arms. Can you let us have, for friendship or money, ordnance and 10,000 stand of arms? Answer me [at the] Saint Charles Hotel, New Orleans."[5]

Blackburn spoke at the public meeting on the same day at Lafayette Square in New Orleans. The gathering honored the Kentucky volunteers for their support of the Confederacy. Blackburn told of his instructions from Magoffin to procure arms from Mississippi and Louisiana. There he also told Southern sympathizers that the center and west of Kentucky would join them as soon as they were armed (eastern Kentucky had stronger Union sympathies). Later, on April 26, he wrote again to LeRoy Pope Walker as an agent for Governor Magoffin: "Can you let Kentucky have four unmounted guns from Baton Rouge?"[6] Another Southern procurer of arms, Benjamin J. Adams, later advised Magoffin that he [Adams] needed an additional $30,000, which Magoffin solicited from another Kentucky bank, again with the promise of Kentucky's neutrality (making the total $80,000 for purchases from Southern sources). Kentucky thus gained some additional weapons, still allegedly for defense only. Indeed, the *Daily Nashville Patriot* declared on May 11 that Blackburn had secured "2,500 stand of small arms[,] seven pieces of heavy artillery[,] nearly six hundred kegs of powder[,] and 12,000,000 percussion caps, besides a vaeuable [sic] machine for [rifling] muskets."[7]

Blackburn was described as an effective orator, and certainly Southern-leaning newspapers received his message with enthusiasm (and called him "a special agent of the Governor of Kentucky"). One report said, "Yes, in virtue of his credentials, he declared to the South that Kentucky did not care to delay *even for the action of her legislature* [emphasis in the original], but was ready and willing if only armed, to rush instantly into the fray in behalf of the Confederate States against the United States."[8] Was Blackburn truly speaking for Magoffin and Kentucky? Magoffin's immediate response is unrecorded. If he in fact had been deputized to promise Kentucky's support for the South if they received sufficient weapons, documentation of such a bold and specific course of action is lacking.

Some viewers saw Blackburn and Magoffin as agents of "perfidy." Blackburn had touted himself as "an accredited representative of Kentucky," suggesting that his words were Magoffin's words. Blackburn had declared that "Kentucky would 'in a few days be, in act, shoulder to shoulder with the states in the Southern Confederacy.'"[9] Political watchers asked how Kentucky could do anything to move into the Confederacy since no state convention had yet been called and no vote of the people had been taken. Blackburn was accused of being part of "wild and reckless passion." Previously he had stated, "The centre and west of the State were ready to leave the Union the moment they had arms."[10]

Supporters of both the North and neutrality agreed that "no matter who may have accredited him to say it, there was no foundation for it in fact. But he was accredited, it seems, to appeal to the South.... We do earnestly hope that he [Magoffin] did not, formally or informally, accredit Dr. Blackburn to say in New Orleans what that gentleman did say."[11] Maybe Blackburn's representation in New Orleans was the start of his own fanatical support for the Southern cause—support calculated to win by any technique, with the end justifying the means. On May 16, 1861, the Kentucky State House of Representatives approved a neutrality proclamation. Not waiting for the state senate to act, on May 20, 1861, Magoffin signed that neutrality proclamation. Perhaps Blackburn's bold and reckless proclamations supporting the South forced Magoffin to act quickly to reinforce his desire for neutrality.

Nevertheless, Magoffin ultimately issued "General Orders #17," a pronouncement acknowledging that the Kentucky legislature supported the North. Magoffin's desire to keep Kentucky a neutral border state by the technique of "armed neutrality" was overruled. General Ulysses Grant had come into Paducah and Southland, Kentucky, for the Union, and General Leonidas Polk had arrived with Confederate troops in Columbus, Kentucky. These troop movements forced Magoffin's hand and the vote of the Kentucky legislature. Magoffin signed that "General Orders #17" on September 13, 1861, stating that the "invaders [the Confederates] must be expelled."[12]

Dr. Blackburn's complete activities later in 1861 are a bit obscure. In mid–November 1861 Brigadier-General Lloyd Tilghman of the Confederate States Army reported that he had encountered a large group of hogs intended for the use of a Dr. Blackburn, whether for trading for other military items or for food for the Confederate troops is unknown.[13] This man was likely the same Dr. Blackburn who had been sent by Governor Magoffin. A physician dealing in guns and hogs simply reinforces the notion that he loved the South and was willing to do anything to further its cause.

Dr. Blackburn also rendered services in 1862 as a volunteer civilian "aide-de-camp" (personal aide; in many situations the chief of staff) to Major-General Sterling Price (former governor of Missouri) of the Missouri State Guard. Some sources say that Blackburn also had the title of "chief surgeon" for Price. The Missouri guard would later be merged with the Confederacy's

6. Early Confederate Service 49

Army of the West. Blackburn worked delivering messages as needed and continued to obtain supplies for the army.[14] On July 31, 1862, Major-General Price sent Blackburn from Tupelo, Mississippi, to deliver a message to Major-General Earl Van Dorn in Vicksburg, Mississippi, regarding the movements of General Ulysses S. Grant's troops and opportunities he believed presented themselves for the Confederates to move troops near Tennessee through to Kentucky. Further, Price next, on August 11, 1862, asked Blackburn to await a message from Secretary of War George W. Randolph in Richmond, Virginia, regarding the transfer of small arms to Price's troops about to advance on Tennessee. Blackburn thus kept busy relaying messages and locating materials that Price needed.[15] On August 20, 1862, Blackburn reported to Major-General Sterling Price that he had obtained 8,000 guns for the Confederacy (to be delivered to Columbus, Mississippi, and Gainesville, Alabama), and that 30,000 more guns had arrived at a Confederate port for the Southern cause. Blackburn in that telegram identified himself as "Aid-De-Camp [sic]."[16]

In February 1863 Blackburn left his duties with Price and accepted an assignment from Mississippi governor John J. Pettus as "Medical Commissioner" (actually one of two commissioners) to direct the treatment of Confederate soldiers recovering from their wounds.[17] Governor Pettus appropriated $50,000 for the task of coordinating this medical care for the Confederate soldiers, the use of the money dependent entirely upon Blackburn's assessment and judgment. Blackburn visited medical facilities in Alabama and Mississippi in early 1863, and he tried to consolidate the medical efforts. However, he discovered that centralization—though a good concept—was not possible because no single facility was large enough or endowed with sufficient resources to accomplish this task. So he was forced to settle for soldiers' rehabilitation at multiple facilities.

Blackburn would later declare that he had become the "Medical Director of the State of Mississippi" in January 1863 and that he considered himself "intimately acquainted with Jefferson Davis," that he had corresponded with Davis, and that he could even identify Davis's handwriting. Blackburn was familiar with the seals used to certify Confederate documents, and he was also acquainted with other members of the Confederate cabinet.

On May 13, 1863, Blackburn wrote to Richmond, Virginia, volunteering his services to "my [Confederate] Government and our Suffering Soldiers" as General Inspector of Hospitals and Camps, "without pay or rank," serving Colonel George Baird Hodge of Kentucky. His offer was transmitted on May 16, along with the recommendations of delegations to the Confederate congress from Kentucky, Mississippi, Arkansas, and Tennessee.[18] Colonel Hodge himself affixed a note approving Blackburn's offer. On May 20 Blackburn received a reply from the Confederate States of America's surgeon general, Samuel Preston Moore, that said, "There is no necessity for this appointment, there being a sufficient number of Inspectors of hospitals in the service."[19] Thereafter, Blackburn helped the Confederacy by blockade-running, purveying supplies for the Confederacy.

On June 23, 1863, Blackburn asked his friend Major General Dabney H. Maury, the commander of the Department of the Gulf in Mobile, Alabama, to appoint him to organize the delivery of supplies from Canada to Mobile. Blackburn wrote, "It is my intention to visit Canada, and if practicable purchase a good sea going vessel from the Northern Lakes, load her with ice, and run her through the Blockade in to this port [Mobile].... If you will give me assurance of protection I will obligate myself to turn over to the Government for Hospital use the cargo of ice after selling sufficient to reimburse me for my outlay of vessel, in and out cargo. I would also request that you will state that the vessel will be permitted to return with cotton, this being the policy of the Government."[20]

Governor Pettus concurred in this plan, and Blackburn became an agent for Mississippi to engage in blockade-running. Maury approved his proposal the same day Blackburn wrote his letter, Blackburn receiving his commission to be a Confederate agent in Canada on June 23, 1863. He planned to deliver whatever was needed in the South, using Mobile as his port. There Confederate ships were available to protect him in his efforts. One of those "needed" supplies in the South was ice! Rich Southerners not only used ice to chill their favorite drinks, they also used it to preserve meat, in primitive air conditioners, and to reduce the fevers of sick patients. They even thought ice killed the germs (whatever they might be) that caused yellow fever. Dr. Blackburn planned to transport ice to Mobile and return to Halifax with cotton. The shipping pattern of taking ice to the South and returning with cotton for the northern United States or the Canadian provinces was actually quite common. Ice was indeed a valuable commodity. Consul Charles Maxwell Allen in Bermuda reported that he paid $3 each month to have four pounds of ice delivered to his house daily (ice sold for 2 pence per pound).

After arriving in Mobile with his first shipment of ice, Blackburn was given 50 bales of cotton by Governor Pettus through the Confederate quartermaster-general of the State of Mississippi, Colonel Absolom M. West. Blackburn was to take the cotton to Cuba, where he would trade it for "arms and munitions of war." (A bale of cotton, weighing about 400 pounds, at that time sold for about $100, though the price would rise to $400–500 by the end of the war.) Blackburn thus sailed toward Havana, Cuba. However, his ship was intercepted by a Union vessel of the West Gulf Blocking Squadron as it left Mobile Harbor. The Union navy didn't recognize Blackburn for what he was—the Confederate agent in charge of this blockade-runner—and thinking that he was just a civilian passenger they allowed him to go free. Blackburn then returned to Canada.[21]

6. Early Confederate Service

Since the summer of 1862 Blackburn's wife Julia had been living in Louisville, which had by then become Union territory. On July 21, 1863, Colonel Marcellus "Marc" Mundy of the "Head Quarters Military Command Louisville" gave Julia permission to join her husband "in the Southern Confederacy" on August 1. She was limited to one trunk of 100 pounds for personal belongings (plus another one of like size for the effects of her children) and no more than $1,000 in cash, with the proviso that she couldn't return to Union territory without being considered to be a spy unless she again received special permission from Major General Ambrose Everett Burnside.[22] On July 24, 1863, she obtained confirmation from Brigadier General J.T. Boyle allowing her to travel to the South to join her husband. Boyle described Dr. Blackburn as a man "who is in the Rebel Army."[23]

Blackburn and Julia traveled to Halifax in August 1863, and from there they moved inland and settled in Toronto at the Queen's Hotel. There he established a small medical practice at 40 Adelaide Street East.[24] Later in 1867 it would be located at Church Street, North of King Street, these two sites being only one block apart.[25] He and Julia then travelled between Toronto and Halifax to obtain additional funding and to organize more supplies to be delivered to hospitals in Mobile. Blackburn was unquestionably a staunch Confederate supporter, and his actions were contributing to the Southern cause.

It had to have been at about this time that Blackburn began thinking about other ways to advance the Confederacy. Furthermore, other Confederate agents began to consider new techniques and schemes to defeat the North. These agents evaluated methods of warfare previously thought to be out of bounds. Patriots on both the Union and Confederate sides of the conflict looked for unique ways to destroy the enemy. Although Dr. Blackburn was a physician dedicated to healing the sick, his skills might be used otherwise. Biological warfare became an option—maybe smallpox, maybe yellow fever.

In 1863 no one understood the transmission of disease, and most experts thought that both yellow fever and smallpox could be passed from person to person by contact with contaminated articles. Doctors had the vague notion that some substance or "miasma" propagated the illness. In reality, germs—bacteria and viruses—caused the epidemics, but decades separated physicians in the Civil War from this knowledge. Physicians simply knew that close proximity to a victim of yellow fever or smallpox increased the chances that one would contract the disease. Spreading a yellow fever or a smallpox epidemic to the North could devastate the Union cause and promote a Confederate victory. Indeed, all epidemics terrorized cities; the panic in the populace that would follow would seriously inhibit the Northern war effort.

By December 1863 Blackburn was perfecting the details of his scheme to spread yellow fever or smallpox throughout the North. It was during this month that Blackburn met Godfrey Joseph Hyams (who would later use the alias J.W. Harris) in Toronto and engaged Hyams' help with the plot.[26] Blackburn had arrived at the idea to distribute infected articles of clothing and bedding throughout Northern cities, especially New York, Boston, Washington, D.C., Philadelphia, Norfolk, Virginia, and New Bern, North Carolina. He chose the latter site not because it was a major city but because New Bern housed a large contingent of Union troops. Furthermore, Blackburn had President Abraham Lincoln in his sights, as well. He planned to attempt the delivery of a "gift" to President Lincoln in the form of a shirt contaminated with yellow fever. Blackburn tried to advance the Confederate cause by incapacitating—or even killing—Lincoln. He would endanger the civilian population, troop encampments, and even the Union's commander in chief.

7

Godfrey Joseph Hyams, Co-Conspirator

Godfrey Joseph Hyams was the antithesis of Dr. Luke Blackburn. One was a commoner, the other an aristocrat; a shoemaker and a physician, a pauper and a wealthy landowner and slaveowner. Implausibly, they would work together—but for very different motives.

Hyams was born in Manchester, England, around 1833 and later was a resident of London. A child of Joseph (or Jacob) and Louisa Hyams, he was the second of five children, having two brothers and two sisters. His father worked as a common laborer, a glasscutter. The younger Hyams' adult life in England began tumultuously. Listed as a shoemaker's apprentice in 1851,[1] he married Hannah Martin in 1854.[2] Both lived repeatedly on the wrong side of the law. Godfrey Hyams appears in the Kent, England, criminal records as a man tried and convicted on October 19, 1854, on two charges of larceny.[3] He was convicted on both counts and sentenced to prison for six months for each of the two crimes. Hannah likewise had arrests for larceny. Most certainly this Godfrey Hyams was the same as the one who came to the United States in 1857. Following his trial, conviction, and jail sentence in England, he abandoned Hannah, a pattern to become common for a man later most generously described as a "scoundrel." He came to the United States from East London, arriving on April 14, 1857, giving his age as 24 and his occupation as shoemaker.[4] Godfrey thus would have been about 30 years old at the time he met Dr. Blackburn in Toronto.

Hyams arrived in the United States via New York on the packet ship *Margaret Evans*, a vessel that made a trip each direction between New York and London every week, carrying packets of mail, passengers, and freight. The *Margaret Evans* weighed 1,000 tons and was 266 feet long and 36 feet wide. Elegant and luxurious, she transported hundreds of passengers, 60 in first and second class, and 300 in steerage.[5] This particular trip of the *Margaret Evans* had 85 passengers, with only one person in first or second class and 84 in steerage.[6] Hyams was in steerage.

Uneducated, Godfrey Hyams later would be described in various terms, some of which were quite unflattering: a "great rascal," a "cross-eyed" man, a "cock-eyed Jew," a "creature," a "low, ignorant, Jew-Christian-Athiest," a "scoundrel," a fellow "of the Jewish persuasion," and the "Israelitish man." Described as having a dark complexion, being short of stature and slight of build, and looking rather weak, he wasn't an imposing presence nor did he seem likely to be either an effective secret agent for the Confederacy or a convincing witness later in his career. Hyams moved inland from New York and soon resided in Richland Township in Jefferson County, Arkansas (near Pine Bluff), and after one year he moved near Helena, Arkansas (St. Francis Township). Helena is a river port city along the Mississippi. Located south of Memphis, Tennessee, about 75 miles downriver, and north of Vicksburg, Mississippi, about 225 miles, it flourished from river traffic that supplied the nearby land and cities, but it also brought the expected vices and crime that accompanied wealth. Ill repute accompanied the economic blessing of the Mississippi River.

Floods from the Mississippi frequently covered the nearby farms. Cotton became a dominant crop. Helena was not a paradise of either pleasant weather or good health. Gastrointestinal diseases—cholera, typhoid, and other forms of dysentery—ran rampant during the hot, muggy months of the summer, and malaria also attacked local residents in the heat. More affluent residents of Helena periodically fled to higher grounds, seeking cooler and more healthful environments. Many diseases were water-borne, and the water supply was obtained from three sources: cistern, well, and the Mississippi River.[7] Water from many local wells had the taste of limestone, causing residents to avoid these sources (although they may have been the best chances for clean water). During the Civil War, troops resorted to drinking water directly from the Mississippi River, muddy though it was. Indeed, officers eventually issued orders prohibiting use of water from any other source.[8]

River trade greatly influenced the life in this small town, and it would be important in the Civil War, as well, when the supply route for troops often took the form of steamboats plying the Mississippi. No railroads existed in Helena in 1860, and only a few roads connected it to the western part of Arkansas. By the time of the Civil War, citizens of Helena had heard many plans of railroad construction but none had materialized. Investment in the railroad had been insufficient in this part of Arkansas, so the river was the only major transportation available. Here Hyams came to support his family and perhaps to make his fortune.

Helena was in the center of Phillips County, one of the richest counties in Arkansas before the Civil War. It had 83,000 acres of farmed land, valued at more than $8,000,000. Plantations were common; 224 were larger than 100 acres, 40 had more than 500 acres, and four had more than 1,000 acres.

7. Godfrey Joseph Hyams, Co-Conspirator

The wealth of Phillips County lay in its land and its slaves. Cash flow was meager, in comparison, explaining the loyalty of the large landowners to the Confederacy. Dr. Luke Blackburn's family owned property in this area, and they owned slaves as well. Just before the war, in 1860, Phillips County boasted a population of about 15,000, more than one-half of the population being slaves. The wealthy dominated the landscape: 25 people owned 57 percent of the property; seven people owned 37 percent of all acreage.[9] Lawyers and newspapers were more common than might be expected for this small town. Lawyers were needed to resolve the many land disputes in the area. The three Helena newspapers—the *Shield*, the *Weekly Bulletin*, and the *Weekly Notebook*—kept the population informed of the events leading to the Civil War.

Hyams found the city of Helena to be an undeveloped western town sitting on the bank of the Mississippi River. Only four north-south streets comprised the footprint of the city—Water, Ohio, Cherry, and Walnut. Water Street would eventually succumb to the forces of its own name, as the Mississippi River would erode it out of existence. Roads in Helena in the 1860s were dirt—dust in the summer and mud in the rainy season. Streets were only two to three blocks long; buildings were wooden, subject to fires. The tallest structures were only two stories high. Floods were common, even expected. Horses, mules, cows, and all kinds of primitive conveyances crowded the city,[10] but during flooding rowboats and canoes replaced horses and buggies. Steamboats, both side-paddle and rear-paddle varieties, plied the Mississippi and stopped at Helena. It was here in Helena, Arkansas, that Godfrey Hyams engaged in his trade as a shoemaker.

Arkansas as a whole comprised 165,465 males, 143,020 females, and 104,375 slaves. Phillips County had a rather small population in 1860: 3,558 males, 2,462 females, and 8,817 slaves. Helena was a town of only 1,555 (both men and women, including 527 slaves). Next-door Desha County, where the Blackburns also had property, had 2,133 males, 1,079 females, and 3,788 slaves.[11] The political situation in Arkansas was similar to the climate in many border states. Arkansas technically was not a border state (and was considered to be a part of the South), but its residents demonstrated the ambivalence of the true border states of Maryland, Kentucky, Delaware, and Missouri. Most wealthy landowners clung fiercely to Southern principles, needing slavery for tending the crops, while some poorer residents tended more toward the sentiments of the North. This southern slave-owning environment constituted the early exposure of Godfrey Hyams to American culture. Here he would begin his connections with the Blackburns, living where mixed emotions might cause him to waffle from one allegiance to another.

In Helena, Hyams would be a "shoemaker and cutter" (leather cutter). Some sources cite Little Rock, not Helena, as his residence. Little Rock, Helena, and Pine Bluff are situated in a triangle only about a maximum of

100 miles apart and a minimum of 40 miles, and he may have lived briefly in those other towns earlier. Shoemakers were in great demand in the Confederacy. Newspaper reports cited extreme shortages of material and supplies for the troops. One paper said, "We are afraid that there will be a great scarcity of leather and shoes next winter, unless more tanneries are established and better care taken by our farmers of the hides or skins of animals."[12] A pair of shoes cost $1.00–3.50, and the demand kept good shoe and bootmakers busy. The *Memphis Daily Appeal* on September 18, 1861, reported, "The men are destitute of everything—shoes, hats, shirts, socks, drawers, pantaloons and coats. Unless clothing is obtained, it will be impossible to make a campaign this winter."[13] Not many weeks later, the *Little Rock Arkansas True Democrat* told local residents that convicts at the Arkansas Penitentiary (about 120 of them) had been pressed into service to make shoes, as well as other items in short supply. The local contractor with the penitentiary estimated that by spring the convicts would be able to produce 10,000 pairs of boots and shoes,[14] although experienced shoemakers guessed that the quality of the product coming from the prison would be quite poor. Soldiers needed either boots or shoes. "If practicable, each soldier should have two good substantial suits of winter clothing—less than this will not enable him to keep clean as well as comfortable—more would encumber him on the march. In addition, he should have a good overcoat, and at least one good blanket! The shirt and drawers may be of soft cotton, but all other articles (of clothing, socks and undershirts) should be of wool. Shoes, coming well up round the ankles, are better than boots. Two good pair are needed."[15] Those heavy, high-laced shoes covering the ankles were called brogans, and they were the preferred equipment. Soldiers could not march barefoot; bootmakers of good quality products were needed by both the North and the South.

As a boot and shoemaker by training and trade, Hyams no doubt saw the advertisement placed by Porter, Richardson, and Company from Helena, Arkansas, in the *Memphis Daily Appeal* on August 14, 1861, that proclaimed, "Shoemakers Wanted Immediately. The undersigned wish to employ twenty-five or thirty good Shoemakers, at their Boot and Shoe Factory, in Helena, Arkansas, and are prepared to give them permanent employment and the highest prices for work. Those wishing a good situation in that line of business, will do well to apply immediately. All work paid for at the end of each week."[16] Hyams needed "permanent employment," "highest prices," and "a good situation" for sure. He needed a reliable paycheck at the end of each week. The advertisement, which ran at least ten times between August 11 and September 5, 1861, must have spoken to Hyams' dreams to improve his financial status. Other businesses also sought large numbers of boot and shoemakers. The "Memphis Boot, Shoe and Leather Manufactory" advertised during the same month for 50 such journeymen workers.[17] Later, a shoemaker in Camden, Arkansas, reported a need for 30 shoemakers.[18] The Civil War had created a great need for military boots for the troops. Scarcely five months later, W. Richardson placed an advertisement in the *Helena Weekly Note-Book*, on January 9, 1862, announcing the "Helena Boot and Shoe Manufactury" was selling "Boots, Shoes and Brogans" and in-home service.[19] Though records from this company have disappeared, Hyams may well have been one of the employees. Workers returning to New York from Helena in early 1862 told of a shoemaking industry in Helena with prices of $3.50 per pair.[20]

Hyams likely moved to Helena sometime in 1861 or 1862 for employment in that bootmaking and shoemaking business. His name appears nowhere on the 1860 U.S. Census, so he may have been in transition when the census was conducted in June and July 1860. Hyams was Jewish, and he moved into an area that was just beginning to have a small influx of Jewish residents. By the beginning of the Civil War, a few more Jewish residents had migrated there. In 1860 about 200 Jewish merchants lived in all of Arkansas, and more than a dozen Jewish merchants were in business in nearby Desha County in the 1850s. During the Civil War about 70 Jewish citizens in Arkansas fought for the South. Helena opened its first synagogue—B'Nai Jeshurun (Sons of Israel)—in 1867, with 65 families attending (the name was later changed to Beth El).[21]

Pay scales during this time in Arkansas were adequate, but they wouldn't make anyone rich. A farmworker in 1850 made enough over his basic board in a day to buy "three pounds of meat, or a peck of corn, or a gallon of molasses." A carpenter made about five times this amount; a shoemaker made about twice as much as the farmworker.[22] By 1860 these numbers had more than doubled. Hyams could survive in this economy if he was willing to work hard, but if he desired riches he would have to seek them elsewhere. "Elsewhere" was not yet defined.

Luke Blackburn's brother James W. Blackburn, a lawyer, lived in West Helena at this time on property he had purchased on February 3, 1859.[23] James, 26 years old in 1860, lived with his wife, Henrietta, who was 26, and three children, William (12), Silley (10), and James Junior (2). This Blackburn family had seven slaves in Helena in 1860, three females and four males.[24] James Blackburn later also owned property in Pine Bluff. James would later encounter Hyams in Canada, where Luke Blackburn conspired with Hyams. Likewise, Luke P. Blackburn co-owned 74 slaves with his brother in Mississippi Township in Desha County, Arkansas, in the 1860 Slave Census.[25] Desha County is next to Phillips County, where Helena is located.

Hyams later said in court testimony that he was married in St. Louis in 1861 or 1862, though no record exists for this marriage. He lived in St. Louis for five months before returning to Helena, likely in 1861 or 1862. The complete name of this first American wife (his second marriage—the first was to

Hannah Martin in England) has been lost to history, though later evidence suggests that it could have been Bridget Sheehan. When the Civil War erupted, Hyams first supported the Union and flew its flag, identifying himself as a "Douglas Democrat." He was accosted and threatened in Helena by Southern supporters, and he was given 12 hours to leave unless he agreed to remove the flag. So he took it down.

• • •

The Union force in Arkansas, the Army of the Southwest, was led by Brigadier General Samuel Ryan Curtis. His troops came from Missouri in early 1862 and marched south to engage the Confederates under Major General Earl Van Dorn at the Battle of Pea Ridge, Arkansas (also called the Battle of Elkhorn Tavern). Winning at Pea Ridge on March 7–8, 1862, Curtis drove farther south, eventually stopping at Helena. General Van Dorn soon retreated east of the Mississippi River. During Curtis's march to Helena water and food were scarce, and his soldiers had to comb the landscape to find supplies. They devastated the countryside, and what they did not take they destroyed. Soldiers were again forced to forage and confiscate food and supplies from the Confederate sympathizers along the way, often employing a "scorched earth" policy on the route, burning and destroying whatever was left behind so that it couldn't fall again into Confederate hands. What hadn't already been pillaged by the retreating Confederate troops was laid waste by the Union forces. One Confederate newspaper reported on the march of Curtis' troops: "Every thing which could be eaten by hungry horses or men has been devoured, and not content with foraging upon the country, almost every thing which could not be eaten was destroyed. Fences and other improvements on farms have been burned. Houses have been robbed, and such furniture and other things as could not be removed, destroyed. Everything which wanton wickedness or thievish minds could suggest has been brought to bear upon our people to grind them into dust by oppression, and to starve such as survived.... All have suffered."[26] Troops were forced to drink water "the color of chocolate."[27] Often the retreating Confederate forces had purposely contaminated the drinking water or destroyed any remaining food that might be foraged by the Union men.

Destruction wasn't just a by-product of the Union occupation of Helena, it became the reason for their existence there: "It became the unofficial goal of the Federal cavalry at Helena to strip the local population of food, agricultural goods, horses and mules, and slaves—any materials that supported the many Confederate bands in the area. Newly-promoted Second Lieutenant John Mann believed appropriating Rebel property, especially slaves, 'was one way we had of whipping the [R]ebels that was almost as effective as fighting, taking their property from them and applying it to the Union cause.'"

7. Godfrey Joseph Hyams, Co-Conspirator   59

The assault on Captain Francis P. Redman's home was described as follows: "The Federal cavalry visited his plantation at every opportunity, and slaughtered the 'old [R]ebel's beef, pork, mutton, chickens[,] geese, ducks, and took his sweet potatoes, corn, honey, pots, kettles, buckets, and everything they could render useful, leaving his household effects alone unmolested.' Many officers encouraged the soldiers to take what they needed." Such activity was considered to be "the bright side of a soldier[']s life."[28] Social structures were breaking down. It was *Lord of the Flies* a century before William Golding wrote the book. In this Helena, Hyams and the Blackburns met each other.

All Confederate possessions were targets, especially food. Other items in great demand were salt, medicines, and items needed for transport, such as horses and mules. Scarcely a beast of burden existed that wasn't confiscated by the Union troops. Later, Hyams' mules would be no exception. Even paper became a rare commodity. Union and Confederate supporters alike depended upon newspapers for their information about the war's progress. Each side had its editorial supporters. Newspapers of that day, like those of today, became both the deliverers of news and the creators of it. Morale often dictated action, and newspapers tried to direct the morale of their readers.[29]

Both education and religion were also dramatically impacted by the war. Many schools closed, and home schooling often became the norm, especially in north and west Arkansas.[30] Church attendance suffered, while soldiers frequently lived lives of debauchery away from home.

Curtis's troops took the town of Helena without a fight on July 12, 1862. Though the entry into Helena was accomplished without a battle, the march across Arkansas itself had been brutal. It was described as "one of the most arduous and fatiguing of any made during the Civil War. While the first soldiers entered Helena on July 12, 1862, many stragglers continued to arrive over the next few days. The weather was intensely hot, and the road lay through the malaria-breeding swamps and fenlands, where the trailing masses of Spanish moss on the cypress trees wave like mourning bands over the reeking lands."[31]

The devastation wrought by Curtis's troops didn't go unnoticed by the Confederate army. Major-General Thomas Carmichael Hindman of the Confederate army—who himself called Helena, Arkansas, home and therefore one who had a vested interest in the welfare of the citizens of Helena—wrote to Major-General Samuel Curtis on July 31, 1862: "Your attention is also called to the reports which come to me directly and from innumerable sources of great atrocities committed by your troops on their march to Helena and since, such as the burning of houses, robbing women and children of their clothing, bedding and last pound of meat and breadstuffs; taking medicines from planters and practicing physicians; in some cases offering personal violence to females even to the horrible extent of ravishing them. These are crimes against humanity and civilization."[32] Curtis responded symbolically by confiscating Hindman's house and possessions and personally used Hindman's house as both his residence and his headquarters. Hindman, a former Helena lawyer in his mid-thirties, a politician, wealthy landowner, and prominent Helena citizen who stood a diminutive 5-feet-2-inches tall, was described as "dapper, jaunty, dandified, addicted to patent leather boots and rose-colored kidskin gloves, frilled shirt fronts and a rattan cane." He was unaccustomed to either defeat or humiliation.[33]

Union troops similarly occupied other mansions in Helena, either as residences for Union officers, as hospitals, as administrative offices, or for other Union needs. One writer said, "Besides the wanton destruction of property in the general devastation of the country, Gen. Curtis, by the time he gets beyond the borders of the State, will have stolen at least two thousand negroes. He has not been content to steal men, who would be useful in working roads, making fortifications, and other work necessary in the army, but he has stolen women and children, who are of no use, and are, besides, a burden and expense to him on his march."[34] The Confederate-leaning *Memphis Daily Appeal* reported the following on July 31, 1862:

> Numerous outrages have been perpetrated in this war, but it remains for CURTIS and his hirelings to overshadow all other atrocities, and entitled themselves to the doubtful honor of being the most heartless freebooters the North has yet to loose upon the people of the South. The ruinous work of wantonly destroying plantations continues, scarcely a single one having escaped. In every instance the useful stock and all provisions and produce has [sic] been seized, and the negroes carried off.... We also learn that numerous outrages have been committed upon unprotected females, some of them so hellish a nature as to almost forbid repeating.[35]

Food in Helena continued to be nearly as scarce as it had been on the march; water was often undrinkable, and disease felled as many of the troops as might have been wounded or killed by opposing Confederate forces, if there had been any. Supplies still hadn't arrived by boat, and it would be days to weeks before adequate provisions would come to the Helena port. Common diseases were dysentery, malaria, typhoid, and typhus. Not only did Curtis have to secure supplies for his troops, of which hundreds were now wounded or sick, he also had thousands of slaves in tow, persons he designated as "contraband." This army of 20,000–24,000 men overwhelmed the small town of Helena's 2,000 residents. Most soldiers upon arrival were in marginal condition to fight, but it wasn't necessary to do battle since most of the Confederate forces had fled to east of the Mississippi River. Even absent the need to fight, the soldiers immediately disliked Helena and dubbed it "Hell In Arkansas."[36] Conditions "increased the sick list fearfully, and fever and dysentery broke out, further decreasing our already reduced force.... Nobody seems to care whether we live or die.... Sickness increased so fast that men die every day, and we have started another private graveyard."[37] Another soldier wrote in 1862, "We have not had the luck to leave this God-forsaken Town yet."[38]

Part of Curtis's daring march to the east had been predicated upon having supplies available to them both before and after they arrived in Helena. Because of continued problems with supply routes, the Union forces were bereft of food and other supplies upon arrival in Helena. Memphis was just north on the Mississippi River, and Union supplies could ultimately be obtained by riverboat delivery. But the army was starving upon its arrival in the eastern part of Arkansas as they approached Helena. Lincoln and the Congress had issued the First and Second Confiscation Acts just prior to Curtis's march from Missouri to Helena. In addition, Curtis's Special Order #150 bolstered the permission for Union forces to strip goods from Arkansas citizens. These acts and the order gave permission for troops to take goods from Confederate sympathizers, although warring armies had used such practices for millennia. The First Confiscation Act (1861) became effective upon Lincoln's signature on August 6, 1861. It allowed the seizure of Confederate property from Rebels participating directly in the "rebellion." The Second Confiscation Act (1862) expanded the seizure powers to include all Confederate property. Neither act, in reality, did much to alter the behavior of Union forces. The Confiscation Acts initially intended to provide needed goods for the Union troops, as well as to free slaves (another form of "property"), but the practices soon degenerated into profiteering as the troops pillaged whatever they wanted whenever they wanted. Goods appropriated included items needed to clothe and feed the Union forces, but the soldiers also took items for their own personal financial gain. What began as a rule allowing rather standard wartime confiscation of needed goods became a license to steal and sell any items of value. (This tactic was not unique to Northern troops, however. Southern forces often robbed spoils from their conquered territories, also.) Even General Curtis himself was accused of having more interest in making money from the sale of expropriated cotton than in providing for his army. Major General Henry W. Halleck issued an order for the Helena troops to confiscate cotton supplies, giving the profiteers additional cover for their activities.[39] Curtis was replaced by Major General Eugene A. Carr in October 1862, the same month that a United States custom house was opened in Helena to deal with legitimate cotton trafficking.[40] Curtis wasn't indicted or convicted for his alleged profiteering, although he later was called on to explain his actions to President Lincoln.

Curtis's counterpart in the Confederate army didn't escape accusations of misbehavior, either. General Earl Van Dorn, commander of the Arkansas Confederate troops, had begun to move his forces eastward on March 17, 1862. Many Southern sympathizers believed he was abandoning Arkansas, although he was really going to western Tennessee to aid Brigadier General Andrew Johnson and General P.G.T. Beauregard. Although Van Dorn was late in arriving, he joined forces with Beauregard in Corinth, Mississippi. Van Dorn was accused of promoting officers without approval from headquarters (filling "unauthorized positions and commands") and of engaging in sexual indiscretions while in command. Jefferson Davis preferred a court of inquiry rather than a trial to explore whether there was any evidence of a crime (this process was similar to a grand jury hearing). After the court of inquiry, Van Dorn wrote to Davis in his own defense: "I have heard from several sources that it has been reported to you that I was a *Seducer* [emphasis in the original] and a libertine—that I had seduced the daughter of a respectable citizen of Vicksburg.... [A]s a Christian and before my God I do most solemnly declare that it is false—that I not only did not seduce the young lady referred to, but that I never seduced *any* young lady *in my life*...." However, he then equivocated about his morals by saying that, with the exception of his wife, "I have never had intercourse with *any* woman, as I believe, who was not alike accessible to others."[41] Recognizing that specifics of his behavior were open knowledge, he continued:

> There was a wild, frolicksome young lady of Vicksburg whose acquaintance I made during the defense [of the Vicksburg siege by Union forces], whose indiscretions as well, probably as some of my own, may have given grounds for the prudish and censorious to slander, and the idle to talk, but that young lady (Miss George) I believe to be as virtuous as any young lady in Vicksburg or in Miss[issippi]—She has been most shamefully punished for hers, as I have been for my thoughtlessness and folly—or pleasantries as they may be called.... I am unfortunately not a good Christian—*but I am not* a Seducer, nor a drunkard—neither am I with all my faults capable of meanness.[42]

In spite of his protestations to President Jefferson Davis, five months later Van Dorn was killed by a Tennessee man who suspected that Van Dorn had acted inappropriately toward his wife. Wartime atrocities and indiscretions weren't limited to one side in this great conflict.

Curtis decided that it was necessary to establish Union fortifications in Helena, and Fort Curtis was the result of this decision. Thousands of slaves had followed Curtis on his march from Missouri across Arkansas. Seeing the Union victories as their immediate chance to escape slavery, they abandoned their fleeing slave masters and marched with the Union troops into Helena, further taxing the tenuous food and supply lines. Trusting the Union army to protect them, the former slaves often became paid workers for the Union soldiers and for Union war projects, such as the construction of those fortifications in Helena. Here Godfrey Hyams would experience the economic hardships of the Civil War.

• • •

7. Godfrey Joseph Hyams, Co-Conspirator 63

Hyams remained in Helena until General Curtis occupied the city and established his dominant and successful campaign in eastern Arkansas. Hyams' wife and family received the ill treatment from the Union troops characteristic of the troops' behavior against all Southern sympathizers. Hyams also had four mules taken from him that were being transported on the steamboat *Meteor* near Helena, Arkansas, between 4:00 and 6:00 p.m. on July 18, 1862. Major John F. Weston, who at that time was also provost marshal general of Helena, delegated the mules to the Union quartermaster for use by the Northern troops. Hyams later sought reparation for this loss, writing two letters protesting the confiscation of his property. The second letter (the first has been lost), written to Assistant Adjutant General E.D. Townsend on December 26, 1862, was posted from Hyams' home at 221 North Ninth Street in St. Louis, where he was living at the time (before he fled to Canada). He complained that Major John F. Weston and the Union provost marshal general of Helena had not reimbursed him for his loss.[43] It's unclear if Hyams was ever paid reparations for this military seizure, but—even if he had been—the episode couldn't have made him think too favorably of Union activities and troops. Union soldiers had burned his furniture, confiscated his home and other personal property, and insulted his wife, cementing—at least for the time being—his conversion to the Confederate cause.

Hyams himself never actually served in the Confederate army in the South, although the Rev. Dr. Stuart Robinson, a Presbyterian minister who was living in Canada, testified in Toronto in May 1865 that Hyams had told Robinson that he [Hyams] had been a captain in the Confederacy.[44] Hyams alleged that he had served 15–16 months in the 13th Arkansas Infantry Regiment Volunteers under the command of a "Colonel Tappen." In fact, Captain James Camp Tappan was the commander of the "Tappan Guards," a volunteer group formed as the 12th Militia Regiment of Phillips County on May 23, 1861, later existing as Company A of the 13th Arkansas Infantry Regiment, a group drawn primarily from the Helena region. Hyams claimed to have suffered a leg injury at the Battle of Shiloh on April 6–7, 1862. This unit did, indeed, fight at Shiloh. But, given Hyams' testimony about his other travels and his propensity to fabricate stories, such service was unlikely, and no Confederate records exist for any soldier named Godfrey Hyams who would fit his description. Furthermore, for Hyams to be injured with a bullet to the leg in April 1862 at Shiloh and to recover sufficiently to be fully active in May and July 1862 in Helena would be highly unlikely. Finally, Hyams' knowledge of the Civil War activity in and around Helena would have given him ample data to concoct such a story, as he was inclined to do.

Hyams had met Dr. Luke Blackburn in Helena, testifying later that he "was acquainted with Dr. Blackburn; first knew him in Arkansas.... I knew Dr. B. by sight."[45] Blackburn's wife's family (both the Gist family and the

Boswell family), in addition to Luke Blackburn's brother James Blackburn, had property there. James Blackburn lived in Helena during the early 1860s, working as a lawyer, county attorney, election judge, and county commissioner, in addition to his farming activities. With both the Blackburn family and Hyams having roots in Helena, a very small town along the Mississippi River, the exact relationship of these two families in Arkansas—if any—is unclear, although Hyams testified later that he had never actually talked with Dr. Luke Blackburn when they both lived in Helena. No doubt in a city as small as Helena, both James Blackburn and his brother Dr. Luke Blackburn had encountered Godfrey Hyams somewhere along the city's muddy streets during this era.

Hyams fled to St. Louis again in August 1862, his motive apparently being simply to escape the rigors of war and harassment by Union troops.[46] Alternatively, Hyams once testified that he was arrested and taken to St. Louis.[47] Whether arrested in Helena or St. Louis, Hyams was imprisoned in the Gratiot Street Military Prison in St. Louis. This prison was a Union facility, and it housed "not only ... Confederate prisoners of war, but spies, guerrillas, civilians suspected of disloyalty, and even Federal soldiers accused of crimes or misbehavior." One St. Louis resident said, "In those stirring war days no man was of importance or standing until he had been locked up in Gratiot Street prison at least a few days.... The citizens referred to would be rounded up about town and locked up without charges, apology, or explanation and after being boarded for from one week to two months they would be called before the Provost Marshal and presented with the oath of allegiance to the United States, which they had to sign without question, no matter how great the effort."[48] The provost marshal was in charge of all such local prisons, and his word was law. He was able to transfer prisoners, keep them, or release them as he saw fit. A provost marshal's charge during the Civil War was to keep "the peace and quiet of [his] respective districts, counties, and sections; and to this end may cause the arrest and confinement of disloyal persons, subject to the instructions and orders of the department."[49] It was martial law, minimally codified.

The Gratiot Prison in St. Louis, located at the corner of 8th Street and Gratiot Street, was in essence a clearinghouse for all types of infractions—or lack thereof. It was built to hold a maximum of 1,200 prisoners, though at times the number swelled to 2,000. Men, women, and children alike were housed there. Far from being a benign site of incarceration, however, the conditions there were horrendous, as they were at all of the prisons used to house Confederate sympathizers. Disease and death were rampant in these poorly maintained jails. Diarrheal illnesses and smallpox were endemic.

Hyams' infraction was not listed—it was written in the jail logbook as "citizen." People arrested simply for suspicions of being Southern sympathizers had their "infraction" recorded as "citizen." Most people interned there were released quickly (days, weeks, or months) or transferred to other facilities—locally to the Myrtle Street Prison, the Schofield and Benton Barracks, the Chestnut Street Prison, or, at a greater distance (and more commonly), the Alton Prison, about 25 miles away on the Mississippi River in Illinois.[50] Hyams probably was suspected of disloyalty to the Union cause (which was, of course, true). He was imprisoned on August 27, 1862; his "regiment" was listed as St. Louis; his military rank was also "citizen," and his place of capture was reported to be St. Louis, belying his one testimony that he had been arrested in Helena.[51] Hyams was quickly sent to Alton Prison in Illinois but with the notation on his disposition that he was released by order of the provost marshal general, probably Captain John Bishop,[52] on September 4, 1862.[53] Likely this brief incarceration further fueled Hyams' anti–Union sentiments.

Hyams remained in St. Louis at least until the end of December 1862, living at 221 North 9th Street. In May or June 1863 he went to Toronto, again to escape the war and because many pro–Confederate refugees used Canada as an asylum. (Hyams' later testimony stated that he was in St. Louis for only 11 weeks before going to Canada,[54] which would have made his departure for Canada in January 1863). It's unclear if his wife went with him initially, but she at least joined him soon thereafter. They first lived at 18 Terauley Street, and Hyams, a shoemaker by trade, joined Hugh Shields, a boot and shoemaker whose shop had been at 35 Queen Street West at least since 1862 (there is no record of Shields in that location in 1861).[55] Shields was a native of England, about 36 years old. He had a wife and four children and lived at the shoe shop on Queen Street West. Previously, in 1862, the landlord at 18 Terauley, James Walker—a tavern keeper, had no renters, but by 1864 Hyams and a Mrs. Mary A. Whelan were listed as living there. The Toronto directory made no mention of Hyams' wife and child or children, although the directories usually didn't mention family members. Likely they were living there with him. Hyams' next residence was 120 York, where he moved on April 8, 1864, apparently into a neighborhood going downhill and likely less expensive, because many of the neighboring homes were empty. His fortunes were certainly deteriorating. The Toronto directory also listed him at 120 York in 1865,[56] but he disappeared from Canadian records thereafter. By 1866 both Hyams' and Shields' names were missing from the Toronto scene. Shields would later live in Wayne, Ohio, where he continued his bootmaking business at least from 1870 to 1880.[57]

By late 1863 Hyams was unable to pay his rent or buy food ("without a cent"), and his wife was six months pregnant with a boy who would be named Thomas Francis Stonewall Jackson Hyams.[58] They had at least one other child at the time, possibly two, and Hyams probably was willing to do just about anything for money. He would soon be approached by Dr. Luke Blackburn and his co-conspirators with a scheme they told him would make him rich and perhaps even famous for bringing down the Union army. It was too good to be true. Hyams was ready to jump at the chance to change his fortune, however implausible the method might seem. The thought of striking it rich would be enough for him to consider doing the unthinkable. Aiding the Confederate cause would simply be an added incentive.

Since Hyams wanted to support the Confederate cause, in November 1863 he wrote to Mr. H.C. Slaughter, a Confederate rebel agent who was enlisting men for the struggle against the Union forces. Hyams was considering returning to the South from Canada. Slaughter answered through the Rev. Dr. Stuart Robinson of Kentucky (the former Louisville Presbyterian minister, then living in Toronto), who arranged a meeting between Hyams and Blackburn at the Queen's Hotel in Toronto in December 1863.[59] Blackburn had heard of Hyams from his brother James Blackburn, the lawyer who also had lived in Helena, Arkansas, but who also spent a brief period of time in Toronto. Perhaps Dr. Blackburn himself remembered Hyams from the time they both spent in Helena in 1861 and 1862. James Blackburn and Hyams had met briefly by chance in Toronto, and James had told his brother Luke about encountering Hyams, then described as an avid Southern sympathizer who by this time was about 30 years old. Hyams was now ready to participate in Dr. Blackburn's schemes.

Blackburn and Hyams began their business arrangement by meeting at the Queen's Hotel in Toronto in December 1863. After a quick discussion in a rather public setting, Hyams and Blackburn retreated to Blackburn's room, where they talked in private about how Hyams could help the Confederacy. Blackburn asked Hyams if he was a Freemason. He wasn't, but Blackburn gave him a Freemason's handshake nonetheless and swore on the honor of a Freemason that he had never deceived anyone nor would he ever deceive or betray Hyams.[60] If Hyams had only known, it was an oath soon to be broken. Blackburn then asked Hyams if he would be willing to go on an "expedition," to which Hyams answered in the affirmative. Blackburn told him that he would be contributing far more to the Confederacy than if he had recruited 100,000 soldiers for the cause. Blackburn informed Hyams that he would likely stand to make $100,000 for his services to the Confederacy (probably one-half of what had actually been allocated for the plan), $60,000 of it to be paid immediately upon his return to Toronto after completing his task delivering clothing contaminated with yellow fever to cities in the Union. (In Toronto, Hyams would later testify that he was told his reward was "guaranteed" to be $60,000, maybe up to $120,000[61] or many times more that figure, up to $1,000,000.)

If Hyams had only stopped a moment to think of the magnitude of that offer, he would have known that it was an impossible prize, but apparently he didn't. If Hyams questioned Blackburn about the source of the money, the answer didn't dissuade him from accepting the job. Thus, Hyams was offered the opportunity to become Blackburn's "agent" in the scheme to deliver infected clothing to the North. Blackburn told him that his only task would be to take charge of a shipment of contaminated clothing infected with yellow fever. Blackburn asked that the clothing be distributed to Washington and other cities, the intent being to cause epidemics, during which the Confederates could gain ground in the war. Hyams would retrieve trunks from Bermuda in Halifax, working under the assumed name of J.W. Harris, and transport them to these select cities of the North. Blackburn gave Hyams $50, and Hyams, both destitute and wanting to help the cause of the South, immediately jumped at the chance to improve his financial status.

Hyams must have considered the risk to his own health. The specter of yellow fever was a scourge throughout the United States and in many tropical climates. The "Yellow Jack" struck fear into the hearts of men and women alike. Perhaps Hyams wasn't very educated about this disease, or perhaps the monetary offer was simply too compelling. He was, after all, down on his luck. He had a wife and children to feed, and he had no hopes for any job that would pull him from poverty. (How many children Hyams had is unclear; the Rev. Dr. Stuart Robinson, in describing him, simply said that Hyams had "children.")[62] In addition, Blackburn had told Hyams that a person would be safe if he protected himself by smoking strong cigars and chewing camphor while he handled the infected garments and bedding. This recommendation flew in the face of Blackburn's later contention that the contents of the trunks would kill a man at 60 yards. Nevertheless, Hyams agreed to the plan. During this time, Hyams' finances remained perilous. Frequently he asked other Canadian Confederates for money, sometimes for food, sometimes for supplies to support his shoe and bootmaking business. On at least two occasions (February 29, 1864, and April 15, 1864) he wrote asking for assistance, once to the Confederate Benevolence Society in Montreal and once to Dr. Stuart Robinson.[63]

Blackburn needed to depart immediately for Montreal, and he instructed Hyams to continue his cobbler's work as usual in Toronto. When the time came for Hyams' part of the plot, Blackburn would inform him. Dr. Stuart Robinson would function as their communication agent. If Hyams needed to move before his assigned job, he would tell Robinson, and Robinson would relay Hyams' new address to Blackburn. Blackburn was next going to Bermuda after his trip to Montreal, and thereafter farther south, though he didn't specify where. Although Robinson was involved in communications, Hyams would later testify that Robinson didn't know the contents of the trunks or their purpose.

8

Nefarious Schemes and Diabolical Plans

The concept of "black flag warfare" included the capture or murder of leaders of the government, but it also encompassed the acceptance of the wounding or killing of innocent civilian bystanders, women and children included. Terrorist plots by definition were calculated to produce fear and panic in the hearts of the general population. These tactics could include the destruction and burning of bridges, roads, railways, homes, and even cities.

Early in the Civil War, schemes against Lincoln himself surfaced. One of the major plots against Lincoln, in which he was to be kidnapped or killed on his trip to his first inauguration in early 1861, was unsuccessful.[1] In September 1861 a citizen of Georgia wrote to Jefferson Davis suggesting assassination as a valid warfare technique.[2] Another discussion regarding kidnapping Lincoln was held in the summer of 1863 in Jefferson Davis's presence. Davis listened and then said, "Gentlemen, you must capture him and bring him, if possible, to Richmond without hurting a hair on his head, but if an attempt is made to recapture him you must see that he never reaches Washington alive."[3] A noncommissioned officer of the Confederacy also wrote to Davis on August 17, 1863, volunteering to raise 300–500 men (or more) to go to Washington to kill Lincoln and Secretary of State Seward.[4]

Historian Edward Steers reported in his book *Blood On the Moon*: "By the winter of 1864, the burdens of a cruel war began to bear heavily on both sides. As the weeks turned into months with no clear resolution in sight on either side, strategies began to change. Targeting the respective heads of state was no longer outside the boundary of acceptable warfare. By the end of 1863 it seems clear that Jefferson Davis and Abraham Lincoln were viewed as legitimate military targets."[5] Blackburn indeed had already formulated his plans for germ warfare by late 1863.

Trying to assassinate the head of state was not uniquely a Southern military tactic. Both Abraham Lincoln and Jefferson Davis were in assassins'

8. Nefarious Schemes and Diabolical Plans 69

cross-hairs. The so-called Dahlgren Affair might have targeted high Confederate officials. It would have terrorized the populace, as well. Colonel Ulric Dahlgren was a Union officer involved in an attempt to free captive Union soldiers from Belle Isle Prison in Richmond in February 1864. Dahlgren was killed, and papers found on his body allegedly revealed an explicit change in war strategy. The papers told of the plan to free the prisoners then burn the city of Richmond (with attendant destruction of Confederate property and death of innocent Southern lives, including noncombatants), and finally to capture Jefferson Davis and his high-level government leaders. Another paper found on Dahlgren talked of killing Jefferson Davis and his cabinet. The Union troops were to "destroy and burn the hateful city [Richmond]; and ... not allow the Rebel leader Davis and his traitorous crew to escape.... The men must keep together and well in hand, and once in the city [Richmond] it must be destroyed and Jeff Davis and Cabinet killed."[6] This was no longer a "gentleman's war." All imaginable tactics were allowable—including that so-called black flag warfare.[7] The men above Dahlgren in the chain of command of the Union army (Brigadier General Hugh Judson Kilpatrick and his superior, the commander of the Army of the Potomac, General George G. Meade) denied that they had anything to do with this type of warfare. The *Richmond Examiner* inflamed Confederate passions by publishing editorials highlighting the turn of events that had led to such changes in tactics. The *Examiner* said that the Union army a few months earlier had been planning an "indiscriminate slaughter of guards and populace."[8] Union military officer Benjamin F. Butler, commanding general of the United States Army, Department of Virginia and North Carolina, had outlined some objectives of his campaign, which included the plan to "destroy the public buildings" and to "capture some of the leaders of the rebellion, so that at least we can have means to meet their constant threats of retaliation and hanging of men white and black. If any of the more prominent can be brought off, I believe a blow will be given to the rebellion from which it will never recover."[9] However, this entire story rested upon letters and papers that were allegedly found on Dahlgren's body. These papers soon mysteriously disappeared, so originals could never be examined for authenticity. Nevertheless, having the concept of black flag warfare exposed served to promote this behavior on both sides of the conflict.

From July to December 1864, Lieutenant W. Alston sent a series of letters to Davis in which he proposed to "rid this country of some of her deadliest enemies by striking at the very heart's blood of those who seek to enchain her in slavery." He added, "I consider nothing dishonorable having such a tendency." Davis read it and referred it "for attention" of the assistant secretary of war, John Archibald Campbell.[10] In December 1864 another such plan was hatched by George W. Gayle from Selma, Alabama, calling for a reward for the murder of President Lincoln. Davis apparently didn't rebuke any of these writers. Indeed, he appeared at least to view these ideas as tolerable plans to consider.[11]

In February 1865 Davis wrote to Canadian conspirators stating that he would approve of any means necessary to win the war. The agents in Canada felt that they needed more explicit directions, so they sent John H. Surratt to Richmond to secure orders. Davis is said to have told him, "'Surratt, there is no necessity for your coming here for any special authority, for the soldiers in the North and in Canada are expected to carry the war to the knife, and they require no more authority to kill Lincoln than they do to kill any Union soldier. Such killing,' he said, 'would be a legitimate act of warfare; for,' said he, 'If a couple of Yankees were to come into my house and kill me they would be lauded for it and rewarded as heroes.'" Surratt then returned to Canada with this news and with papers that allegedly approved of such plans.[12] Illegitimate tactics against Lincoln and the North expanded as the Civil War progressed.

A letter from Williamson Simpson Oldham, a senator from Texas, to Jefferson Davis on February 11, 1865, suggested that Davis might have been aware of many of the plots for black flag warfare and that the prevailing sentiment simply required that Davis not actively obstruct the plan. Oldham told of "the project of annoying and harassing the enemy, by means of burning their shipping, towns, etc." ... He claimed "there is no necessity for sending persons in the military service into the enemy's country, but the work may be done by agents." Oldham predicted that such plans would "devastate the country of the enemy, and fill his people with terror and consternation."[13]

William W. Cleary would later testify that Jefferson Davis was aware of Blackburn's plot and passively assented to it. No record exists of Davis's approval, but neither did he give orders to stop it or any of the other black flag schemes. Davis had received two letters from friends (one of them the Episcopal minister Rev. Dr. Kensey Johns Stewart) who told him of the plans, and Stewart pleaded with Davis to abandon such tactics against the North. Stewart served many roles for the Confederates in the Civil War. He was one of many agents who worked at least part of his time in Canada performing secret functions. Stewart wrote to Davis in December 1864 complaining about the ineffectiveness of some of the Canadian Confederate operatives. He advised Davis that some of the activities were immoral and offended the sensibilities of the North, serving only to incite further hatred against the South:

> I cannot regard you as capable of expecting the blessing of God upon, or being personally associated with instruments & plans such as I describe below. As our country has been and is entirely dependent upon God, we cannot afford to displease him. Therefore, it cannot be our policy to employ wicked men to destroy the persons & property of private citizens, by inhumane & cruel acts. I name only one. $100 of

8. Nefarious Schemes and Diabolical Plans

public money has been paid here to one "Hyams" a shoemaker, for services rendered by conveying and causing to be sold in the city of Washington at auction, boxes of small-pox clothing.... There can be no doubt of the causes of the failure of such plans. It is only a matter of surprise that, God does not forsake us and our cause when we are associated with such misguided friends.[14]

There is no positive certainty that Davis actually saw this letter, though one might assume that he read it. He thus may have known of Blackburn's plans at least by December 12, 1864, if not before then, but he did nothing to thwart them. Davis remained silent, and—at the very least—his henchmen considered his silence to be his approval.

• • •

The Civil War had been turning against the South. Confederates needed additional leverage in the struggle, and about the only remaining tactics available were the unconventional, the revolutionary, and the black flag variety. Some thought that submarines were the answer. Submarines were stealthy vessels that could attack Union naval and shipping vessels without being seen. But the *Hunley*, a revolutionary new Confederate submarine being prepared as an attack instrument against the North, was neither ready nor did it prove to be useful to turn the tide of the war. Furthermore, many military officials considered submarine tactics to be out of bounds. Submarines were "invisible"; they didn't involve face-to-face combat. They were "ungentlemanly." But, in reality, only tactics such as black flag warfare remained as options to bolster the chances for the Confederacy. Blackburn would become a part of such tactics, including germ warfare, poisoning water supplies of the North, wrecking dams that provided water to the North, burning Northern cities, and rescuing Confederate troops from their prisons in the North.

Jefferson Davis had begun organizing Confederate activities in Canada on March 16, 1864, by sending Captain Thomas Henry Hines, of the Ninth Kentucky Cavalry, a former member of Morgan's Raiders, to gather Confederate forces who had escaped to Canada and regions of the northern United States. James A. Seddon, the Confederate secretary of war, wrote to Hines on Davis's orders, instructing him to go to Canada, organize soldiers there, and coordinate with the other agents Davis would send as part of the Confederate Secret Service. Seddon wrote on March 16, 1864, for Hines to "view the possibility, by such means as you can command, of effecting any fair and appropriate enterprises of war against our enemies, and will be at liberty to employ such of our soldiers as you may collect, in any hostile operation offering, that may be consistent with the strict observance of neutral obligations incumbent in the British Provinces."[15] Hines was given rather wide latitude in choosing what the "hostile operations" might be.

The Confederate war efforts thus officially expanded into Canada long after Blackburn had begun his own activities there. Jefferson Davis established and approved a contingent of Confederate loyalists, primarily in Montreal. The first person considered by Davis to be chief for the Canadian operation was Alexander Hugh Holmes Stewart. Davis asked Stewart to come to Richmond to discuss a matter "too delicate for correspondence." Some Confederates believed that tens of thousands of Southern sympathizers were ready to rise up in the North both to fight for the South and to pursue peace. Stewart likely thought that the projects envisioned by Davis were too ambitious and had too likely a chance of failure, so Stewart rejected Davis's offer, thinking that "success hinged on a 'remarkable delusion' about the extent of the Northern peace movement."[16] Stewart cited family obligations as the reason for his rejection of the job, but his real reason was probably his disbelief that the endeavor had any chance of success.[17] Jacob Thompson was Davis's second choice for the command. On April 7, 1864, Davis wrote to Thompson, saying, "If your engagements will permit you to accept service abroad for six months, please come here [to Richmond] immediately."[18] Davis and Thompson were good friends. Thompson accepted. Other major Canadian Confederate operatives included Clement Claiborne Clay from Alabama, Professor James Philemon Holcombe from Virginia, and Captain William Walter Cleary of Kentucky. These four men would soon play an important role in Luke Blackburn's plots and schemes. Blackburn was already in Canada, and there he would work with the other Canadian Confederates, though he wasn't involved in many of the other ill-fated projects.

Confederate money funded the men sent to Canada who were charged with disrupting the Union's war effort. Davis and Thompson verbally discussed the means to this goal, though no specific written instructions from Davis survive. Thompson's team, however, considered many options to accomplish their task: inciting Northern sympathy for the Confederacy, attempting to sabotage Lincoln's reelection in 1864, organizing groups otherwise supportive of the South's goals, liberating Confederate prisoners held in the North, burning cities, destroying or poisoning water supplies, raiding and burning Northern cities or outposts, and engaging in germ warfare. Alexander H.H. Stuart would recall that the written charge from Davis was to "foster and give aid to the peace sentiment then active among the border states."[19] Jacob Thompson and Clement Claiborne Clay were in charge; William W. Cleary and James Holcombe assisted them. The Confederate congress authorized funds for the Canadian operations on February 15, 1864, specifying the creation of the Confederate "Secret Service." One million dollars was to go to Canadian operations out of the five million appropriated to the Confederate Secret Service overall. Thompson was immediately given $100,000 in gold on April 25, 1864. Furthermore, Thompson's orders did not include any need to account for the expenditures from the funds given to him. He could spend them as he wished, which turned out to be extravagant allocations toward questionable causes, most all of which would turn out to be dismal failures. Davis commissioned the men with a letter to Thompson dated April 27, 1864, that read, "I hereby direct you to proceed at once to Canada, there to carry out such instructions as you have received from me verbally, in such manner as shall seem most likely to be conducive to the furtherance of the interests of the Confederate States of America which have been entrusted to you."[20] The verbal "instructions" would be a matter of debate for all time. Did it include coordinating an assassination? A germ warfare plot? Bombing of Northern cities? Poisoning of Northern water supplies? The letter to Thompson was purposefully vague, with the specifics clear only in the context of their prior discussions. For history, however, it has remained maddeningly imprecise.

Davis would execute orders for many disbursements of money for this group over the next year. He most frequently disguised the payments as going toward "Necessities and Exigencies," though rarely he would be more direct and request monies for "Secret Service." Neither category really explained what projects the monies were funding. Furthermore, agents would receive rewards in direct proportion to the amount of damage they inflicted on the North. Not everyone involved saw the enterprise as a golden opportunity. Former Alabama Congressman Clement C. Clay wrote, "I am on my way to Canada. It is a very difficult and delicate duty, for which I am not suited by my talents, tastes or habits. I cannot enjoy secret service. I have accepted it with extreme reluctance"[21] And he did not enjoy it.

• • •

Jacob Thompson was a wealthy lawyer and former Mississippi planter, born in North Carolina on May 15, 1810. Supremely intelligent, fluent in both French and Italian, he was a strong supporter of education. Thompson was one of the founders of the University of Mississippi and a devout Christian. While he had academic credentials, his "people skills" may have been somewhat lacking. Friends described him as being rather too trustful, undiscerning, and willing to believe whatever a man told him. He believed that others were as honest and true to their word as he tried to be. He was loyal to friends and family, and he expected the same in return.[22] He would soon learn that well-intended plans would go awry more often than not; rogues, saboteurs, and spies would thwart his schemes meant to advance the South.

Thompson was a United States congressman from 1839 to 1851, and early in his career he amassed great wealth including two plantations, extensive land holdings, a hotel, a sawmill, and three cotton gins.[23] He was a member of James Buchanan's cabinet as secretary of the interior from 1857 to 1861 but resigned in January 1861 to support the Confederate cause. Thompson and

Abraham Lincoln were actually friends, and a mutual respect had developed between them as they both served in the Congress in Washington before the outbreak of the Civil War. But Thompson's devotion to the South overshadowed his friendship with Lincoln.

When Thompson was away from his home in Oxford, Mississippi, on December 4, 1862, Ulysses S. Grant and his army advanced to Oxford and commandeered the Thompson home, converting it to a military hospital. In the process, the troops also confiscated over 400 bales of cotton from the plantation.[24] These events might have influenced Thompson to accept assignments later from President Jefferson Davis. Thompson became inspector general of the Confederate army but later entered the military proper and quickly rose to the level of lieutenant colonel. He was an assistant to General Pierre G.T. Beauregard and participated in actions of the Army of the Mississippi at Shiloh, Vicksburg, Corinth, and Tupelo. He later was the inspector of troops for Lieutenant General John C. Pemberton.[25] After the Confederates were defeated at Vicksburg, he returned briefly to Oxford, Mississippi.

Thompson was appointed by Davis to be "commissioner" to Canada. He began this duty in May 1864, and he was effectively the leader of the "Canadian Confederacy." Blackburn interacted with Thompson, though he didn't seem to be directly under Thompson's supervision. While Thompson was in Canada, Union troops again waged an assault on Thompson's home in Oxford. They looted his house, and just two weeks thereafter, on August 22, 1864, Union forces under the command of General Andrew Jackson "Whiskey" Smith stormed Oxford. Smith ordered Officer William S. Burns to torch the Thompson home. On that day, the Union troops additionally burned and looted 34 stores and businesses in Oxford.

Confederate reports of the siege of Oxford said, "General Smith's conduct and that of his staff was [sic] brutal in the extreme, they having been made mad with whiskey. The soldiers were licensed for any crime—robbery, rape, theft and burning."[26] These events likely helped to steel Thompson's resolve to continue to follow Davis's assignment to lead the Canadian Confederates in their plans to mobilize terrorist groups and secret societies in the North. While their ultimate goal was to achieve peace, if they were initially unsuccessful in this quest they would utilize guerrilla warfare to disrupt life in the North—burn cities, free Confederate prisoners, commandeer Northern governments, raid Northern strongholds, and introduce germ warfare.

• • •

Clement Claiborne Clay was a lawyer and former United States senator from Alabama, elected in 1853 at only 35 years of age (and reelected in 1857, serving from 1853 to 1861). A land and slave owner, he became a senator in the Confederate senate from 1861 to 1863.[27] He was a close friend and confi-

8. Nefarious Schemes and Diabolical Plans

dant to Jefferson Davis. Clay's wife Virginia would later say, "From their first meeting, Secretary Davis was the intimate friend of my husband."[28] Clay helped to attend Davis in 1858 when Davis suffered the illness that robbed him of sight in his left eye.[29] Clay was the godfather to Jefferson Davis's son Joseph Evan Davis, born in 1859. Joseph died at age 5 after an accidental fall from a third-floor balcony at the Confederate White House. Tragically and coincidentally, Lincoln's son William Wallace "Willie" Lincoln also died, at the Washington White House during Lincoln's first term.

Davis offered Clay the post of secretary of war in the new Confederate government, but since Clay suffered severe and at times incapacitating asthma, he declined the offer.[30] Clay was less active than the other members of the Canadian commissioners. His ill heath kept him from the vigorous duties and travel that the others pursued, and he was once described as "an ailing, indecisive aristocrat."

In January 1861 Clay resigned his post in the U.S. Senate, rebelling at Lincoln's policies and responding to the secession of the Southern states, allying himself with the Confederacy. He became a member of the Confederate senate but requested a military post in the Confederate army in November 1863, after he was defeated for reelection to the Confederate senate. Davis appointed him instead to the post of a "commissioner" in Canada. There Clay promoted the Southern cause from both outside the borders of the United States as well as in the North itself.

Although Thompson and Clay were unofficially the codirectors of the Canadian Confederate activity, Thompson was clearly the leader. Thompson worked out of Toronto, while Clay centered his activity along the border at the town of St. Catharines, near Niagara. They worked poorly together, so the geographic distance between them was perhaps an advantage.[31] Captain Thomas Henry Hines from Kentucky had been both men's commander before they went to Canada. He said that they "were not harmonious, from the inception of their mission, on many material points connected with it. This fact was the source of constant embarrassment, and proved one of the most potent obstacles to success."[32] The two constantly disagreed. Whatever their respective personality faults, they couldn't work well together. John Breckinridge Castleman, ultimately another Confederate serving the South in Canada, said of Clay, "Clay was not a practical man. He lacked judgment and was in ill health, was peevish, irritable and suspicious."[33] Thompson was more independent, clearly the leader of the commissioners, and communicated with Clay mostly by written correspondence rather than in face-to-face meetings.

Early during the operations of the Canadian Confederate group, Clay asked—even demanded—that he have his own bank account with the ability to spend as he saw a need. Thompson finally assented, giving him $93,614.[34]

Thereafter, Clay and Thompson worked even less together. There certainly was no serious collaboration between them, in part because of their personal differences, in part because of frequent geographic separation, and in part because of Clay's ill health. Clay preferred to work with Professor James P. Holcombe.

• • •

James Philemon Holcombe was a lawyer and professor of law at the University of Virginia. His father was a physician who had freed his slaves and moved to Indiana from Virginia in 1843. The younger Holcombe remained in Virginia and was an ardent supporter of slavery, states' rights, and secession. On February 19, 1864, President Davis assigned his special commissioners to Canada to direct the Confederate sympathizers there. Davis gave Holcombe, 43 years old at the time, an initial task of directing efforts to claim the steamship *Chesapeake* for the Confederacy. Men supportive of the South had captured the *Chesapeake* at sea on December 7, 1863, but the legality of their possession of it was questioned. This Chesapeake Affair, as it was called, had been settled by the time Holcombe arrived in Nova Scotia, but Holcombe stayed in Canada to help Confederate soldiers, many of them escaped from Union prisons, to return to the South, and to assist in the organization of Confederate schemes against the North. John Hay, Abraham Lincoln's personal secretary, unflatteringly described Holcombe, a fervent Southerner, as "a tall, solemn, spare, false-looking man, with false teeth, false eyes, and false hair."[35]

• • •

William W. Cleary's identity was confused in many Civil War documents and later reports, including—of all things—the indictment charging the conspirators for the Lincoln assassination. The person indicted by the government with Booth, Herold, and the other conspirators was listed as "William C. Cleary." In fact, William *Walter* Cleary was the person they sought in connection with the assassination plot.[36] Furthermore, some sources cite him as "*Walter*" W. Cleary.[37] Even the revocation of the rewards for Thompson, Tucker, Sanders, Cleary, and John Surratt had him listed as William G. (not "C." or "W.") Cleary.[38]

William W. Cleary was born in September 1831 in Lexington, Kentucky. He graduated from Transylvania University in 1849 and received his law degree from there in 1851, the school both Blackburn and Jefferson Davis had attended. Cleary was admitted to the bar of Kentucky and settled in Cynthiana, Harrison County, Kentucky, in 1852. He served in the Kentucky General Assembly. William Cleary had a unique appearance. Detroit lawyer, and later Sixth Circuit Court judge, Halmer H. Emmons would describe him as "about

8. Nefarious Schemes and Diabolical Plans 77

30 years old, five feet 7 or 8 inches high, sandy hair grey eyes fair complexion red beard. Head little on one side, one shoulder higher than the other."[39]

During the Civil War, Cleary was briefly a member of Company D, 3rd Kentucky Infantry, Local Defense Troops. In the middle of June 1862, when he heard that he was about to be arrested by Union officers, and knowing that it wasn't possible for him to escape farther to the South, he fled to Canada. There he stayed at the Clifton House in Clifton, Ontario, and two weeks later he went to the Queen's Hotel in Toronto, places soon to become Confederate haunts in Canada. In September 1862 he returned to Kentucky. Cleary was briefly the clerk of the Council of the Confederate Government of Kentucky, and thereafter on January 20, 1863, he became a clerk in the Claims Division for the second auditor's office of the Confederate State Treasury Department in Richmond. Cleary then joined the group of Confederates that included Thompson, Clay, and Holcombe, serving in Canada at Jefferson Davis's request. Cleary was also considered to be a close friend of Jefferson Davis, and his diary records that he met with Davis on March 8, 1863, without further notation ("Called on the President").[40] Cleary was never completely sure about the wisdom of his joining the group of Confederates going to Canada. He, however, initially had wanted to be a part of the Canadian project. He wrote to Richard Hawes, the Confederate governor of Kentucky, on March 16, 1864, asking to be a member of the team going to Canada to promote the Southern cause. Cleary was interviewed on March 24 and April 7, and it seemed that he was still a candidate for the position. As late as June 15, 1863, he would record in his diary, "Am not certain yet that there is anything in it [the Canadian venture], trust there is for then I could arrange for my family."[41]

Cleary was informed of his own acceptance on the Canadian team on April 20 ("Saw Mr. Benjamin this morning, and I am to go," Cleary's diary recorded).[42] We glean many details of the operations of the Canadian Confederates from Cleary, who was commissioned as the secretary of this group. He was considered to be an honorable man, and his later testimony against Dr. Luke Blackburn would bear much weight in the assessment of the veracity of the other witnesses. Cleary expected to begin his travels via Nassau 7–8 days after his assignment, but soon the trip would take another turn.

• • •

Jefferson Davis dispatched Thompson, Clay, and Cleary to Canada on May 3, 1864 (Holcombe was already there). They first went to Wilmington, North Carolina, where they boarded the *Thistle*, a 636-ton iron side-wheel, two-masted steamship that took them to Bermuda. Thereafter, they boarded the *Alpha* for Halifax, Nova Scotia.

Cleary thought that the route they would be taking to Canada would be via Nassau, but the ship they used was going to Bermuda. They left Richmond on May 3, 1864, and departed from Wilmington on May 5 on the *Thistle*, a 201-foot blockade-runner. Stopping for a night at the mouth of the Cape Fear River Inlet near Fort Fisher, they waited until May 6 to enter the Atlantic. The Confederate ship CSS *Raleigh*, a naval ram vessel, accompanied the *Thistle* and lured the Union boats away from it at the beginning of its 674-mile, 72-hour trip to Bermuda. Running the Northern blockade of the Wilmington port, they eluded the 13 Union naval vessels guarding the harbor, in part by steaming with all lights out and a hood covering the furnace to shield Union lookouts from seeing the glow of the fire. The *Thistle* could travel 14 knots per hour and was "a long, narrow side-wheel steamer, lying low in the water, painted grey or nearly white, so that she could scarcely be seen at night." Tension was high as the *Thistle* worked its way through the blockade. "It seemed at times as if a stone could have been pitched from our vessel into one of these dangerous neighbors [the Union pursuers]. If we were detected we might expect a broadside.... A blockade-runner was not built to fight, but intended to trust to her heels."[43] The Union boats spotted and pursued the *Thistle*. "We could see the black smoke pouring out from the chimnies of the pursuer, and our Captain said she was gaining on us—in a few hours she would be near enough to fire into us. This was pleasant intelligence to gentlemen going out on diplomatic business. I thought I might as well have remained and have been shot in the regular way on land.... We made all arrangements to burn our mail and papers, and to distribute the money. Each passenger began to prepare his little story, that he might be able to properly entertain his captors.... The chase lasted five hours."[44] Cleary reported that the passengers "fortified themselves with 'Dutch Courage,'" gin taken from the captain's stores.[45] Abruptly the Union vessel slowed—perhaps it had encountered some mechanical failure—and the *Thistle* escaped on its trip to Bermuda. The British flag was displayed at the fort at St. Georges, and the Confederate flag on the *Thistle* was welcomed at this island refuge. They had achieved safety.

Enjoying a brief respite from their close call with the Union gunboats, the trio met with Major Norman Walker, the Confederate agent at St. Georges in Bermuda whose office would later be involved with Dr. Blackburn. Walker's wife Georgiana Gholson Walker was a Confederate socialite (she was also good friends with Jefferson Davis's wife Varina) who kept a detailed diary of her life on Bermuda during the Civil War. The Walkers had previously entertained Dr. Luke P. Blackburn at a dinner on February 11, 1864: "To-night we had to dinner, Col. Kane of Baltimore, who was imprisoned so long by the Yankees & Dr Blackbourne [sic] of Kent'y. The latter gentleman had brought me from Canada a magnificent haunch of venison, which would have delighted the hearts of those old gentlemen of yore, who feasted on 'venison pastry.'"[46] In her diary for early May 1864 Mrs. Walker also described meeting with Thompson and Clay, though Cleary wasn't mentioned.[47] She was the hostess for a dinner in honor of Thompson and Clay, and she described the gathering and the meal she served to her guests: "Turtle soup, boiled fish, boiled potatoes, cucumbers, fillet of boeuf au champignons, oyster patés, mutton chops, tomatoe sauce, croquettes on rice, roast saddle mutton, boiled chickens, egg sauce, asparagus, green peas, tomatoes, baked potatoes, duck with truffles, plum pudding, cocoa-nut pudding tartlets, salad, macaroni omelette, cheese, bread & butter, ice cream, fresh peaches, ambrosia, jelly, blanc mange, bananas, oranges, citron, strawberries, table set 'a la Russe,' coffee. *Dishes all handed.* Champaign, sherry Maderia, claret, cherry cordial, noyau, curacoa."[48] At least the higher-ranking members of the Confederacy didn't languish in poverty and privation in Bermuda.

In Bermuda the entourage of Thompson, Clay, and Cleary boarded the British mail steamer *Alpha* on May 10 (or May 16, according to the *Bermuda Gazette*, which listed only Thompson and Cleary as passengers)[49] and continued to Halifax, where they arrived on the 19th. They rendezvoused with Professor Holcombe, who had already been living in British North America, as it was called then, for three months pursuing the Chesapeake Affair and assisting Confederate prisoner of war escapees to return to the South. British North America comprised five provinces—Canada East, Canada West, Nova Scotia, Newfoundland, and Prince Edward Island. Each province had independent sets of laws and jurisdictions, a detail that would become important for Dr. Blackburn in a few months. Holcombe had engaged the services of Benjamin Weir, a businessman in Halifax, to both ship goods to the South and aid in the transportation of the repatriating soldiers. Their business was tricky because they had to appear to abide by neutrality laws while all the time supporting the Southern cause.

Clay had to remain in Halifax for 10 days because of illness,[50] but Thompson and Cleary continued to Canada (Nova Scotia was not a part of Canada then, becoming a part of the Dominion of Canada in 1867). Cleary first went to Toronto then Montreal. Thompson arrived in Montreal on the 29th of May, where he and Cleary again met Professor Holcombe. Clay would finally arrive in Montreal on June 11.[51]

• • •

Thompson began by organizing the resistance movements in the North, trying to recruit various organizations such as the Knights of the Golden Circle, the Sons of Malta, the Order of the Sons of Liberty, and others who would be called Copperheads (named for the emblem they wore on their lapels— the head of Liberty, cut from copper pennies). Thompson, who had joined the Sons of Liberty as an infiltrator to learn of their plans, led Confederate officials to believe that he had thousands—or even hundreds of thousands—

of Southern supporters in the North, many of whom were Copperheads ready to rise up and overthrow the North. Southerners felt that Confederate supporters, especially in Ohio, Illinois, and Indiana would coalesce to overthrow Northern governments in support of the South. Thompson touted the numbers and strengths of groups supporting the opposition to the North, only one of which was the Sons of Liberty. Mr. Clement L. Vallandigham was the "Grand Commander" of this organization, and he claimed that it numbered as high as 300,000 members in all of the territory controlled by the North. Specifically, he cited 85,000 in Illinois, 56,000 in Indiana, and 50,000 in Ohio.[52] Another report from one J.W. Tucker in a note to President Jefferson Davis claimed that 490,000 members of a secret society in the North were ready to support the South. These members allegedly wanted to organize resistance to the North and cause a rising of Southern sympathies in Iowa, Illinois, Michigan, Wisconsin, Ohio, and Indiana.[53] The numbers of participants were grossly overestimated, however, as the Confederates in Canada would soon learn when they tried to organize them into a functioning unit.[54]

It wasn't long before Thompson, Clay, Holcombe, and Cleary began attempting to negotiate with the North. Holcombe and George Nicholas Sanders were staying at the Clifton House in Niagara Falls. Sanders wrote to Horace Greeley, informing Greeley that Sanders, Thompson, and the other commissioners were accredited by Jefferson Davis in Richmond to discuss peace efforts for the Confederacy (they weren't). Thus they began an aborted attempt to negotiate peace with agents of President Lincoln. They failed.[55]

Thompson wasn't present for these negotiations, and he even instructed Cleary to avoid using his name during the discussions. This separation effectively signified the rift between Clay and Thompson. Their goals and methods were different, and they had a difficult time working together. It was reported, "Unfortunately the Commissioners were not harmonious, from the inception of their mission, on many material points connected with it. This fact was a constant source of embarrassment, and proved one of the most potent obstacles to success. All of them were very estimable gentlemen, but Messrs. Thompson and Clay found it impossible to agree." Thompson "was inclined to believe much that was told him, trust too many men, doubt too little, and suspect less." And he couldn't keep confidences. Clay, on the other hand, "gave too much confidence to parties whom he had known previously and under conditions altogether different from those he was required to meet. As a consequence, he was much under the influence of men who were honest, doubtless, but over sanguine and impracticable."[56]

Another player in the Confederate schemes was George N. Sanders, who was characterized as a narcissist, a pathological liar, and a "con man."[57] Furthermore, Clay's health remained poor, "making him restless, impatient, and

8. Nefarious Schemes and Diabolical Plans

impulsive." So the Confederate operations in Canada had three very separate prongs: Thompson attempted to foment uprisings and chaos in the North; Clay and Holcombe continued to organize repatriation of escaped Confederate prisoners; and Sanders promoted ill-devised and unauthorized peace efforts. Blackburn's schemes were included in Thompson's endeavors, although Blackburn operated mostly independently. The group's efforts were splintered and destined to fail.

• • •

Thompson organized many raids into Union territory. First, he needed to free the Confederate prisoners held in the North. Johnson's Island Prison held nearly 3,000 Confederate soldiers. This facility had a complex of thirteen two-story wooden buildings constructed on an island of about 300 acres located three miles north of Sandusky, Ohio, on Lake Erie. In the summer, a half-mile of water separated the island from the mainland; in the winter, the water became ice, but escapes were uncommon (the Union reports gave the number at 12, though the real number was likely higher). Opened as a prison in April 1862, it processed 10,000–15,000 Confederate captives—mostly officers—over the course of the war. At its peak it housed 3,256 prisoners; the monthly average was 2,549. This prison was actually quite humane; death rates were less than 2 percent per year, compared with 10–12 percent in other Northern prisons.[58] Two previous attempts to rescue the Confederate prisoners (in 1862 and 1863) had failed.

Thompson devised a third plan to rescue those Confederate prisoners on Johnson's Island that would require very few assistants, using a Confederate takeover of the Union ship *Michigan*, a gunboat stationed nearby. Scheduled for September 19, 1864, and later dubbed the Lake Erie Raid, it would be led by John Yates Beall and would occur almost simultaneously with the attempt to disrupt the local government in Chicago. Beall, a blockade-runner with experience piloting ships, schemed to take the small steamer vessel *Philo Parsons* and use it to capture the USS *Michigan*, the only gunboat on Lake Erie, under the command of Captain John C. Carter and anchored at Sandusky, Ohio. After taking the *Michigan*, then the prison, then the arsenal at Sandusky, the Rebels were supposed to sack cities along the northern waterway—Detroit, Cleveland, Buffalo, and others. This grandiose plan seemed good in theory, but it failed miserably. Johnson's Island would continue to hold its prisoners until the end of the Civil War. Beall would soon be captured and arrested at Niagara Falls after he tried unsuccessfully to sabotage Union trains. He was taken to a jail in New York City then transferred to Fort Lafayette in New York Bay. He was tried on February 10, 1865, for being a Confederate spy. Claiming that he was acting under direct orders from the Confederate command, on February 21 he wrote to a Confederate commissioner asking to be a part of a prisoner exchange, but he was too late. He was executed on February 24.[59]

• • •

Not dissuaded by the sad turn of events with the *Michigan* in September 1864, the Rebels planned another raid into Union territory at St. Albans, Vermont, on October 19, 1864. Residing in St. Lawrence Hall in Montreal, Clement C. Clay proposed to take about 20–25 men to attack St. Albans, about 40 miles south of Montreal. Thompson, who directed all large expenditures from Rebel bank accounts, financed the scheme with $100,000 of Confederate money.[60] The precise goal of the raid was not clear, other than to punish the Union sympathizers and to bring the understanding of the horrors of war to Northerners in Vermont. They succeeded in robbing three banks (the First National, the St. Albans, and the Franklin County) of a total of $208,000, killing one man and wounding three others. The leader of the raid, Lieutenant Bennett H. Young from Kentucky, was quickly captured, and fourteen men from his band were either captured or surrendered. At the trial in Canada, George Sanders and Jacob Thompson supported the men on trial. The accused argued that they were performing "legal" acts of warfare since they were sanctioned, even financed, by the Confederate government. They were not spies, thieves, thugs, or murderers; they were men waging war, and as such they weren't subject to the charges levied against them by the Canadian government. Though they lived in Canada, they claimed that they were not violating Canadian neutrality by using it as a base of operations. Astoundingly, their defense worked, and they were released without receiving any convictions or punishments.

• • •

The Canadian Confederates tried multiple other approaches to the disruption of Northern activities. Ultimately, Thompson allocated $25,000 to Captain Thomas H. Hines for a two-pronged attack in the Chicago area. One element promoted disorder at the Democratic National Convention in Chicago on July 4, 1864. There they tried to cause fires and foment riots in the city. However, the convention was delayed and so was the anticipated disruption. The other element was an attack at the Confederate prisoner of war camp at Fort Douglas near Chicago. The Canadian Confederate agents planned to free the 9,000 prisoners there who were under the guard of Colonel Benjamin J. Sweet and about 800 Union soldiers at the Fort Douglas camp. The planned breakout was set for November 8, 1864, Election Day. But Colonel Sweet had identified the majority of the Confederate infiltrators, some of whom were members of the Sons of Liberty. Both events were poorly organized. Their pretentious schemes went nowhere, as Sweet and his men

8. Nefarious Schemes and Diabolical Plans 83

performed a counter operation the day before, on November 7. Union soldiers captured the Confederate leaders and "106 bush-whackers, guerillas, and rebel soldiers," along with 142 shotguns, 349 revolvers, and thousands of bullets. Spies and infiltrators in the Confederate ranks had informed the Union about the plans, so the project went nowhere. The feckless Confederates had failed again.[61] They desperately tried to accomplish foul deeds. Their malevolence was real. Their competence was not.

Canadian Confederate ineptitude was exceeded only by their infighting, inability to keep their plans secret, faulty espionage, infiltration of Union spies within their ranks, and unrealistic expectations from schemes that were always destined to fail. The Blackburn yellow fever plot was only one of many. Jacob Thompson would lament in a letter to Secretary of State Judah P. Benjamin, "The bane and curse of carrying out anything in this country [Canada] is the surveillance under which we act. Detectives, or those ready to give information, stand at every street corner. Two or three can not interchange ideas without a reporter."[62] Soon thereafter Benjamin would write to Thompson: "We are satisfied that so close an espionage is kept upon you that your services have been deprived of the value which is attached to your residence in Canada. The President thinks that it is better that you return to the Confederacy."[63] Thompson had outlived his usefulness, and even his personal couriers were unable to travel to Richmond without being intercepted. Benjamin decided to replace him with General Edwin Gray Lee, the second cousin of Robert E. Lee, hardly an obscure person himself. His identifiable ties to well-known Confederate higher-ups would hamper his effectiveness, just as incompetence had hindered his predecessor.

• • •

Other schemes had similarly prominent targets. In September 1864 one such plan involved kidnapping President Lincoln, which, of course, had to have contingencies considered in which Lincoln or his guards or associates might resist and result in the injury or death of the president. Thomas Nelson Conrad scouted the White House for the purpose of kidnapping the president and taking him to Richmond. Conrad was sent out from Secretary of State Judah Benjamin's office, funded by the Confederate Secret Service, and it's likely that Jefferson Davis knew of this plot, too.[64] Some of Conrad's funds were paid in gold, and Davis had to approve all distributions in gold from the Confederate treasury. James A. Seddon, secretary of war for the Confederacy, wrote to Conrad at least twice about his kidnapping plan, and Seddon directed Lieutenant Colonel John S. Mosby and Colonel Charles H. Cawood to help Conrad, however necessary, to achieve his task.

• • •

Canadian Confederates hatched other projects designed to produce terror and mass destruction. One such plan was to destroy the Croton Dam at New York. The Croton Dam supplied water to the City of New York from 41 miles away with 30,000,000 gallons per day (it had a maximum delivery capacity of twice that amount). Considering that the local reservoirs held only a 2–3 day supply of water, destruction of the dam would cause the city of New York to find water to be "as scarce and expensive as whiskey in Richmond."[65] Since the "foundries and factories engaged in the manufacture of munitions of war and army supplies" would be stopped, the support of the Union army would be seriously impaired. Furthermore, without water to fight fires, another plan to burn New York City would become more feasible. The dam easily held 500,000,000 gallons of water, and dynamiting the dam would also destroy mills, foundries, towns, bridges, and manufacturing plants along the course of the river. This black flag operation was ideally suited to accomplish many goals. But it never materialized.

• • •

Another objective involved poisoning that same water supply. Dr. Luke Blackburn calculated the quantity of various poisons—strychnine, arsenic, prussic acid, and others—needed to be effective. He believed that the project was feasible, but Jacob Thompson, the keeper of the purse strings, thought that it might not be possible to obtain enough poison to do the job. Another physician, Dr. Montrose Anderson Pallen of Mississippi—a surgeon in the Confederate army, was present for some of the meetings, and he approved, suggesting that the poisons could be purchased in Europe.[66] He would later deny his involvement.[67] Like many other schemes, this project was never pursued.

• • •

Confederate terrorism plans also included the plot to burn New York City. Robert Kennedy, one of the firebombers, said, "We wanted the people of the North to understand there are two sides to this war and they can't be rolling in wealth and comfort while we in the South are bearing all the hardships."[68] It was retribution; it was terrorism. The conspirators attempted the scheme on the eve of the presidential election, November 7, 1864 (the day before Col. Benjamin Sweet foiled the Chicago escapade). But because the incendiary devices weren't ready the plan wasn't executed until November 25, 1864, after Lincoln had already been elected to his second term. A Confederate agent distributed about 48 bottles of an inflammable and spontaneously combustible liquid to eight Confederate fire-bombers, led by Robert M. Martin and John William Headley. They planned 32 fires, including 19 hotels, a theater, and P.T. Barnum's American Museum. Many of these bombs in New York City didn't successfully ignite fires, though 15 hotels and the Barnum Museum were damaged, and several hay barges burned along the river. Overall, however, the entire plan was unsuccessful. Most of the fires were small; firefighters successfully extinguished them quickly, and the blazes caused no deaths. (Ironically, and probably not a part of the plot, John Wilkes Booth was performing at the Winter Garden Theatre next to the Lafarge House. As a fire was started next door, he calmed the audience, telling them that they were in no danger. The show continued.)[69] Seven of the eight arsonists escaped, but Robert Cobb Kennedy was captured and ultimately hanged on March 25, 1865, at Fort Lafayette in New York Harbor.

Headley wrote a long memoir about the Confederate effort to sabotage Northern cities. He believed that Godfrey Hyams was responsible for traitorously revealing the plan for the New York fires to Northern agents.[70] However, Headley didn't know Hyams well, nor had he been told accurately about Hyams' past, for Headley described Hyams as a man "who had escaped from prison [perhaps referring to Gratiot Prison or Alton Prison, though Hyams had been released and didn't need to escape] and was reputed to be wealthy."[71] Given his close association with the Canadian Confederate conspirators, Hyams did indeed have access to some of the plans for Confederate attacks on the North, and he could have been a double agent even then. More likely, he simply followed the money; if he thought that a course of action would yield him a fortune he would pursue it. Headley thought that Hyams had also revealed the plans for the capture of the *Michigan* to free Confederate prisoners at Johnson's Island, the plans to storm the prison at Camp Douglas in Chicago, and other Confederate schemes. Headley reported that Blackburn was to be the agent for a similar fire attack on Boston,[72] although any other evidence against Blackburn for such a role is lacking. Headley attributed the failure of that fire, and one in Cincinnati, to Hyams' treachery as well. None of these schemes worked.

9

Plans for the Importation of Pestilence

The First Shipment of Articles Contaminated with Yellow Fever

Originally Blackburn schemed to spread both yellow fever and smallpox throughout Union territory by distributing contaminated articles obtained in Bermuda. The yellow fever scourge of 1863–1864 was one of the four major epidemics of the mid–1800s in Bermuda. Bermuda was accustomed to such visitations, but no one knew how the disease was spread, and there was no cure.[1] In 1864, four hundred seventy-one people, 3.5 percent of the entire population of Bermuda, died from it. By contrast, in 1843 there were 496 (5 percent) deaths and 281 (2.5 percent) in 1856. The worst year was 1853, when 814 (7 percent of the Bermudian population) succumbed to yellow fever. Blackburn earlier might have been able to obtain articles of clothing of victims of smallpox, but in 1864 smallpox in Bermuda was uncommon. Fortunately for the people of Bermuda and the North, yellow fever was the only epidemic Blackburn could try to export from Bermuda during the years 1864–1865. Rare cases of smallpox appeared sporadically there but not in a frequency or severity Blackburn could use successfully as a means of biological warfare.

The 1864 yellow fever epidemic in Bermuda was one of many that had ravaged those islands in the 19th century. Between June 1864 and January 1865, over 3,000 cases of yellow fever appeared in Bermuda, and over 500 deaths occurred.[2] St. Georges was the principal port city of the Bermudian islands in its role as a hotbed of Confederate blockade-running. However, the city of St. Georges itself was quite primitive. Surgeon-Major T.W. Barrow of Bermuda wrote as follows:

9. The First Shipment of Articles Contaminated 87

> The sanitary state is such as may be expected in so miserable a place. Most offensive odours prevail on all sides from the various cesspits, and filth of all kinds thrown into the streets. There are no sewers or drains. The only way in which the streets are cleansed is by the heavy rain which occasionally falls, the quantity being greatly augmented by the drainage from the surrounding heights. Thus, here is a small town lying as it were in a basin, cut off from all winds, without sewers, full of cesspits rarely emptied, with no water-supply beyond what is collected from the roofs of the houses, and with the streets unscavengered. When I add that the houses are excessively overcrowded, is it surprising to find that yellow fever here runs riot, and is of a far more deadly type than elsewhere in Bermuda?[3]

The military barracks in St. Georges needed extensive upgrading. The hospital attached to the barracks was built for 24 patients, though the norm was 48. The "waterclosets" most often had no water in them, making their function close to useless. The hospital during the epidemic wasn't sufficient for the demands:

> Seventy men ... were thrust into a place which could not properly accommodate thirty-five.... The sick were not only lying around the wards, but may be said to have covered the entire floor.... I do not know any sight more appalling than the wards of an hospital crowded ... with yellow fever patients.... Here a strong man is seen in violent convulsions, rapidly followed by black vomit and death; there may be seen one lying in a state of calm and utter indifference to everything around him; a sudden turn of the head, followed by a forcible ejection of inky vomit, indicates his approaching end.

The fate wasn't much different for the doctors and nurses: "In fact, between the 5th and 15th of September [1864], all the medical officers in St. Georges were either dead or prostrated by fever."[4] Dr. Blackburn worked under these conditions.

• • •

Blackburn had accomplished many of his blockade-running deals and supply of the Confederate troops from Halifax, Nova Scotia. His headquarters there was the Halifax Hotel on Hollis Street. In February 1864 he met with Alexander "Sandy" Keith, Jr., the nephew of a local brewer and a brewer himself.[5] In addition, others likely colluded with Blackburn there. One report in the *Halifax Sun* newspaper, written by the editor A.J. Ritchie, suggested that two members of the Dalhousie Medical School faculty, Dr. Edward Jennings and Dr. John Slater, were involved in the planning to bring the infected materials into Halifax from Bermuda. Ritchie claimed that Premier of Nova Scotia Sir Charles Tupper (also a medical doctor), had told him of Jennings and Slater's involvement. Tupper denied that he had said anything of the sort, and Jennings and Slater threatened to sue the newspaper. The entire scandal languished as the Medical Society investigated the charges, and it quietly disappeared from view, never reaching any definitive legal action.[6]

Shipping by sea would be important for Blackburn, both for his own travel and for the delivery of his articles contaminated with yellow fever. In addition, many Confederate supplies came by ship from Europe, were transferred to smaller ships in Bermuda, and then were sent to Southern ports. Vessels from the United Kingdom (mostly from London and Liverpool) and other European cities supplied the ports of St. Georges, Bermuda; Nassau, Bahamas; Havana, Cuba; and Matamoros, Mexico. Guns and ammunition were the most valued commodities. Britain was officially neutral, but British-built (though not British-approved) ships carried many of these cargoes. The North needed fewer supplies from Europe, so the Confederate business dominated Bermudian wharves and sailing activity. Cargo was transferred in Bermuda from larger, slower sailing ships to steam-powered ships running to Southern ports because the steamers were faster, more maneuverable, and could elude the blockade by the Union navy. The Union's "Anaconda Plan," the attempt to squeeze the life out of the Southern war effort by isolating and blocking Southern ports with Northern gunboats, would have been even more successful if it hadn't been for these sleek Confederate blockade-runners.

Halifax, Nova Scotia, was also a port frequented by Confederates, but mostly for passenger traffic and mail delivery. Halifax had been an integral part of Bermudian life since the late 1700s.[7] Much food and lumber came from Halifax, so shipping routes were well established by the time of the Civil War. British shipping from Falmouth, England, through Bermuda served New York City as well in the early 1800s.[8] Bermuda began designing and advertising for contracts for building Her Majesty's Dockyard on Ireland Island in 1809; construction began in 1810.[9] During the War of 1812, a Halifax-Bermuda mail service was established. Cunard Shipping was a standard mail and passenger carrier between Halifax and Bermuda during the Civil War. One particular Cunard vessel, the *Alpha*, played prominently in the transportation of Confederate rebels, including Blackburn, between Halifax and Bermuda. Its usual route was Halifax-Bermuda-St. Thomas-Bermuda-Halifax. The Halifax-Bermuda portion of the *Alpha*'s journey took about five days; the Bermuda-St. Thomas portion was about five or six days. A trip from Halifax to Bermuda was made about every two weeks.[10] Blackburn and his fellow Confederates would frequently use the *Alpha* (often incorrectly called the *Alphia* by the Southerners) for their trips from Halifax to Bermuda. Then they would board a blockade-runner to the South, most often arriving at the port in Wilmington, North Carolina.

The *Alpha* was 514 tons (some sources say 653 tons), measured 222 by 27 feet, and had 32 men as crew. It had one steam funnel and three masts for sails (Figures 9A, 9B, 9C, 9D, 9E and 9F). The steamship was made of iron, and the main propulsion was a single screw driven by a two-cylinder, direct-

9. The First Shipment of Articles Contaminated

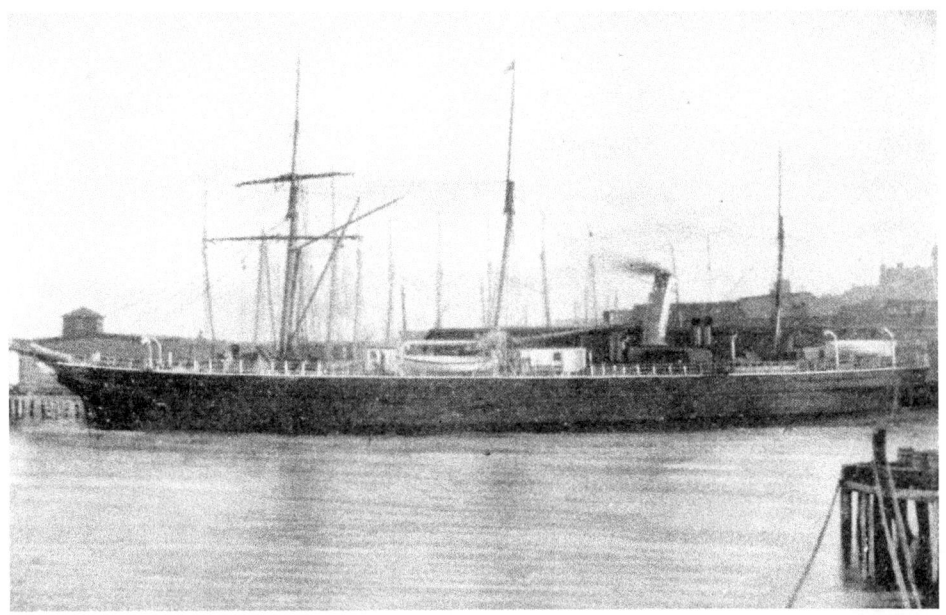

Figure 9A. First known photograph of the steamship *Alpha*, taken in 1863 shortly after the christening of the vessel on March 17, 1863. The *Alpha* was put into service in 1863 after its construction at the Clyde Shipyards in Glasgow, Scotland, by Barclay, Curle, and Company. Being a single-propeller steamship and weighing 653 tons, it was first owned by William Cunard, the younger son of Samuel Cunard, famous owner of the Cunard Lines. It was 221.8 feet long and 27.6 feet wide, with a depth of 14.9 feet, and was powered by a two-cylinder, 112-horsepower engine, carrying both passengers and cargo on the Halifax-Bermuda-St. Thomas route. It was sold in 1888 to Robert Pickford and William Anderson Black, of Glasgow, who, having formed the company of Pickford and Black, operated a mail and passenger service running to Halifax-Bermuda-Grand Turk Island and Kingston, Jamaica. Subsequently, the *Alpha* was sold in 1899 to Samuel Barber, a banker turned shipper in Vancouver and Victoria, British Columbia. Its career ended on December 15, 1900, when it ran aground and was completely wrecked on the edge of Yellow Island Lighthouse near Vancouver Island, killing nine men onboard, including Barber (Mariners' Museum, Newport News, VA; *Alpha* Steamship 1863; photograph #PB29373; photographer unknown).

drive engine. Launched in 1863, the new ship carried about 25 first-class passengers and 150 third-class passengers.[11] The ship had only seven first-class staterooms, and two dozen first-class berths: "Many passengers had to sleep in the first-class saloon, which doubled as a sitting room and dinning [sic] room. The handful of stewards and stewardesses had their hands full with the many passengers, including women and children, who were constantly seasick. The deck was crowded with cattle and sheep."[12] Lifeboats were limited. Death from sickness during the journey was not uncommon. During the

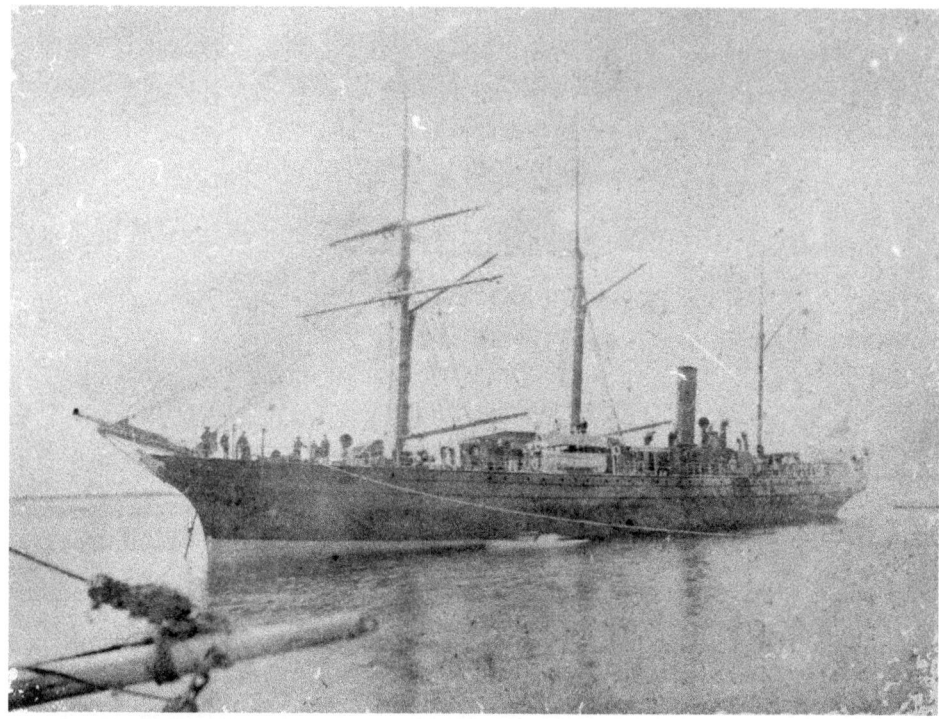

Figure 9B. Photograph of the *Alpha* anchored in the St. Georges, Bermuda, harbor, circa mid-1860s (Bermuda Archives, Photographic Collection, Negative #2543).

time of Blackburn's travels, David Hunter was the captain of the *Alpha*.[13] Although the *Alpha* was relatively new, that doesn't mean the accommodations were necessarily good or the trip was enjoyable.[14] Often overcrowded, frequently tossed about by stormy seas, the *Alpha* was a source of seasickness for many, if not most, passengers. Sanitary conditions were marginal. So while Blackburn and his colleagues used this route, then connecting to Wilmington as the second leg of their journey, the voyage certainly was not a vacation.

Travel on the *Alpha* invariably included a mass of "deck passengers." These often included cows, sheep, and other animals, as well as humans. The small poop deck was a gathering place for passengers before the gong rang, which it did three times daily, announcing the meals served in the "saloon." Passengers would then walk single file into the saloon for their food. As the *Alpha* approached Bermuda, Union navy blockading vessels would sometimes be sighted outside the coral reefs that surrounded the island, but they almost always let the *Alpha* pass untouched.

One Colonel James H. Burton, an officer in the Confederate States Army,

9. *The First Shipment of Articles Contaminated* 91

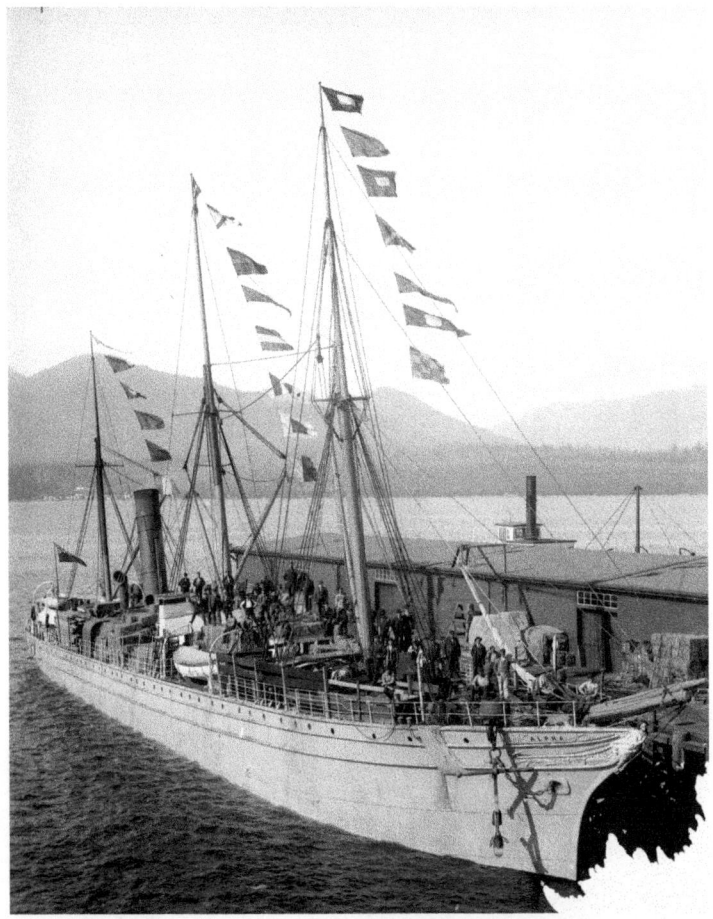

Figure 9C. The steamship *Alpha*, commonly reported incorrectly in Civil War era communications as the *Alphia*, was the mail steamer that plied the route Halifax-Bermuda-St. Thomas. It was an uncomfortable ship for passengers, with little room above deck (photograph by Stephen Joseph Thompson, likely taken in the late 1800s. From Caledonian Maritime Research Trust: http://www.clydeships.co.uk/view. php?exact=1&year_built=&builder=&ref=1258&vessel=ALPHA#v; and the City of Vancouver Archives, British Columbia, Canada, Archives Box 208-D-6, CVA 137–106, *S.S. Alpha* at dock: http://searcharchives.vancouver.ca/uploads/r/null/1/3/1379432/c3bba1fc-ec5d-4fc3-9097-7b38c9fb6b32-A20130.jpg).

kept a diary of his travels in 1863.[15] He recounted his experience on the *Alpha* from Halifax to Bermuda:

> **Tuesday, Sept. 15th** ... Deposited trunks &c. in Cunard's warehouse, engaged passage in the Screw Steamer "*Alpha*," Capt. Hunter, to Bermuda; and drove with Mr. Regnault to the "Halifax Hotel" and took rooms there. Spent the day in walking

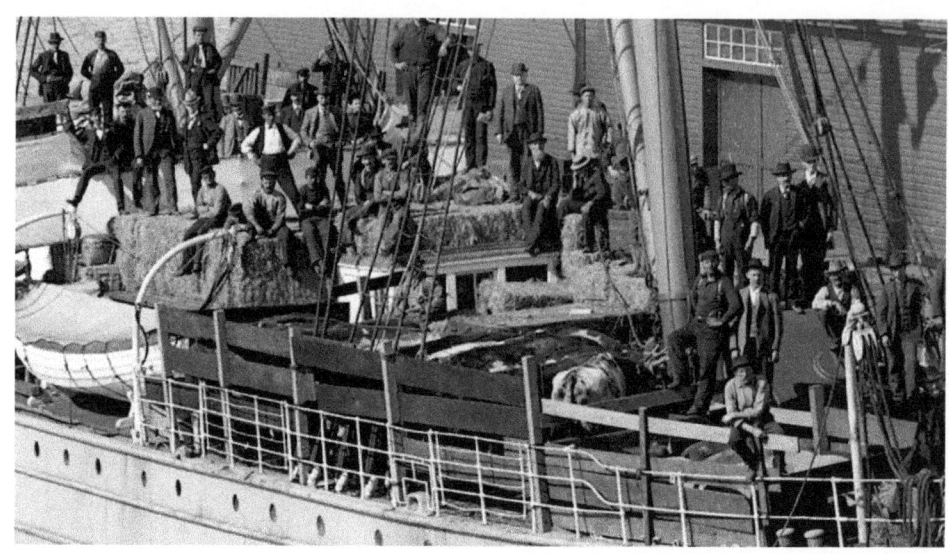

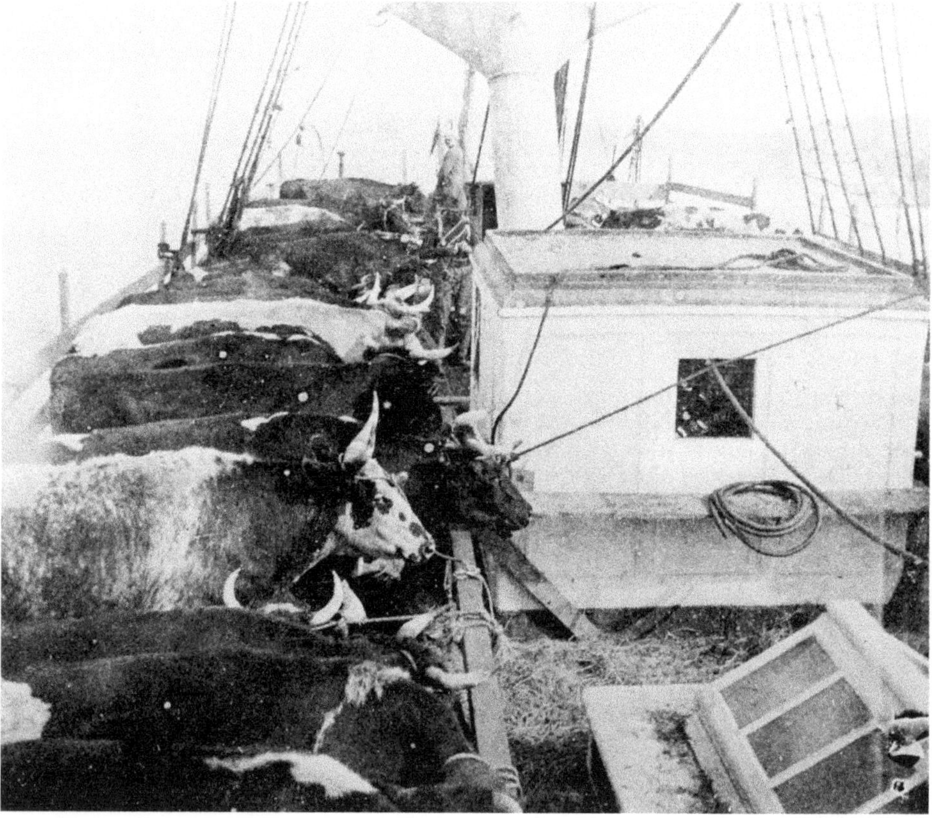

9. The First Shipment of Articles Contaminated

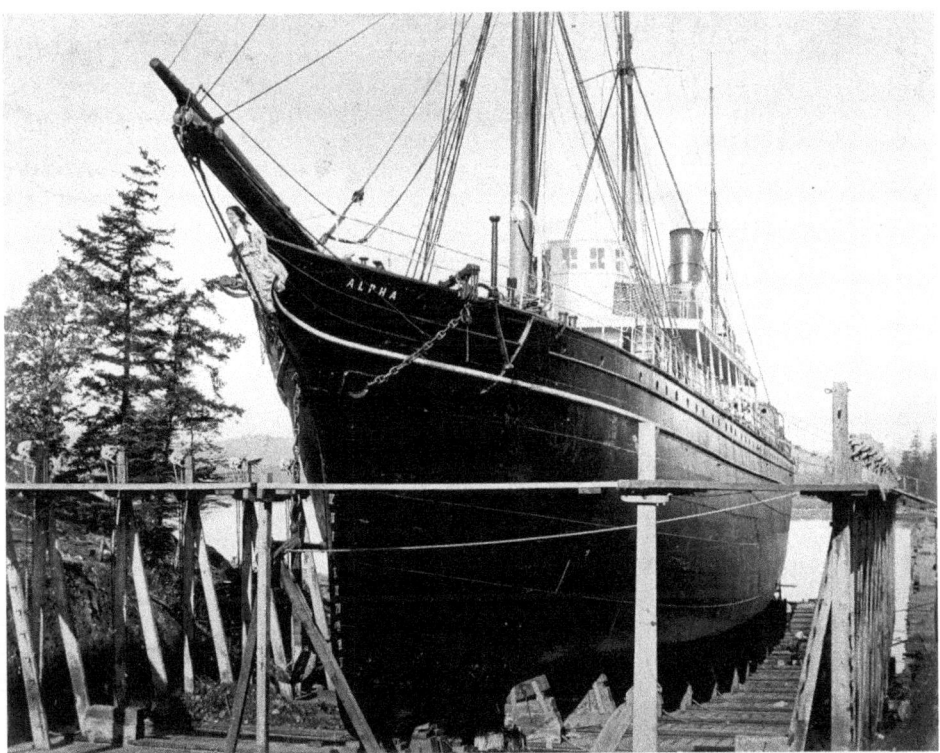

Opposite top: Figure 9D. Enlargement of the central portion of the Figure 9C, shows cattle being transported on the deck itself (photograph by Stephen Joseph Thompson, likely taken in the late 1800s. From Caledonian Maritime Research Trust: http://www.clydeships.co.uk/view.php?exact=1&year_built=&builder=&ref=1258&vessel=ALPHA#v; and the City of Vancouver Archives, British Columbia, Canada, Archives Box 208-D-6, CVA 137–106, S.S. *Alpha* at dock: http://searcharchives.vancouver.ca/uploads/r/null/1/3/1379432/c3bba1fc-ec5d-4fc3-9097-7b38c9fb6b32-A20130.jpg). *Opposite bottom:* Figure 9E. The quarters onboard the *Alpha* remained cramped, as it again carried livestock (courtesy New Westminster Public Library. Photographs by P. Jones, likely taken c. 1899. Accessed at www.nwheritage.org, photograph #2453). *Above:* Figure 9F. The *Alpha* was refitted and upgraded in the late 1890s. This photograph was taken while it was still in drydock. Even after many improvements, it was still used as transport for cattle, as well as people (courtesy New Westminster Public Library. Photographs by P. Jones, likely taken c. 1899. Accessed at www.nwheritage.org, photograph #2454).

around the town, making some purchases of dry goods, boots & shoes &c. in company with Mr. regnault [*sic*].

Wednesday, Sept. 16th, Halifax, N.S. Spent the most of the day in company with Mr. regnault walking about twon [*sic*, meaning "town"], and making purchases of various articles to take home.... In the evening remained home at my hotel writing....

Thursday, Sept. 17th, Halifax, N.S. Made further purchases of boy's violin, blankets, candles, starch &c. Completed the packing of my case of goods purchased in Halifax and sent it down to the Steamer "*Alpha*," for shipment to Bermuda....

Friday, Sept. 18th, Halifax, N.S. Completed all preparation for leaving this city for Bermuda, settled hotel bill, and drove with Mr. Regnault down to the Steamer "*Alpha*," and went directly on board. At 12, noon, the gun fired, and we cast off from the wharf and steamed out to sea. Decks covered with cattle, to the great annoyance of the passengers. There are 90 head of beef cattle and 120 head of sheep on board. The sheep and about 20 head of cattle being in the hold. There are about 26 passengers in all on board, including several ladies, some of whom came over with us from Liverpool in the "*Arabia*...."

Saturday, Sept. 19th, S.S. "*Alpha*" Sea rather rough—ship rolling considerably—and most of the passengers very uncomfortable, self included. Cabins very badly ventilated—keep out the air, but let in the sea and the rain.

Sunday, Sept. 20th, S.S. "*Alpha*" Rev'd Mr. Terry volunteered to read the church service, but did not finish because of the rough weather and uncomfortable condition of the passengers. My cabin is about 7 feet square, and in this small space 5 passengers are stowed away in small berths—and bunks fitted up for two more, which fortunately are unoccupied. One wash basin &c serves for all. Many of the passengers sleep on the seats in the saloon in preference to their berths, including several ladies. The table, and the entire accomodations [*sic*] on this ship are villainous.

Monday, Sept. 21st, S.S. "*Alpha*" Head winds so far all the way from Halifax, and progress of the ship slow. Passengers growing tired of their voyage, and wishing for a fair wind, but none comes.

Tuesday, Sept. 22d, S.S. "*Alpha*" Wind becoming more favorable, and progress of the ship more satisfactory. Dr. Hoge and Mr. Terry slept on deck last night. Atmosphere growing milder as we progress to the south. Beautiful moonlight nights. Begin to look for the appearance of Bermuda.

Wednesday, Sept. 23d, S.S. "*Alpha*" Land sighted at 8 a.m. Signaled for a pilot who came off to us at 10 o'clk. Wind blowing very fresh, sea rough, indications of a storm. Ship struck by a wind squall last night, but did not do much damage. Pilot took the ship safely into St. Georges Harbor, and dropped anchor at 11 a.m. Soon after a severe storm of wind and rain set in which lasted all afternoon with more or less intensity. Commenced landing the cattle at once. They were each slung over the side of the ship by the horns into the water, and then made fast to a large barge, which towed them ashore in squads of about a dozen. Engaged a small boat and went ashore with my light luggage. Got caught in a rain squall, but managed to stay tolerably dry. Went to the house kept by Mrs. Heyward, where I stopped when I came out; but could get no room. Storm too severe to allow of my seeking about for lodgings, so Mr. Terry kindly allowed an old, lumpy sofa to be put in one corner of his room, on which I slept, or rather did not sleep, for the night.

The *Alpha* continued on to St. Thomas and returned to Bermuda on Sunday, October 4, an 11-day round-trip. It was a difficult journey, but Dr. Blackburn and other Confederates took this route on more than one occasion.

• • •

9. The First Shipment of Articles Contaminated 95

The yellow fever epidemic starting in the spring of 1864 in Bermuda was devastating. Charles Monck, the governor general of the United Provinces of Canada (British-controlled), enlisted Dr. Luke Blackburn's help in combating the outbreak that was killing so many on that British island. Staff-Surgeon Major T. W. Barrow, the deputy inspector of hospitals, wrote of the epidemic, and a commission was appointed by Great Britain's Colonial Office to investigate the extent of the contagion and its cause. Many deficiencies of the St. Georges environment were cited as contributors, including vapors, low tides, filthy conditions, absence of sanitary conditions in the town (no sewers or drains, cess-pits overflowing), odors and stenches in the town, "dissipated, dirty sailors," a constant flow of ships from diverse locations where yellow fever abounded, refuse thrown from the ships, entrails of fish and animals thrown into the harbor, poor air circulation, crowding of the population, poor freshwater supply, brackish water, general intemperance, and overall filth.[16] The list of offending agents was huge.

In early 1864 Blackburn made his first pilgrimage to Bermuda from Halifax. He volunteered to help the patients in Bermuda who had contracted the disease. Everyone dreaded yellow fever: it caused nausea, vomiting, diarrhea, gastrointestinal hemorrhaging, delirium, seizures, coma, and death. It was an ugly picture, and Blackburn was familiar with its ravages. Neither he nor anyone else knew how to treat the disease properly, but he was a compassionate physician, willing to expose himself to the dangers of the disease. This exposure constituted an unknown risk, for no one knew exactly how the illness was transmitted. It seemed that close contact was necessary for the disease to pass from one person to another. Little else was known except that over one-third of the patients would die. In the process of death, patients soiled their bedclothes, sheets, towels, and blankets with vomitus and excrement. Dr. Blackburn reasoned that he could collect soiled bedclothes and garments and send them by ship from Bermuda to infect the cities of the North. So he went to Bermuda, treated the sick, and collected these soiled items. His purpose was to start an epidemic in the North, though he had advertised his goal to very few people. He had described his subterfuge to his confidants as "an infallible plan directed against the masses of Northern people solely to cause death."[17] Blackburn had already enlisted the help of Godfrey Hyams, who was ready to complete the transport of the contaminated items to the northern United States. He would assure that the trunks were delivered to target cities, and then the items would be sold at auction or otherwise distributed.

Dr. Blackburn first arrived in Bermuda on February 10, 1864. The manifest of the steamship *Alpha* from Halifax had both Blackburn and "Colonel Marshall [sic] Kane," another Confederate agent, listed in the group of passengers travelling in the first-class cabin. Colonel George Proctor Kane was a former chief of police of the City of Baltimore, who was arrested on June 27, 1861, for his Southern-leaning tendencies. He was a rabid secessionist suspected of being a Confederate agent, and he was considered to be a real threat to the Union forces in Baltimore at the start of the Civil War. Often called Marshal (or Marshall) Kane, sometimes "Colonel Kane" because he had been a colonel in one of the Baltimore militias, he was imprisoned first at Fort McHenry. Government officials then moved him successively from there to Fort Lafayette in New York, Fort Columbus in New York, and, finally, Fort Warren in Boston. Ordered released on November 26, 1862, he then fled to Canada, as did many Confederate sympathizers.

Kane's presence on the ship carrying Blackburn to Bermuda couldn't have been an accident. This route was the one frequently used by blockade-runners as part of their passage to the South. Since the *Alpha* was rather small, and both were travelling first class, Kane and Blackburn no doubt conversed during the five-day journey, perhaps even plotted together. They were accompanied by about 13 other "Southern gentlemen," some of whom had congregated for a few days in Halifax before departing for Bermuda. The *Bermuda Gazette* described them and their compatriots as holding Halifax "in grateful remembrance. A day or two since they were treated to a jolly sleigh ride, and to-day Kane and the several officers of the party were the guests of the Halifax Club, who gave them a complimentary dinner."[18] (Kane would later return to Baltimore and be elected its mayor in 1877.)

Some evidence suggests that Blackburn had two "medical students" working with him.[19] One might have gone to Bermuda with Blackburn, as a reference is made of Blackburn's "servant" who accompanied him. Blackburn, briefly residing in Bermuda, soon became known as an ultra-Confederate. He wasn't secretive during his stay on the island; he even touted himself as an "agent" of the Confederacy to friends there.[20] Described as portly and middle-aged, he was viewed by some in Bermuda as a savior, by others as a meddler.

Dr. Blackburn registered at the Hamilton Hotel, one of the island's best guesthouses in the 1860s. There in Bermuda he volunteered to help the victims of yellow fever. Though allegedly on a humanitarian mission, he wasn't uniformly accepted by the other doctors on the island. Consul Allen reported that Bermudian physicians "did not believe he was a physician because he was so coarse and illiterate, and one of the hospital nurses said that whenever one of his patients was sick he would stretch out a handkerchief to catch the black vomit, and afterward wrap up the handkerchief and carry it away with him. This, together with his close connection with the resident Confederates, led me to mention my suspicions to some of the officials, but they laughed at me."[21] Locals often described Blackburn as a blustering fool, but the Bermudian physicians had a right to be suspicious, and they probably had the natural tendency to believe that they needed no outside help fighting the epidemic.

9. The First Shipment of Articles Contaminated

To Let.

THE CORPORATION OF HAMIL-TON have now much satisfaction in offering FOR RENT the Two Story STONE BUILDING, lately erected by them in the Town for a Hotel. It is 150 feet by 36 feet, with a wing added in the rear 36 feet by 24 feet—and contains, vizt.:

2 Large DRAWING ROOMS, 26 feet by 18 feet each,
2 Large SITTING ROOMS,
1 Large DINING ROOM, 34 feet by 22 feet,
1 Smaller DO. 22 feet by 14 feet,
1 READING ROOM,
1 BAR ROOM,
26 BED ROOMS,
BATH ROOMS and WATER CLOSETS,
3 CLOSETS for Glasses. &c.. &c.,
2 CORRIDORS, extending the whole length of the Building,
A Commodious KITCHEN, with Pantry, Store Room, and Lift Room,
1 Commodious CELLAR,
A TANK, of sufficient size for Hotel purposes.

WINDOWS protected by Blinds,
Each BED ROOM is furnished with, a Bedstead, a Table, a Wash-Hand Stand with Marble Top, a Dress Bureau, a Towel Horse, 2 Chairs and one Rock Chair.
The Large DINING ROOM is furnished with Tables, Chairs, Side Boards, and a Lift.
The KITCHEN is furnished with a Kitchener of the most improved American pattern, with a large Water Boiler attached, and Cooking Utensils necessary for it.

THE BUILDING is situated on a healthful and beautiful spot, and commands extensive views of the Surrounding Country. It affords many facilities for strangers visiting Bermuda, is spacious, well arranged and well ventilated.
In front it has a stone Balcony 64 feet in length, affording a delightful promenade.

TENDERS for Renting this Building as it now stands, will be received until
The 1st day of October Next,
when the highest offer, if otherwise approved of, will be accepted.
For further information apply to
H. J. TUCKER,
Mayor.
Bermuda, July 25, 1861.

A CARD.

THE Undersigned having just made some Additional Comforts to her Dwelling House,—next West of the Royal Bermuda Yacht Club,—begs respectfully to inform the Public generally that she is now prepared to take a few BOARDERS or LODGERS on Moderate Terms. She hopes by strict attention she will still continue to receive a share of the Public Patronage which has hitherto been so liberally bestowed on her.

CATHARINE SLATER.
Hamilton, March 22, 1864.

Left: Figure 10A. Lacking a medical office in Hamilton, Bermuda, Dr. Blackburn treated patients at both the Hamilton Hotel and at Catharine Slater's Boarding House. Neither was adequately equipped for medical purposes. The Hamilton Hotel was newly constructed when Dr. Blackburn came to Bermuda. Having 26 guest rooms, it was a modern facility and the most lavish of the rooming houses on the Bermudian islands. Here Dr. Blackburn both stayed and treated some of his patients who had yellow fever (*Royal Gazette*, Hamilton, Bermuda; August 20, 1861). *Right:* Figure 10B. Catharine Slater's Boarding House was a more modest establishment slightly closer to the water's edge in Hamilton. Here Dr. Blackburn also treated patients who had yellow fever (the correct spelling of Ms. Slater's name was likely "Catherine") (*Royal Gazette*, Hamilton, Bermuda; March 29, 1864).

After all, they were experienced with yellow fever in their own right, and a certain pride may have pitted them against an outsider, especially one who charged nothing for his services, while the local doctors needed to charge a fee to stay in business. Blackburn initially met with some of these local physicians at the Hamilton Hotel. There he talked of his experience treating yellow fever in the South and proposed to help fight this epidemic in Bermuda. Though some were skeptical, others welcomed his help and expertise.

Blackburn began to see patients at both the Hamilton Hotel and at Catharine Slater's Boarding House just a few blocks away (Figures 10A, 10B,

10C, 10D and 10E).[22] This arrangement was highly irregular, but he had no Bermudian medical office, and apparently the local hospital wasn't available for his use.

The Hamilton Hotel was new (opened in 1861) and had taken almost a decade to construct. The cornerstone had been set on August 19, 1852. Public

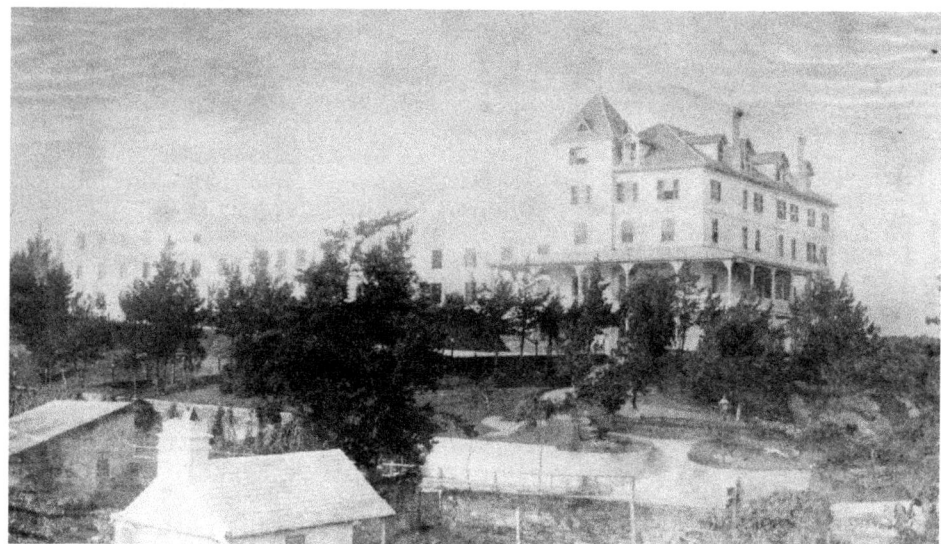

Above: Figure 10C. Hamilton Hotel, circa 1860. The front of the hotel was a grand and imposing structure, while the rear of the hotel—rather indistinct in this photograph—was lower, three stories high with about twenty columns of windows (Bermuda Archives, Photographic Collection, "Hamilton Hotel from Burnaby Street," Bermuda Historical Society, N.E. Lusher Album, Box 2, number 9, BHS/02/001/009). *Opposite top:* Figure 10D. Front Street, Hamilton, Bermuda, circa 1860. In this photograph, there are seven major buildings facing the waterfront. Slater's Boarding House was the third from the left, the darker structure in the photograph, next to the first narrow building. This view corresponds to today's buildings between Burnaby Street (on the left) and Parliament Street (outside the right border of the photograph). The Victoria Hotel later occupied the space of the third building from the left, and the Emporium subsequently replaced it (Bermuda Archives, Photographic Collection, "Front Street and Burnaby Hill from Hamilton Harbour," Bermuda Historical Society, N.E. Lusher Album, Box 2, number 3, BHS/02/001/003). *Opposite bottom:* Figure 10E. Front Street, Hamilton Bermuda, circa 1860. The first building on the left housed W.T. James' Groceries and was then 41–42 Front Street (before a later renumbering of the lots). Also located in this building on the second floor was the N.E. Lusher Photographic Gallery. The second building's occupants are currently unknown. The third building (the one with a single person standing in the portico, or veranda) was Slater's Boarding House (old 47 Front Street; now 69 Front Street), where Dr. Blackburn treated some of his patients with yellow fever (Bermuda Archives, Photographic Collection, untitled sepia print, Bermuda Historical Society, N. E. Lusher Album, number 2/12, DAP/01/23/002).

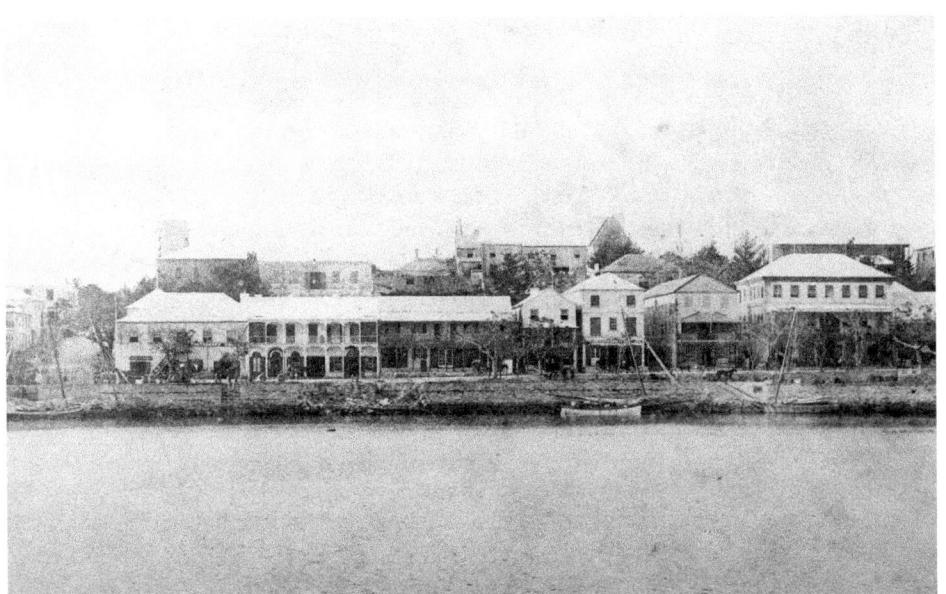

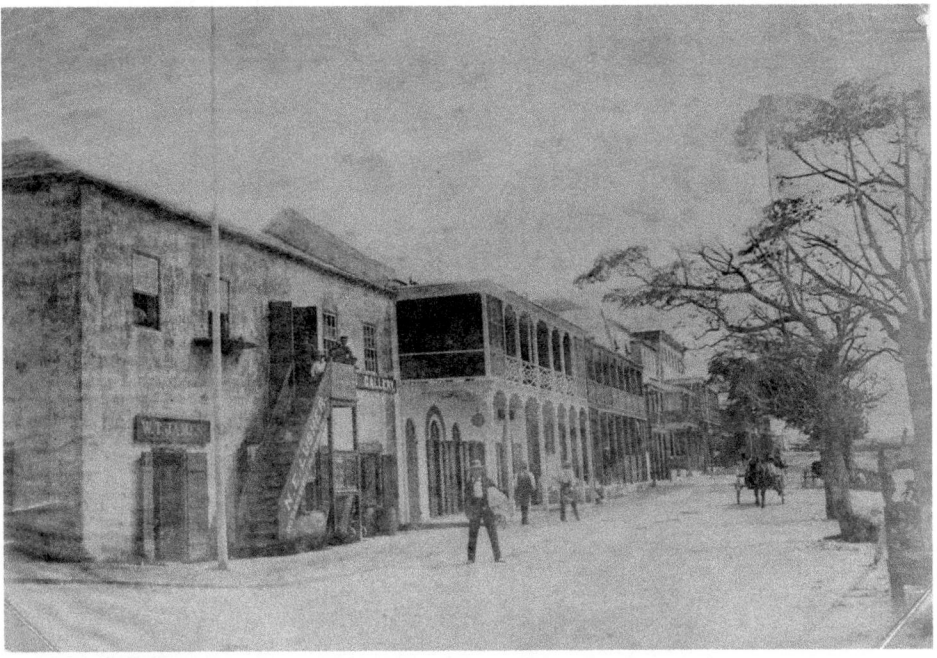

money had been promised for the construction of the hotel to provide "better accommodation of Strangers visiting these islands."[23] The hotel was originally slated to have 36 rooms, and off-duty British Army soldiers were paid to help dig the foundation. Newspaper ads had requested bids for the supply of the 41,000 stones needed to construct the foundation. When completed nearly nine years later, it had only 26 rooms, not the 36 planned, though it would continue to grow over the next 100 years, until a fire largely destroyed it on December 23, 1955. It boasted a building 150 feet by 36 feet, with a wing in the rear measuring 36 by 24 feet. There were two large drawing rooms, 26 by 18 feet each, and two large sitting rooms, one large dining room 34 by 22 feet, and a smaller one at 22 by 14 feet. It had a reading room, a bar room, 26 bedrooms with bathrooms and water closets, "windows protected by blinds," and even touted its large water tank, "of sufficient size for Hotel purposes." Each bedroom had a bedstead, a table, a washstand with a marble top, a dresser bureau, a "towel horse," two chairs and a rocking chair. It was quite the modern establishment. The front balcony spanned 64 feet, with a "delightful promenade."[24] To this grand structure completed nine years later, Blackburn came to try to bolster the fate of the South.

Other rooming houses and small hotels existed in the town of Hamilton. The Bermuda Hotel, also called the Hamilton Hotel until the larger and more elaborate one was built, and Oldfield's Royal Hotel Hamilton, also occasionally referred to as the Hamilton Hotel, were just two of them. Mrs. Catharine Slater's establishment was a much more modest boardinghouse on Front

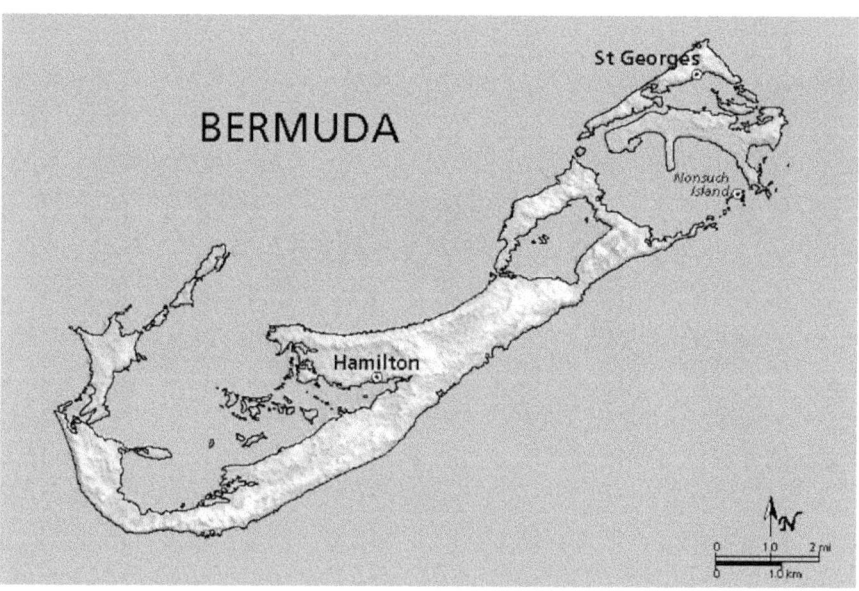

Figure 11A. Major Bermudian cities and ports. Hamilton and St. Georges were the two major port cities in this small island nation. St. Georges was the seat of blockade-running for the Confederacy. Nonsuch Island became a quarantine station for sailors ill with communicable diseases and for contaminated items likely to cause sickness (Kulshan Cartographics, Bellingham, Washington).

Street closer to the water and a few hundred yards from the new Hamilton Hotel (Figures 11A, 11B and 11C). As her competitor the new Hamilton Hotel opened, she quaintly advertised in British style that her house had "some Additional Comforts," and that she "begs respectfully to inform the Public generally that she is now prepared to take a few BOARDERS or LODGERS on Moderate terms. She hopes by strict attention she will still continue to receive a share of the Public Patronage which has hitherto been so liberally bestowed on her."[25]

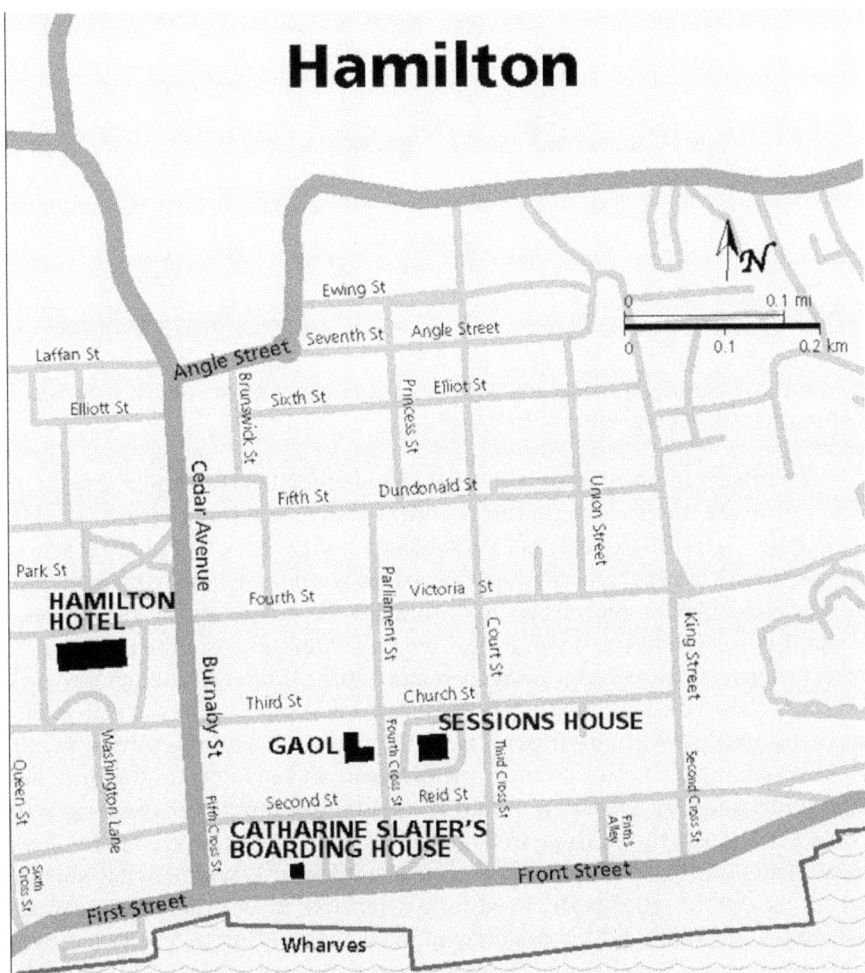

Figure 11B. The Hamilton Hotel and Catharine Slater's Boarding House, where Dr. Blackburn treated patients with yellow fever, were located in Hamilton (Kulshan Cartographics, Bellingham, Washington).

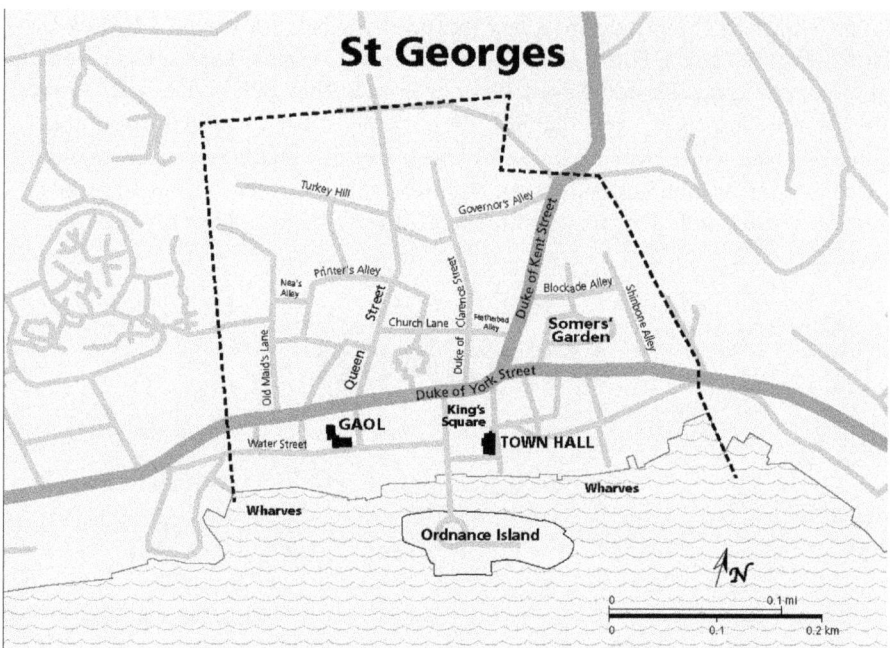

Figure 11C. Confederate blockade-running was centered in St. Georges (Kulshan Cartographics, Bellingham, Washington).

The Bermudian government quickly and wholeheartedly welcomed Dr. Blackburn; the medical community continued to accept him more slowly. He treated the Bermudian patients with skill and compassion, and in the absence of ulterior motives such unpaid service would seem far beyond reproach. But he had those hidden reasons for his courage and generosity, his goal to decimate the North and wrest victory for the Confederates from the tentacles of defeat that seemed to be looming over the South. While Blackburn devoted himself to the compassionate care of yellow fever victims, he also tirelessly and assiduously collected garments from his victims, the more soiled by vomit and excrement the better. Items from the dead and dying were the best. He attempted to create a weapon of mass destruction even before the term was coined, gathering the clothing in large trunks soon to be delivered to his enemies in the North. Finally the epidemic abated, and Blackburn was able to breathe a sigh of relief as the need for his services in Bermuda diminished. No longer did he spend the majority of his day attending to febrile patients who were trying relentlessly to die. As he saw the needs diminish, he made plans to leave Bermuda and to send his warfare trunks to the North.

It's unclear if Blackburn had required any approval from Confederate headquarters to attempt his nefarious deed. Perhaps Secretary of War John

9. The First Shipment of Articles Contaminated   103

A. Seddon or Secretary of State Judah P. Benjamin was aware of Blackburn's plan. Kensey Johns Stewart, the Episcopal minister, later wrote to Jefferson Davis, on December 12, 1864, informing him of the plot.[26] Hyams' promised exorbitant payment of $100,000 (or even more) for his role in the plot was likely to be paid in gold since it was such a large transaction. This suggested that Davis might have been aware of the entire plan earlier, since such payment in gold required his approval.[27] Such allocations were usually disbursed as "Necessities and Exigencies," with notations of Davis's knowledge and permission.[28]

Blackburn remained in Bermuda until March 9, 1864.[29] By then, he had loaded five trunks with contaminated clothing and bedding, and he had an additional three trunks containing his personal items. These eight trunks would eventually find their way to Halifax for their rendezvous with Godfrey Hyams. Blackburn himself journeyed first to St. Thomas, carried by the steamer *Alpha*. The same *Alpha* would take Professor James P. Holcombe from Bermuda to Halifax on March 29, 1864, and also would transport Jacob Thompson, Clement C. Clay, and William W. Cleary from Bermuda to Halifax, arriving on May 19, 1864. It would appear that none of their Bermuda stays overlapped.

The story of Blackburn's travels and how the trunks made their way from Bermuda to Halifax becomes a deep mystery. Blackburn left for St. Thomas in the Virgin Islands on March 9, and the next direct and personal word of his travels came in the form of a letter to Hyams allegedly sent from Havana, Cuba, dated May 10. The letter was sent through the Rev. Stuart Robinson, Hyams' contact person, who was residing in Toronto at the time. Blackburn instructed Hyams to go to Halifax, and Hyams had to ask Robinson for money for his travel expenses.

Blackburn would not arrive in Halifax aboard the *Alpha* until about July 12. The trunks that had originated in Bermuda came to Halifax at about the same time, in mid–July, and Blackburn allegedly had also shipped them to Halifax on the steamer *Alpha*. They could have even come on the same ship taken by Blackburn himself from Bermuda, since a round-trip of the *Alpha* from Halifax-Bermuda-St. Thomas-Bermuda-Halifax occurred only every two weeks. However, Hyams' version of the story had the trunks and Blackburn arriving on different days. Many logistic explanations could satisfy this shipping sequence for the trunks:

- Blackburn could have stored the trunks with someone in Bermuda who upon letter from Blackburn put them on the ship *Alpha*.
- Blackburn himself might have returned to Bermuda between March and July and could have taken the trunks out of storage somewhere in Bermuda and shipped them on the *Alpha* to Halifax.

He could have travelled either ahead of, or behind, them to Halifax since he and the trunks arrived on different days, according to Hyams. However, the interval between Blackburn's arrival and the trunks' arrival would seem to be less than the two weeks required by the *Alpha*'s itinerary.

- Blackburn could have taken the trunks to St. Thomas and Havana and then transported them himself to Halifax, presumably from Cuba. However, that scenario doesn't mesh with Blackburn's statement that the trunks arrived in Halifax on the *Alpha*, as the *Alpha* didn't travel to Cuba.
- The final, and most likely, possibility is that Blackburn kept the trunks with him for a few weeks, traveling to St. Thomas then to Cuba and subsequently back to St. Thomas. Then he finally shipped them to Halifax from St. Thomas on the *Alpha*, maybe even on the same run of the *Alpha* he himself took to Halifax or on a run before or after his own trip.

It seems from all the testimony that Hyams did indeed retrieve the trunks from the *Alpha*. However, the *Alpha*'s manifest outbound from Bermuda to Halifax on the trip in early July listed no trunks as cargo. That's not unusual, however, as the cargo reported for ships of that era had very few entries (Figure 12). It was common to have the entire contents of a ship listed by a single word: "Ballast." Rarely did a captain record, or the Bermudian customs office require, any detail beyond a few lines of description. The contents of the *Alpha* recorded by Captain David Hunter for the Bermuda-Halifax run in question out of Bermuda on July 8, 1864, included only "arrowroot" ("1 half Bbl" and "1 Box" with a value of "£612" and weighing "110#"), "Tobaco [sic]" ("2 Boxes," weight and value unrecorded) and "52 Empty Cask [sic]" (value "£20.0.0," weight unrecorded). No trunks or other cargo was listed.[30]

Adding further to the mystery is the more basic question of why Blackburn went to both the Virgin Islands and Cuba. Speculation has always been that he was raising funds or procuring more supplies for the Confederacy. But his activities and travel schedule have never been documented in detail. Nassau and Havana were other ports to which Southerners freely shipped goods for the Confederate cause, and it is reasonable to assume that Blackburn could have transported the trunks effortlessly through any of these ports. However, testimony had the trunks arriving in Halifax onboard the *Alpha*, which plied only the Halifax-Bermuda-St. Thomas route, and no record can be found to support a claim that the trunks were stored in Bermuda from March to July.

An intriguing article in the *Bermuda Royal Gazette* on July 26, 1865, suggested that Blackburn might have actually taken the trunks with him as

9. The First Shipment of Articles Contaminated

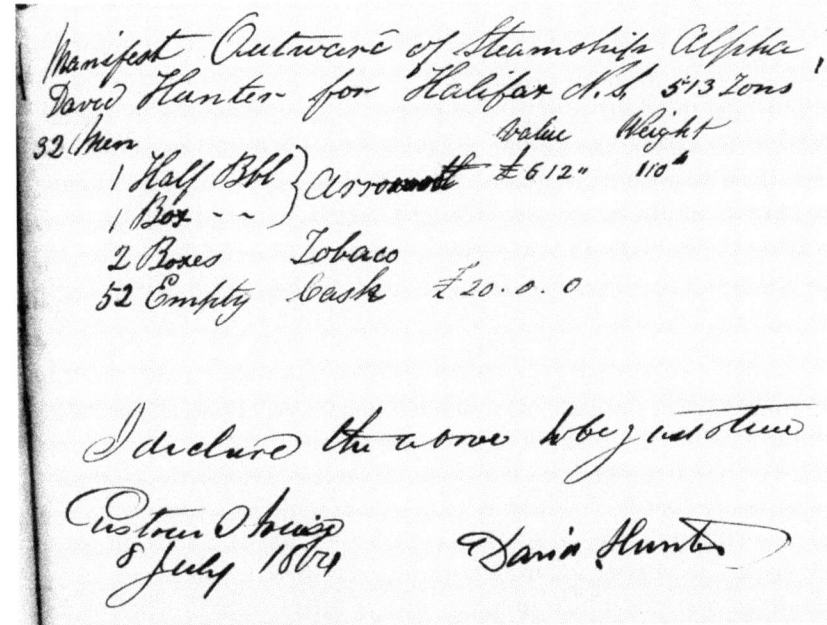

Figure 12. Original page from Bermuda Customs Office documenting the cargo on the vessel *Alpha* on its voyage from St. Georges to Halifax, July 8, 1864 (Outwards Shipping Manifests, 21 July 1863–26 July 1864, Customs Records, unpaginated. Bermuda Archives, Hamilton, Bermuda).

he traveled to St. Thomas and then went on to Cuba in May 1864. The Havana reporter for the *New York World* wrote that "the goods, *in trunks* [emphasis in the original], were brought [to Cuba] from Bermuda; taken from the vessel to the hospital of Dr. [Charles or Edward] Belot by Mr. Hopkins, and placed in the laundry or linen rooms; from thence they were taken by Mr. Hopkins in his boat to some other vessel bound to Nassau, or somewhere else, very clear and satisfactory."[31] Documents attesting to these facts were sent to the office of the Honorable William T. Minor, the consul-general of the United States in Havana. Dr. Charles M. Belot was a physician in Havana who also specialized in yellow fever. Some 20 years earlier the Belot family had established a hospital in Havana (the Regla District) for victims of yellow fever.

Further supporting the notion that Blackburn might have taken the trunks with him as he left Bermuda in March 1864 is information that surfaced only in 1879, not surprisingly around the time of the vote for the governorship of Kentucky, for which Blackburn was the Democratic candidate. The *Cincinnati Gazette* was doing an extensive investigation, trying to determine if the Dr. Blackburn of the yellow fever plot of 1864–1865 was the same man as the Dr. Blackburn of the governor's race. Their conclusion was that this was the same man. Newspapers carried the newly rediscovered testimony of the vice-consul general of Havana, Cuba, Thomas Savage (William T. Minor was the consul general), as well as the sworn statements of those in charge of the hospital in Cuba where Blackburn had reportedly stored the trunks.[32] These men had written the documents in 1865. Despite the rather curious and suspicious timing of the "rediscovery" of this evidence at the precise moment Blackburn was waging a heated political battle for the governorship of Kentucky, the facts and details of the revelation exactly corroborated the stories circulating in 1864–1865, even down to the number of trunks and their contents. The reports, sent via four letters and sworn affidavits from Vice-Consul General Savage to William H. Seward, the secretary of state, C.A. Seward, the acting assistant secretary of state, and H.N. Conger, the acting secretary of state, documented Blackburn's presence in Cuba and both his plot and the logistics of his scheme.[33]

Two French brothers, both of them physicians, Dr. Charles (Carlos) and Dr. Edward (Eduardo) Belot, were in charge of that Cuban yellow fever hospital, the Hospital San Carlos (also called the Casa de Salud), in Regla in 1864. Carlos Belot had established this hospital in 1821 (some sources report 1823). Regla was one of the municipalities of the province of Havana, occupying the eastern side of the Port of Havana and across the water from "Habana Vieja," Old Havana. The Belots gave sworn testimony in 1865 regarding trunks Dr. Blackburn had carried to Cuba. Other witnesses included John D. Hopkins, an American working at the Hospital San Carlos, and Mr. John B. Belt, a highly educated and reportedly reliable witness who lived in Cuba. They all told a consistent story, one that also incriminated an Englishman (though he may also have been a naturalized American citizen) in Cuba, William K. Johnson, a watchmaker who had become a destitute bartender and sometimes drunkard. Reportedly Dr. Blackburn had solicited help in his yellow fever plot from Johnson, much as Hyams had been recruited in Canada. Blackburn may have brought the trunks with the contaminated clothing to Cuba with him and needed both a place to store the goods as well as a source to augment the number of items infected with yellow fever. He employed Johnson to hide the trunks in a linen room of Hospital San Carlos. However, both Drs. Charles and Edward Belot denied complicity in the plot.

Dr. Charles Belot testified that Blackburn had approached him with a scheme to do some "research" on yellow fever, since both Blackburn and the Belots were recognized experts in the disease. Blackburn told Belot of his theory that clothing and articles soiled by the excreta and effluvia of patients dying from yellow fever could themselves transmit yellow fever. Blackburn wanted to gather more soiled articles from the Hospital San Carlos, where patients with yellow fever were housed. He proposed either collecting new items or putting the items already in the trunks into the beds of yellow fever

9. The First Shipment of Articles Contaminated

patients in Hospital San Carlos to augment the degree of contamination. Blackburn proposed then to take the soiled garments to Halifax, where he would arrange to experiment upon an as yet unidentified prisoner convicted to die by execution. Since the convict would be under a death warrant anyway, Blackburn thought it to be ethical to expose him to the contaminated garments to see if they would transmit yellow fever. If the convict came down with the disease, Blackburn's theory would be correct, and both Blackburn and the Belots would gain additional fame from the discovery. Of course, then Blackburn would have added information that would entice him to send yet more contaminated articles to cities of the North. Dr. Carlos Belot refused this plan on ethical grounds.

Blackburn then plotted with William Johnson, and perhaps with John D. Hopkins, at least to store the trunks from Bermuda in the Cuban hospital, where they were placed in the linen room. Later, as sworn by Dr. Edward Belot, John D. Hopkins, the hospital employee, opened one trunk and removed clothing that had originated in Bermuda and had already been soiled by patients suffering from yellow fever. These articles were placed near some patients with mild cases of fever, though it wasn't certain yet that these Cuban patients even had yellow fever. Hopkins then moved the garments to the room of a patient who had died that night of yellow fever (specifically identified as patient "No. 16 of the second ward"), and he subsequently returned the soiled garments to the previously opened trunk. How Hopkins protected himself from catching the disease is not recorded. Hopkins' sworn testimony denied his own role in gathering further contamination, although he admitted to knowing about Blackburn's plot to infect a convict in Halifax.[34] Hopkins wrote, "Dr. Blackburn ... was writing a book on yellow-fever, and he wished to convince the world that he could cause yellow-fever at high latitude; that he intended to take the clothing to Halifax, and there wait until some criminal was sentenced to death, and then request the Governor to allow him to try the experiment upon the criminal.... He further stated that he owed it to mankind to lay his knowledge before the world." The testimony of John B. Belt corroborated other witnesses. Hopkins, of course, denied participating in gathering any additional contaminated clothing. Dr. Edward Belot, however, implicated Hopkins in the exposure of that patient in Hospital San Carlos to soiled clothing from one of Blackburn's trunks.

William Johnson assisted Blackburn in placing the trunks for storage in Hospital San Carlos and in taking them to the wharf for shipment to St. Thomas, likely where Blackburn himself went to accompany or to meet up with the contaminated goods. It's also probable that Blackburn then shipped the trunks to Halifax from St. Thomas, which would indeed have been on the steamship *Alpha*, the transport required if the rest of the story told by Hyams was true. By separating his trip from the transport of the contaminated items, Dr. Blackburn wouldn't be connected with the trunks if they were intercepted by any agents of law enforcement.

Cuba's vice-consul general, Thomas Savage, also claimed that Cuban consul William Minor discovered the plot surrounding these events and took some documents as evidence to Washington, D.C. However, the evidence was never presented at the trial of the Lincoln assassination conspirators. Nevertheless, in spite of the apparent political motivation for all of this information to resurface in 1879 during Blackburn's campaign for governor, the data seem accurate and valid, consistent with all of the other evidence. Blackburn had taken the trunks with him to Cuba, and they were now about to arrive in Halifax (Figure 13).

• • •

Hyams worked his usual shoe repair job in Toronto until June 8, 1864. On that day he received the letter from Blackburn through the Rev. Dr. Stuart Robinson. The letter was postmarked from Havana on May 10. Hyams claimed Robinson had opened the letter, so Robinson would actually have learned what the letter revealed about the plot. Robinson would later vehemently deny that accusation and would continue efforts for over a decade to try to clear his name, presenting Hyams as a liar and describing him as that "Jew-Christian-Athiest perjurer."[35] Robinson knew that Hyams was often associated with other unreliable and disreputable Lincoln assassination witnesses, such as Charles A. Dunham (aka Sanford Conover and James Watson Wallace) and Dr. James B. Merritt.

The letter from Blackburn told Hyams to obtain money from Dr. Robinson in Toronto to travel to Montreal, where he was to obtain more money from a Mr. Slaughter (perhaps the same Mr. H.C. Slaughter who had earlier been involved in the introduction of Hyams and Blackburn). Dr. Robinson refused to fund Hyams' trip on the grounds that the activity Hyams was about to undertake was immoral (and thereby confirming Robinson actually knew of the yellow fever plot). Robinson told Hyams that he "did not want to know anything about this and I did not want Dr. B. to write to me about it. I do not want to do any overt act."[36] Thereafter, Hyams went to a Mr. S.S. Preston, a tobacco manufacturer, who loaned him $10 but only on the promise that Mr. Slaughter would reimburse it and only at the insistence of another agent, Mr. William Lawrence McDonald. Hyams proceeded to Montreal, where Mr. Slaughter gave him $25 for the trip to Halifax. The additional $25 was not enough, so Hyams asked Professor James P. Holcombe for an additional $15,[37] making the total $50 (including the "loan")—a far cry from any grand sum that should have been available if Blackburn's promise had been legitimate to fund Hyams with at least $100,000 from the Confederate bank account. (Holcombe would later claim that the money wasn't a loan but that he had

9. The First Shipment of Articles Contaminated   109

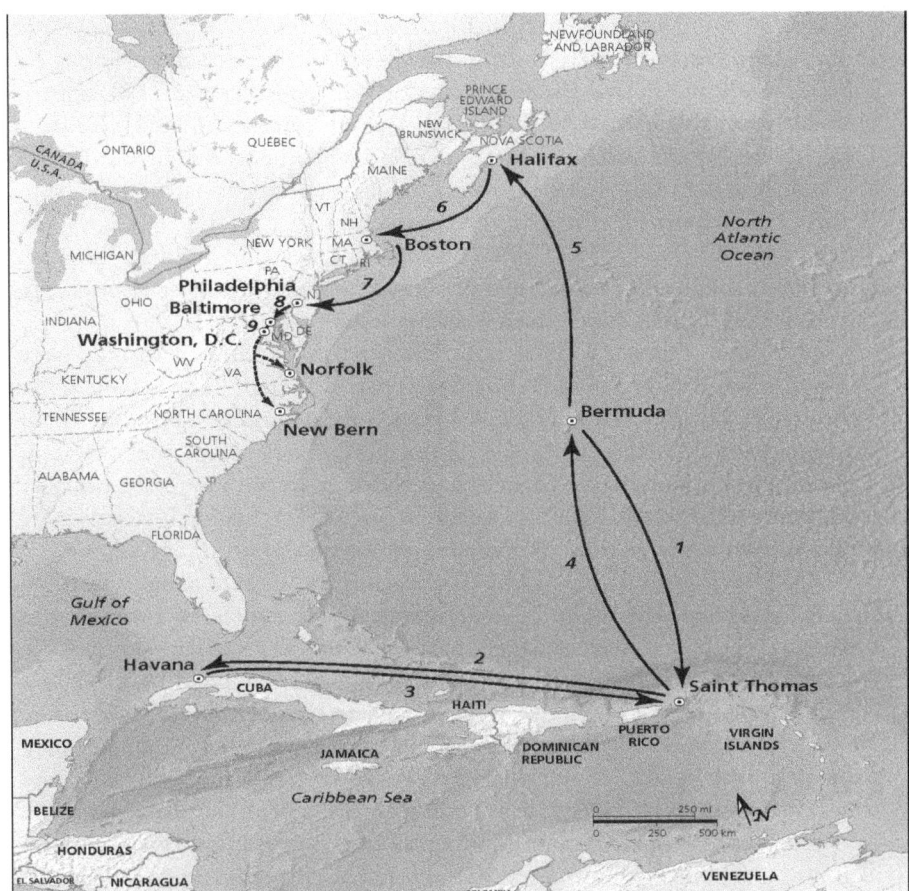

Figure 13. Route of the first shipment of trunks containing goods contaminated with yellow fever. Dr. Blackburn departed from Bermuda to St. Thomas, probably with the trunks, thereafter traveling to Cuba. He apparently tried unsuccessfully in Havana to augment the number of soiled items before returning to St. Thomas. Likely he shipped the trunks back to Bermuda then sent them on to Halifax. Hyams met the trunks in Halifax and had them transported successively to Boston, Philadelphia, Baltimore, and Washington, D.C. In Washington he sold some of the items through an auctioneer, and the rest he shipped toward Norfolk, Virginia, and New Bern, North Carolina. The fate of the trunks headed to Norfolk and New Bern has never been discovered (Kulshan Cartographics, Bellingham, Washington).

been "swindled" out of the money by Hyams. Slaughter said Hyams claimed to be a Confederate soldier escaped from a prisoner of war camp and in need of money to return to the South through Halifax.)

Hyams went to the Halifax Hotel on Hollis Street as directed, where he arrived on June 22, 1864. This hotel was described as "the one decent hotel that Halifax could boast of."[38] Hyams' testimony about this trip was somewhat inconsistent. During one cross-examination, he said he arrived in Halifax on June 18, not June 22. That would have made it three weeks before Blackburn would arrive. Hyams had been directed to look for Alexander H. Keith, a local brewer. Hyams and Keith met at the Halifax Hotel, and Keith confirmed the plans but said they needed to wait for more detailed instructions from Blackburn. Suspecting detectives were watching him at the Halifax Hotel, Hyams moved to the Farmers' Hotel on Argyle Street. Keith told Mr. Michael Doran, the hotelkeeper at the Farmers' Hotel, that he would pay Hyams' bill, knowing that Hyams' funds were woefully inadequate.

Indeed, Hyams was still destitute. His wife and children in Toronto were starving, even though Hyams' shoemaker partner Hugh Shields helped the family, and the Rev. Dr. Stuart Robinson occasionally supported them through hard financial times. On January 15, 1864, Hyams had written, according to Dr. Robinson, "My wife and children are with me—she near her confinement [labor and delivery]—without [a] cent to help her—in my state of destitution I rely on your [Robinson's] benevolence."[39]

Blackburn himself arrived in Halifax on July 12 (Hyams later testified that the date was July 4), informed Hyams that the infected clothing was coming on the screw steamer *Alpha* (again, Hyams repeatedly referred to the ship incorrectly as the *Alphia*), and that there would be eight trunks and a valise. This statement implied that Blackburn arrived before the trunks. The valise was intended for President Lincoln personally and contained fancy shirts, supposedly also contaminated with yellow fever. At about this same time, Hyams received a letter from Dr. Robinson that was hardly reassuring. Robinson reported that Hyams' family was starving and that Hyams should abandon Blackburn's plan and return to his family. Blackburn assured Hyams that the "damned fine Southern men" in Toronto would take care of his wife and children.[40] Hyams was fully aware of the degree of poverty in which his family was living, his wife having pawned her dresses and household goods for money to survive.

The second officer of the Steamship *Alpha*, one Mr. Hill, helped Hyams retrieve the trunks from storage on the boat. Hyams and Hill went to the boat with an "express wagon" driven by John Doran, the son of the owner of the Farmer's Hotel on Argyle Street (Doran was likewise unaware of the contents of the trunks or their purpose).[41] They located the eight hidden trunks and valise on the steamer and transported the luggage to the Farmers' Hotel, where the trunks remained unopened in a private first-floor room to the right of Mr. Doran's private sitting room. Three of the eight trunks were Blackburn's personal property and were not infected, leaving five contaminated trunks (two large-sized and three medium-sized) and the valise intended for President Lincoln. The five infected trunks were tied with ropes as markers of their contents; the three uninfected trunks had no ropes tied around them. Hyams took the three uninfected trunks and the "very nice valise with some very elegant shirts and other things infected with fever or small pox"[42] to Blackburn at the Halifax Hotel, Hyams telling Blackburn that he couldn't be part of a scheme to kill the president. The valise contained the fine new linen shirts (in the president's size) and a letter addressed to the president, supposedly explaining the gift as a goodwill gesture from a secret admirer. The shirts were placed on the top, and a blanket soiled by a yellow fever victim in Bermuda lay under the shirts. Blackburn believed that not only the president but also many people nearby would contract the disease if the valise were opened in the White House. Though Hyams seemed to have had no qualms about importing pestilence to the North and potentially killing thousands of innocent civilians, including noncombatants, women, and children, he balked at the thought of delivering anything directly to President Lincoln that might be contaminated with disease. His scruples were warped, but he still couldn't bring himself to attempt to murder the president. Hyams later would claim that he was unaware of what ultimately happened to the valise (and there is no record of its ever having arrived at the White House). Blackburn gave Hyams another $120 in gold (six $20 gold coins); Hyams' total payment thus far was $170, counting the $10 given to him as a "loan" by Preston. By now, Hyams should have begun to suspect that the riches he had been promised might not be coming his way.[43]

Hyams then needed to find a ship's captain willing to smuggle the trunks into Boston under the ruse that they contained gifts for Hyams' family and friends. The first captain Hyams and Hill approached, a Captain McGregor (or McGreggor or, in other reports, McGriffin), refused to consider the task. Next they asked the help of another mariner, a Newfoundland captain Hyams identified as John O'Brien of the barque *Halifax* (Figures 14A, 14B and 14C). The captain's real name was Bryan O'Brien; he agreed to the plan for a fee of $70 in gold[44] (in the trial testimony of the Lincoln conspirators, Hyams said it was a single $20 gold piece). They left the goods with O'Brien that evening, with the barque scheduled to set sail on July 18 (Hyams would later testify that the *Halifax* sailed on July 24 or 25). However, the ship's departure was delayed five days in Halifax because the weather was bad. It finally arrived in Boston on about August 3. The customs agent missed seeing the trunks because they allegedly were hidden behind some sliding doors where O'Brien was accustomed to putting items that he routinely smuggled. He was experienced in this trade, but he didn't know that the trunks contained contaminated clothing. Hyams kept his story consistent and told O'Brien that the trunks held presents—silks, satin dresses, etc.—to give to his friends and family.

Hyams himself, relieved that he had been successful in finding a vessel

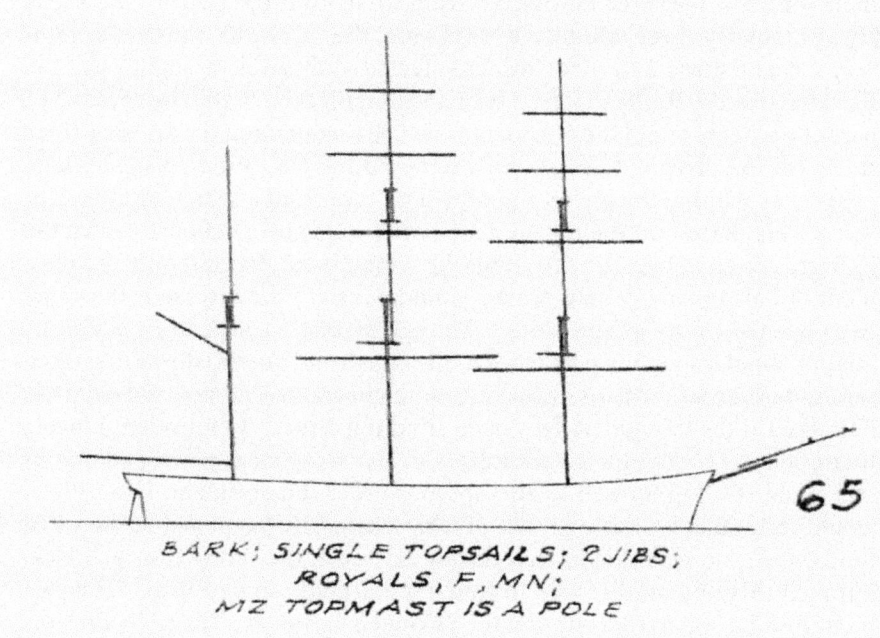

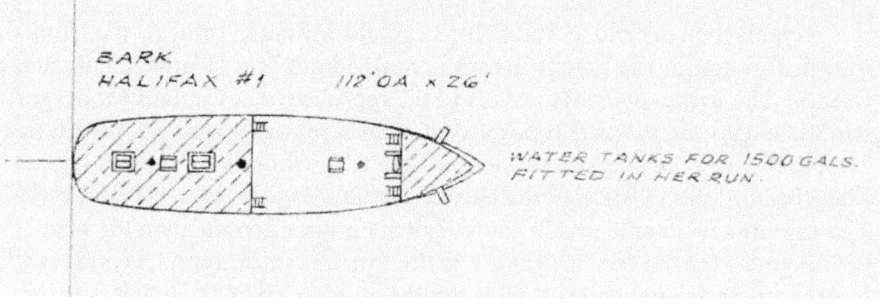

Figures 14A (*top*) and 14B (*bottom*). The Barque *Halifax* was a three-masted ship that sailed from Halifax to Boston. No photographs of it exist from the Civil War era, although the design is depicted in this figure. The *Halifax* was 112 feet long and 26 feet wide and had a depth of 12 feet. Weighing 300 tons, it was built in 1855 by C.W. Connors in Cornwallis, Nova Scotia. The first owner was Clark and Jones in Halifax, Nova Scotia. The interior of the barque *Halifax* was said to contain some secret panels behind which Captain Bryan O'Brien would hide smuggled goods from customs agents. Captain Bryan O'Brien was also commanding the ship *Halifax* close to Green Island, near Cape Sable, Nova Scotia, on February 17, 1866, when it ran aground and could not be recovered (*The Masting of the American Merchant Sail in the 1850s: An Illustrated Study,* by William L. Crothers [McFarland, 2014], p. 121; *American-Built Packets and Freighters of the 1850s: An Illustrated Study of Their Characteristics and Construction,* by William L. Crothers [McFarland, 2013], p 306).

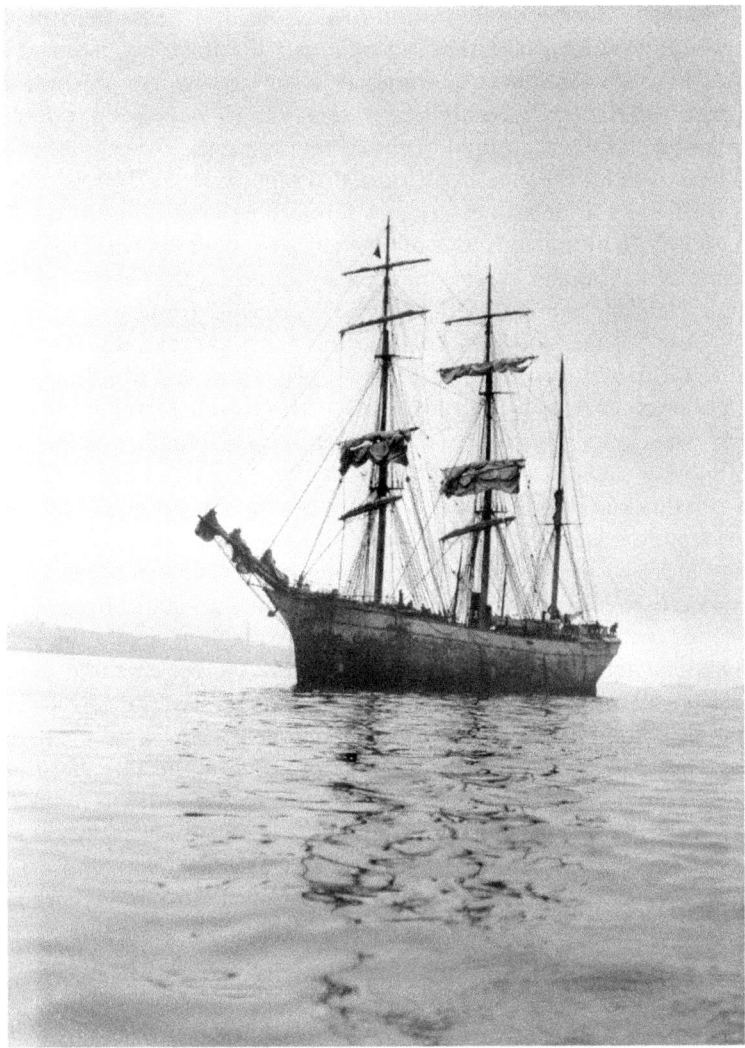

Figure 14C. "Unidentified barque at anchor, Halifax Harbour." While no confirmed photograph of the barque *Halifax* exists today, the ship pictured has characteristics very similar to it (Nova Scotia Archives, Nova Scotia Archives accession no. 1987-453 176; photographer, W.R. MacAskill).

to transport the trunks, traveled to Boston on July 24 or July 25 on a different ship and checked into the Parker House, using his alias J.W. Harris (he would later testify in another trial that it was the Astor House,[45] yet one more rather minor discrepancy in his stories).

Perhaps not just coincidentally, Hyams may have met up with John

Wilkes Booth in Boston on or around July 26, for Booth was then staying at the Parker House. Cordial Crane, an official at the Boston Customs House, wrote on May 30, 1865, that he found it "a remarkable circumstance" that Booth and "J.W. Harris" (the alias for Hyams) might have been in Boston at the same time. Crane examined the hotel register at the Parker House to see if both had stayed there together. Crane also reported that "Harris" allegedly landed his trunks in Boston on August 3. Booth was registered at the Parker House on July 26 along with four other men, one of whom was H.V. Clinton from Hamilton, Canada West, a name also found on the register of the St. Lawrence Hall in Montreal. Others were Charles R. Hunter from Toronto, Canada West, A.J. Bursted (or Rursted) from Baltimore, and R.A. Leech from Montreal.[46] (Also, not coincidentally, both Blackburn and Booth would register a few lines apart at St. Lawrence Hall in Montreal in October 1864. These Confederate agents' paths crossed frequently, whether they were actively scheming with each other or not.) Neither Hyams' name nor his alias "J.W. Harris" was on the Parker House Register that day or other days in July or August, though it is known that he was in Boston at the time.[47] Hyams' identification of his residence as the Astor Hotel may have been correct.

Hyams then took the trunks to an express office on State Street in Boston and shipped them to Philadelphia, where they were to be held until he called for them. The actual chain of possession of the trunks en route remained unclear from all of Hyams' testimonies. In the Lincoln trial transcripts, Hyams said that Captain O'Brien "finally succeeded in getting them off the bark [sic] for me, and expressed them to Philadelphia."[48] In the late 1860s many observers were prone to disbelieve Hyams' stories. He testified many times, and newspapers reported his tales frequently. His inability to be consistent with dates and exact locations where he alleged events happened made his testimony subject to skepticism. Supporters of Blackburn used these inconsistencies in his reports as reason to impugn and disbelieve his entire account.

Hyams was seeking to arrange transportation for the trunks ultimately to Washington and Norfolk. These cities were chosen because an epidemic in large population concentrations would devastate the Northern war effort. Hyams noted that one of the trunks labeled with a large "2" was the one specifically destined to go to Washington (he and Blackburn would refer to it as "Big #2"). There the clothes would be put up for auction for the widest distribution possible.[49] Hyams travelled from Boston to New York on the ship *Commonwealth*. When in New York he lodged at another Astor House. Then he went to Philadelphia by railroad and thereafter to Baltimore. In Philadelphia he met the trunks. First, he had the items taken to the American Hotel, where he was staying (testimony in Toronto was vague about whether he personally took the trunks to Baltimore or had them shipped there). In Baltimore he stayed at the Fountain Hotel (alternately called the Fountain Inn or the

9. The First Shipment of Articles Contaminated   115

Fountain House), and he also had the trunks delivered there. In Baltimore, Hyams bought five other new trunks for $12 and repacked the goods in the five new trunks and three of the old ones, apparently to make them appear more salable and to aid the distribution of the contaminated items. So, after the repacking, there were eight trunks. No doubt Hyams chewed camphor and smoked strong cigars while handling the garments as recommended by Blackburn to avoid catching yellow fever himself.[50]

Solomon Hyams, Godfrey Hyams' cousin, who lived in Baltimore and worked as a tobacconist at 68 North Howard Street, tried to dissuade Godfrey from continuing his mission, but Hyams wouldn't relent. (In one testimony Hyams reported his cousin Solomon to be a lawyer; in another, he said the cousin was a cigar and tobacco manufacturer. Maybe he was both, although he more likely sold tobacco goods than manufactured them.) Perhaps the promise of fortune from Dr. Blackburn's scheme was simply too great for Godfrey to give up the effort. Given his shifting allegiances, it's unlikely that any real devotion to the South drove him or kept him going. His goal was money. Furthermore, in Baltimore he again depleted his already-meager resources. He needed a new infusion of both cash and courage. He returned to Toronto on money borrowed from this cousin Solomon. From Toronto he sent a note to Blackburn, telling him that he needed more money to complete the complicated transaction. Hyams then went to the Clifton House, where he met Blackburn, Clement C. Clay, James P. Holcombe, George W. Gregor (Hyams referred to him as "McGregor"), S.S. Preston, and others. Jacob Thompson wasn't there. Blackburn gave Hyams $150 (other reports said $100) to return to Baltimore and complete his deadly task. Nevertheless, his grand total was now $320, covering only expenses and with nothing left for profit to support his family. Blackburn and Gregor again told of riches that would be coming Hyams' way, naming again his fee as $100,000 and suggesting that Hyams might receive an interest in either a tobacco business or a jewelry business as further reward for his daring work. Blackburn spoke of yet more jobs importing infected clothing that would generate a fee of $1,000,000 to the man who successfully transported these goods. The two wanted immense quantities of clothes to be distributed to the North to assure widespread dissemination of disease. Blackburn also again assured Hyams that his wife would be well treated and supplied. She had been "selling everything" the family owned to keep the children and herself fed. Dr. Blackburn said he was going to rent two houses in Montreal, and Mrs. Hyams and the family could use one and have $20,000 for living expenses until the job was completed.[51] Almost assuredly, this promise was never kept.

After Hyams returned to Baltimore from Canada he distributed the trunks. Again, the testimony here is inconsistent. In the deposition given to lawyer Halmer H. Emmons in Detroit, Hyams said that he first went to Washington, back to Baltimore, and then toward Norfolk. In the official testimony in the court in Toronto, he said he first went toward Norfolk, was turned back, returned to Baltimore, and then went to Washington. The exact details are unimportant, except that skeptics refused to believe Hyams' entire story because of these errors in his testimonies. He left "Big #2" with four other small ones in Baltimore to be taken later to Washington. He took the remaining three on the trip to Norfolk. However, General Benjamin F. Butler intercepted Hyams' transport steamer *Star*, and all persons not directly connected with the Union military had to disembark. Hyams then made arrangements with a sutler named Myers from Boston to distribute the clothing. A sutler was a private businessman who sold items such as clothing, food, tobacco, sugar, and coffee to the troops.[52] "Myers" was likely G.L. Myres, a sutler from Wellsburg, New York, for the Army of the Potomac, who would later work in Annapolis, Maryland, according to an anonymous tipster as revealed in a letter to Secretary of War Edwin M. Stanton.[53]

Hyams told the sutler that the trunks contained "fancy flannel shirts and fatigue coats for non-commissioned officers."[54] He went on to tally the contents: 70 shirts and 6 coats in one trunk; 150 shirts and 25 coats in the others. Myers agreed to distribute the clothing in Norfolk (one trunk) and New Bern (two trunks), both Union strongholds at the time (New Bern was repeatedly called "Newbern" in period newspapers). Myers likely was unaware of the purpose of the transaction, as Hyams instructed him to forward the profits from the sale of the articles to Hyams at the Fountain Hotel in Baltimore, as though it was an ordinary business deal.

Hyams returned to Baltimore, where he retrieved the remaining trunks. He took them to Washington, where he checked into the National Hotel. In Washington he found an "auction and commission merchant" under the direction of W.L. Wall and Company at Ninth and Pennsylvania, where he took the five trunks (two large and three small). Dates of these movements and transactions were also inconsistent. Using his alias "J.W. Harris," Hyams negotiated for the sale of the goods. Wall was out of town on that day, so Albert Bremier (or "Brenner"),[55] an employee and bookkeeper at Wall's company, advanced Hyams $100 on the expected sale of the clothing. Hyams was now up to $420 of his promised $100,000. Apparently the goods sold the next morning. Wall would later testify that he was personally unaware of the contents of the trunks or their intended purpose. Hyams subsequently wrote to Wall from Toronto on September 1, 1864, stating that he hadn't been able to return personally to Washington, D.C., since going back to Canada. Hyams asked Wall for an accounting of what had happened to the clothing—whether it had been sold, and the details of such sale. Hyams said, "I beg most respectfully that you send me an account of sales, and a check on New York for the proceeds.... I shall come over in October, about the 10th, with some five or

9. The First Shipment of Articles Contaminated   117

six thousand pairs of boots and shoes." Hyams listed "Post-Office Box No. 126" in Toronto as his address. Brenner testified that the transaction had involved 96 shirts and 9 coats packed in 5 trunks; the 96 shirts had been sold to Stiegler and Siegel for $184.40; the 9 coats to a Mr. Walker for $4.50; and the trunks themselves (10 were listed, not 5) to William Smith and a Mr. Hand for $4.00. Brenner's testimony was detailed and documented, and the bill of sales of the infected clothing was admitted into evidence in the Lincoln assassination conspiracy trial as Exhibit Number 74.[56]

At about this time in early September, Thompson advanced Hyams $50 on a meager payment of a promised $100, which would be distributed only when Hyams produced evidence of a successful mission. About ten days later, Hyams received the note forwarded from Hamilton from W.L. Wall confirming that the clothing had been sold and distributed. Thompson gave Hyams the "final" $50. Hyams' payments were now up to $520. He was not yet rich and likely was beginning to feel used.

Hyams would testify at the Lincoln conspirators' trial proceedings because prosecutors thought that the many plots in Canada had some connection to the actual assassination of the president. Indeed, Blackburn had planned to attack Lincoln by delivering him the shirt contaminated with yellow fever. At that trial, the military tribunal alleged that the yellow fever epidemic in New Bern, North Carolina, was caused by the Blackburn plot, and that it killed 2,000–3,000 people. The most damning evidence for the entire scheme would later come from the testimony of W.L. Wall. He was a respected businessman, while the other witnesses—like Hyams himself—might have had ulterior motives or something to be gained by perjured testimony (like the pardon Hyams ultimately received). Hyams was considered to be a reprobate. Wall was upstanding, but his testimony almost exactly matched Hyams' story.

Hyams returned to Hamilton, Ontario, Canada, and soon learned of an outbreak of yellow fever at New Bern, North Carolina, confirming in his own mind that he had been marvelously successful. In Hamilton, Hyams met with Clement C. Clay and Professor James Holcombe, who congratulated him on the success of his mission and again reinforced the notion that he would soon be rich and famous. They told him that $200,000 (not $100,000) had been allocated for the job. Clearly, they both knew of the plot, although the alleged future payment details were confused and contradictory. From Hamilton, Hyams sent telegrams to Blackburn at the Donegana Hotel in Montreal and to his wife in Toronto telling her that he had returned safely and would be coming home soon. He left for his home in Toronto, where Blackburn came a day or two later. Hyams reported that he had completed his mission, including delivering "Big #2" to Washington. Blackburn again said that it would kill men at 60 yards, ignoring the fact that Hyams had rearranged the clothing in new trunks and hadn't suffered any illness from doing so. Perhaps that camphor and those cigars had worked.

Hyams then asked for his reward money, and Blackburn told him to go to see Jacob Thompson, the keeper of the Canadian Confederate purse strings. Of course, when Hyams went to Thompson (who allegedly knew all about the purpose of the importation of the clothing), the money wasn't forthcoming. All the time, Hyams' wife and children were still starving. Thompson and Holcombe supposedly told Hyams again that his reward would be $200,000, sometime in the future. Likely at this point Hyams didn't know if he should believe them. If he hadn't become impatient and skeptical, he soon would. He would see Blackburn later in Montreal, and there he again asked Blackburn for his largesse. Blackburn laughed at Hyams, telling him to be patient, that after a while he would be rich, be able to travel to Europe, and be introduced to influential people who would change his life. Blackburn then told of yet greater schemes to introduce yellow fever and smallpox into the North. Blackburn was ready to embark on another trip to Bermuda to collect more yellow fever articles, and—if he were fortunate—some with smallpox.

10

The Second Shipment of Articles Contaminated with Yellow Fever

Yellow fever epidemics in Bermuda and elsewhere continued to be quite common. Yet another one arrived in Bermuda on June 30, 1864, by way of two sailors aboard the blockade-runner *Fannie* from Nassau. It developed into a major epidemic that lasted until January 1865. It was this epidemic that prompted Dr. Luke Blackburn to make his second "mercy mission" to Bermuda.

Blackburn's recruitment of Hyams was not the only attempt to engage another person to assist in the transportation of contaminated goods to the North. He had received similar help in Cuba in March 1864 from William K. Johnson. In June 1864 Blackburn also tried to convince John Cameron, Jr., of Montreal to assist in the delivery of additional trunks in a second shipment to cities in the North of the United States.[1] Blackburn offered Cameron several thousand dollars, supposedly again to be brokered by Jacob Thompson: "[Thompson was] the moneyed agent; the others drew on him for what money they required." Cameron refused on the grounds that he was afraid that in the process of spreading the pestilence he himself would contract whatever disease Blackburn was trying to spread. Cameron, in sworn testimony in Montreal on June 9, 1865, said that the story of his recruitment by, and collusion with, Blackburn was untrue: "I never told Conover or Wallace [two aliases used by Charles A. Dunham, a perjurious witness], nor any one else, that I was to get compensation for aiding, abetting, or assisting in any such infamous deeds, or anything of like character.... [T]he whole statement by Conover in reference to myself and yellow fever and Dr. Blackburn is an infamous fabrication and falsehood."[2] However, others were aware of the plan, including Jacob Thompson, William Cleary, and George Sanders. Sanford Conover, in his sworn testimony at the Lincoln assassination, said, "They all favored it, and were all very much interested in it."[3]

After refusing personally to pay Hyams, Blackburn was already heading back toward Halifax to travel again to Bermuda to collect yet more contaminated items. Again he would work under the guise of helping the yellow fever victims, still accepting no payment for his medical services in Bermuda. This time he arrived in Bermuda on September 4.[4] Blackburn resumed his "humanitarian mission" working to fight the epidemic, with his base again at the Hamilton Hotel. He registered there with his home once more listed as Natchez, Mississippi. From this location he toiled against yellow fever—and collected more tainted items to ship to the North. Acting Colonial Secretary James Tucker reported that Dr. Luke Pryor Blackburn, "a visitor from the Southern States of America ... announced his intention of inviting a meeting of the Medical Officer and Practitioners in Bermuda" to discuss the treatment and containment of yellow fever. He added that "such discussions may be highly beneficial to these islands" and that all practitioners should attend the meeting held in the Hamilton Hotel on September 29 at 3:00 p.m. (Tucker of course was unaware of the real reason Blackburn was offering his services to Bermuda.) On October 4, 1864, the *Bermuda Gazette* reported that Blackburn had met other medical personnel on that Thursday "for the purpose of adopting one fixed rule for treating the prevailing fever."[5] Dr. Henry J. Hinson, Sr., from Pembroke Parish in Bermuda presided over the meeting. There Blackburn discussed with military and civilian doctors his techniques for controlling the latest epidemic of yellow fever.

Few physicians practiced in the Bermudian islands; only about 17 were available for the entire population of 11,451 at that time—one in St. Georges, five in Hamilton, and the rest scattered throughout the islands.[6] (Applying the ratio of doctors to population today in the United States would have meant Bermuda needed about 28 physicians.) Physicians at the meeting heard Blackburn tout his extensive experience in dealing with the disease. He urged consistency in the approach by all physicians, especially the imposition of effective quarantines, in part to calm the patients who might be confused if they heard differing methods of treatment and quarantine from different medical sources. The doctors in attendance at the meeting proposed to detail their own treatments and their success rates at the next gathering; in the future all medical personnel would apply uniformly whichever appeared to be the best approach.

Reception of this "foreigner" from the South was mixed. Some doctors were insulted; others were appreciative of Blackburn's efforts. Dr. Park B. Tucker later questioned Blackburn on the "usefulness of such applications as Tobacco, and Onions; as remedies in Yellow Fever." The author of a letter to the editor in the *Royal Gazette* calling himself "Practitioner," said, "I quite concur with Dr. B. against the non-administration of Calomel Podophyllon [a cathartic agent], or any drastic purgatives in this fever."[7] Another report

10. The Second Shipment of Articles Contaminated

was more personal: "The address of Dr. Blackburn was characterized by good feeling, and by its sound, liberal, and judicious tone. Whether the benevolent object of his visit be in any wise fulfilled or not, the entire community cannot otherwise than cordially appreciate its motive."[8]

• • •

But for Hyams, the situation was becoming even more desperate. He hadn't yet been paid for his delivery of the yellow fever trunks to the North in the summer of 1864. His job as a bootmaker in Toronto wasn't yielding much profit, or perhaps he was even out of work by the fall of 1864. His wife had been forced to sell his bootmaking tools while Hyams was gone from Toronto, as well as her own dresses and other personal family items. She would soon deliver another baby—probably their third—on February 22, 1865. The first had been named Jefferson Davis Hyams and was born about 1863. Their second boy, named "T.F. Stonewall Jackson Hyams," died on March 20, 1865, at the age of 12 months and 28 days.[9] In January 1865 Hyams had at least two children (Jefferson Davis Hyams and T.F. Stonewall Jackson Hyams), for he wrote, from 400 Queen Street, Toronto—a new address, to the Confederate Benevolence Society in Montreal at that time about his wife, who was nearly ready to deliver their third child: "My wife and children are with me, my wife being near her confinement [the labor and delivery of Henry Michael Hyams], not knowing the moment she may be confined, and positively declare I have not a cent to help her through her troubles, I have tried a long time to get something to do that I might make a living, but failed in every effort.... I am now in a state of destitution, relying on your benevolence."[10] He was desperate. Maybe it was time for Hyams to turn toward the authorities of the North for help.

• • •

Blackburn soon had filled three additional trunks for shipment to the North, as yet unaware whether the previous shipment had been successfully distributed or not. He then enlisted the help of a hotel worker in St. Georges for the temporary storage and later shipment of these new trunks.[11] Blackburn's new hire was Edward Cork Swan, a "lodging house keeper." Why he had chosen this particular hotelkeeper in St. Georges to help in his yellow fever plot is unknown. St. Georges had at least seven hotels at the time[12] and many additional rooms that were rented out of private residences.[13] Apparently he chose Swan because the man lived in the port city most used by the Confederates and had a reputation for honesty and reliability, although he lived on Shinbone Alley,[14] an area in St. Georges filled with bars and brothels.

Swan was apparently unaware of the purpose of his job for Dr. Blackburn, but he should have been suspicious at being promised such a large payment for virtually no work. He was to be given $150 per month to store the three trunks and an additional $500 when it came time to send them by ship either to Halifax or New York. To the observer in the 21st century, this sum may not seem outlandish. However, considering that the average commercial sailor in 1864 earned about the equivalent of $500–750 *per year*, the magnitude of Blackburn's offering should have alerted Swan that his fee might be illicit payment for something nefarious.

Newspaper accounts would later suggest that the original plan had been to fill ten trunks instead of the three found in Swan's home.[15] Blackburn instructed him to wait until the spring of 1865 to ship the trunks, presumably because Blackburn knew that epidemics of yellow fever spread more rapidly in warm spring weather. Blackburn must have thought that he had sufficient time to wait, even though the South's fortunes in the war were dwindling very rapidly. The target this time would be New York City. Blackburn left Bermuda in mid–October 1864.

Swan ultimately began to have doubts about ever being paid, and he wrote a letter to George P. Black, another Confederate operative in Bermuda working for Major Norman Walker, the Confederate in charge of shipping for the blockade-runners. In this letter, Swan requested his payment for the services of hiding and protecting the trunks. He wrote as follows on April 11, 1865: "Aware of your knowledge with respect to the importance of the trunks remaining in my charge and also the interest manifested by you concerning the same, I beg to call your attention to the fact of my not having heard or received any answer to my previous letter of the thirty first of March respecting payment of promised remuneration I therefore deem it imperative to notify my intentions to you to seek *undoubted* [emphasis Swan's] remuneration from another source should I not hear from you within the space of twenty four hours."

Black reported that Swan demanded money, even saying that his insistence was blackmail. In the letter, Swan was threatening to go to the Union officials if the Confederates refused to pay him. Black referred to the letter as "one that was issued for the purpose of extorting money from parties under threat for an alleged offence."[16] News media of the day suggested that if the Confederacy were truly behind the yellow fever plot it would not have refused to pay the relatively tiny sum of money at issue between Swan and Blackburn. Keeping the secret a secret would have been worth what Swan was demanding. Perhaps the plot was all Blackburn's doing, and there never really was any Confederate money backing the endeavor. To this day, the funding of the entire plot remains unclear. Some believe the plan was financed from the Confederate treasury, and indeed at least some of it might have been. Other monetary sources mentioned for funding this plot include Blackburn's own

10. The Second Shipment of Articles Contaminated

wealth, Confederate money from Havana, fees realized from the sale of cotton pushed through the blockade, or a combination of all three.

• • •

Germ warfare was nothing new. In 1763 General (Lord) Jeffrey Amherst wrote to Colonel Henry Bouquet regarding the conflict near Fort Pitt in what is now western Pennsylvania. He suggested using blankets contaminated with smallpox to attempt to decimate the Delaware, Shawnee, and Mingo Indians. Amherst wrote, "Could it not be contrived to Send the Small Pox among those Disaffected Tribes of Indians? We must, on this occasion, Use Every Strategem in our power to Reduce them." Bouquet wrote back, saying, "I will try to inoculate the [Indians] by means of Blankets that may fall into their hands, and take Care not to get the disease myself." Amherst replied, "You will Do well to try to Innoculate the Indians, by means of Blankets, as well as to Try Every other Method, that can Serve to Extirpate this Execrable Race." Indeed, William Trent later wrote that the Indians had received two blankets, one silk handkerchief, and one "linnen" from the smallpox hospital, perhaps even given by soldiers on their own accord, irrespective of the communications between Bouquet and Amherst. These "gifts" transmitted smallpox to the Indians, and outbreaks of the disease were recorded among these tribes in the summer of 1763.[17]

Southern-leaning newspapers tried to minimize the atrocity of the alleged plot by reminding its readers of the tactics used in the War of 1812 in which blankets from smallpox victims in New York and Philadelphia were distributed among Indians who were cooperating with the British at Munceytown, near Chatham in Ontario. The resulting epidemic eliminated these Indians from existence. These Southern sympathizers chided Northerners for expressing outrage, as their own government had used similar tactics half a century earlier. Furthermore, the report suggested that the North had already attempted to introduce smallpox into the South by similar methods. The paper concluded with this statement: "As yet we know of but a tithe of the hideous crimes which have been committed in the name of liberty." Nevertheless, the newspaper claimed that if the Blackburn story were true "he is certainly the greatest scoundrel unhung."[18]

• • •

The Union U.S. consul in Bermuda, Charles M. Allen, first became aware of Blackburn's activity in September 1864, but his suspicions weren't aroused then, except for his noting that Blackburn was a Southern sympathizer. Allen reported that Blackburn ostensibly was a humanitarian working without pay to help yellow fever victims and even refused compensation for his own expenses. Allen said Blackburn was "desirous only of benefitting this community, who had manifested so much sympathy for their holy cause." However, Allen also saw that Blackburn "never neglected on all possible occasions to advocate the cause of the rebels."[19]

The real reason for Blackburn's yellow fever benevolence in Bermuda was finally exposed in early 1865 when a Swiss former employee in the office of Major Norman Walker, CSA, in Bermuda became an informant when he approached Consul Allen. This former employee had been summarily fired from Walker's office, and he had a score to settle. Seeing an opportunity to gain intelligence about Confederate activity and having a suspicion that something was amiss with Dr. Blackburn's ministrations to the sick in Bermuda, Consul Allen interrogated the informant, who told Allen that Blackburn's expenses had been paid by the Confederate treasury. He revealed that the "sole object" of Blackburn's one-month stay had been to collect clothing from yellow fever victims to send to Washington, D. C., Norfolk, Virginia, and New Bern, North Carolina (Blackburn had returned to Halifax before this report surfaced). The informant immediately demanded $500 himself to divulge further information about the deal between Blackburn and Swan, saying it was certain he would be unable to find a new job if he revealed anymore details of Blackburn and Swan's plot. Major Walker would know the source of the leaked information, and it would mean that the informant would have to leave Bermuda.

Consul Allen finally came up with $200 to bribe the informant, but only on the guarantee that the story proved true and the trunks were found as described. Allen was told who had the trunks—that man named Edward Swan. The informant described the trunks in great detail, and he told Allen where they were hidden in Swan's house. Allen's fears were confirmed: Blackburn was collecting clothing and linens from infected patients to send to the North to produce epidemics of yellow fever. Allen learned that "when a patient died, he [Blackburn] had his [the patient's] clothes stripped off and cast through the hospital window. His [Blackburn's] manservant was waiting below and carried the things away. With a hint from this Swiss I learned where they were taken to, and with some difficulty procured a warrant to search the place. At first the officials laughed at my application, but I was very earnest, and in a day or two I succeeded in obtaining the warrant, with two policemen to assist me in the search."[20]

Allen went before the meeting of the Corporation of St. Georges on April 12, 1865. It was gathering that day in its function as the board of health. The corporation addressed reports that one of its citizens was harboring a health nuisance. Present were James H. Thies, the mayor, and R.W. Outerbridge, John Fox, and W.S. Trott, aldermen. G. Wainwright, G.S. Rankin, and Joseph M. Hayward were present as the Common Council. Hayward was the secretary.

10. The Second Shipment of Articles Contaminated 125

Allen reported the story of the infected trunks, and he identified Edward C. Swan as the suspect. As the discussion proceeded, a spy and Southern sympathizer at the meeting gave a signal to another Southern agent outside the room to warn Swan of what was happening and to do something with the incriminating evidence. Swan was in the process of trying to remove and burn the contaminated articles when the authorities arrived to search his house.[21] Mayor James Thies, Alderman John Fox, and the town "nuisance inspector," Nathaniel Jackson, had quickly proceeded to Swan's home, along with Consul Allen, arriving before Swan had time to dispose of the evidence. The officials told Swan of the purpose of their visit. Allen and the others found three trunks in the room indicated by the Swiss ex-employee. They were hidden under a table covered with a large oilcloth that reached to the floor. One of the trunks made of leather had labels: "St. Louis Hotel, Upper Town, Quebec," and "Clifton House, Niagara Falls, Canada Side."[22] The other two (a "shoe trunk lashed with rope" and a "green travelling trunk open[,] the facing of lock broken") had no markings on them. After "some demur," Swan handed over the trunks to the officials but only on the agreement that the trunks would be returned to him if nothing dangerous were found within them. He still harbored the hope that he would be paid for his storage of the material; therefore, he demanded that they be returned to him and he requested a receipt for the goods. Clearly it seemed that Swan was unaware of the gravity of his agreement with Dr. Blackburn and likely didn't know the contents of the trunks. Dr. Benjamin Burland, the health officer responsible for inspecting such items, was unavailable that day, so the trunks were given to the local police and taken to the police station for safekeeping.

James Thies, the mayor of St. Georges, wrote on the same day, April 12, 1865, to Harry St. George Ord, "His Excellency, the Governor of Bermuda," stating that he had "undoubted information" that trunks had been "secreted" in Swan's house containing "clothing of persons who are deceased from fever and collected by persons of respectability for an atrocious purpose."[23] Thies also sought the advice of S. Brownlow Gray, the attorney general for Bermuda. The next day, April 13, Dr. Burland was available to inspect the contents of the trunks. First, before the trunks were opened, government officials carried them to the quarantine station on Nonsuch Island in Castle Harbor with the suspicion that articles dangerous to the community's health might be found.

In 1865 many different quarantine stations located on multiple islands in Bermuda were used for sick sailors. Many quarantine sites were needed to protect Bermudians from diseases imported from the ships that came to the islands from locales where yellow fever, cholera, malaria, smallpox, and other contagions flourished. In early 1865 sufficient facilities existed for Nonsuch Island to be considered safe as the recipient of contaminated articles such as Blackburn's trunks.

On Nonsuch Island the officials opened the trunks and found within them a mix of new underclothing and clothing contaminated with vomit and excrement. There were blankets, sheets, underwear, handkerchiefs, all mixed with some new garments and apparently stacked in alternating layers—clean, soiled, clean, soiled. The alternate layering may have been an amateurish attempt to conceal the filthy rags and soiled clothing and handkerchiefs, or it was simply a method of infusing the contagion from the dirty garments to the clean ones. After a listing of the contents was made, the trunks were buried on Nonsuch Island and their inventories carefully recorded (Figures 15A and 15B):

No. 1—Green trunk (open): Contained on top several articles
  a. of clothing, such as, shirts, guernseys etc. etc. quite new, not worn, & unwashed,
  b. A Blanket, covered with dark stains, large & small, rather new, but evidently having been used in a sick room. The stains like those from "black vomit"
  c. Clothes—Bag/yellow/old but not stained
  d. Several guernseys etc. all new or unworn
  e. A sheet at the bottom of the trunk, extensively stained or soiled, stains of a dark color, with others of a yellow tinge from mustard. Used beyond doubt by a sick person.

No. 2—Large Leather portmanteau (locked)
  a. A woolen shawl, old or unstained on top.
  b. Drawers, dirty & stained with mustard
  c. Socks, pocket handkerchief, Coat & Trousers, all worn & dirty & also a Guernsey
  d. Sheet, on bottom, stained all over, some dark, other of a lighter colour, also used in a sick chamber mustard stains
  e. Between these & the shawl on top were a quantity of Guernseys, shirts flannel & cotton etc. all new and two pillow slips & a shirt all very dirty & stained, some of the stains as from port wine, all apparently having been used in a sick chamber

No. 3—Black Trunk (corded & locked/
  a. shirts (cotton & flannel/perfectly new
  b. shirt & guernsey, stained & very dirty
  c. Pocket handkerchief, stained all over with darkblood & a few spots as from "Black vomit"
  d. a fillet deeply stained by mustard
  e. Two Blankets, free stains, but apparently having been in use

10. The Second Shipment of Articles Contaminated 127

f. Drawers & socks, stained & worn
g. Two pillow slips on bottom, deeply stained.

> Signed/ B Burland /M.B.
> R[oyal] Artillery
> Health Officer
> East End
> 13/4/65"[24]

The team then buried the trunks. Records show that the trunks had been carried to Nonsuch Island in a small boat for the fee of one British pound sterling, paid on May 19, and the job of burying them was performed by "a boy," paid 6 pence on June 3, 1865.[25] S. Brownlow Gray, the attorney general, then wrote, on April 17, 1865, to James Thies, the mayor of St. Georges, saying,

> The Corporation should immediately lodge a complaint & charge against the person or persons in whose custody the suspicious articles were found for causing a nuisance by keeping and having in possession within the town certain articles of clothing and bedding infected with injurious matter dangerous to the health of the community and to the common nuisance of all the liege subjects of Her Majesty.... Besides Dr. Burland's testimony it would be well to secure other medical evidence of the danger to the health of the community of the contents of these trunks.[26]

Later, upon considering the degree of potential threat to public health, the health officer sent other workers back to Nonsuch Island. There they bored holes from above ground into the trunks and then poured vitriol (sulfuric acid), purchased by the board of health from Dr. W.R. Higinbothom at the Medical Hall of St. Georges, into them.[27] Confusing matters, Allen wrote in one diplomatic dispatch dated April 14, 1865, "The trunks, which were taken yesterday [April 13, 1865] to the Quarantine Station, [were] opened

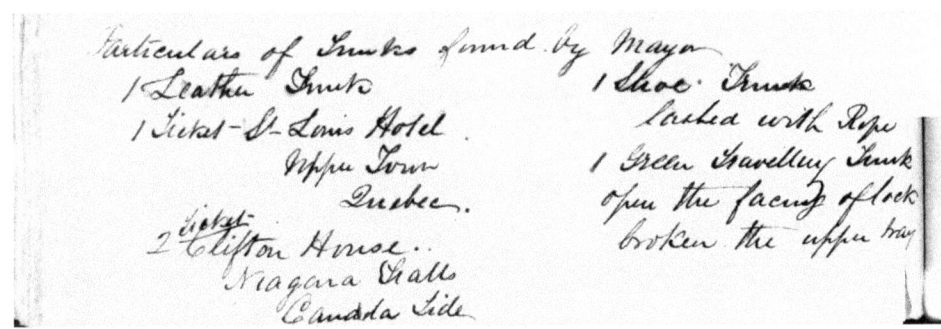

Figure 15A. Page from St. Georges Corporation Book, listing the trunks found in Edward Swan's home (St. Georges Corporation Minutes, Book 3, 1834–1870, unpaginated. Bermuda Archives, Hamilton, Bermuda).

Description of Articles found in three Boxes inspected, on Nonsuch Island, 13th April 1865.

No 1. Green trunk (open)
  a. Contained on top several articles of Clothing, such as shirts, Guernseys &c &c quite new, not worn, & unwashed.
  β. A Blanket covered with dark stains, large & small, rather new, but evidently having been used in a sick room. The stains like those from "black vomit".
  γ. Clothes-Bag (yellow) old but not stained
  δ. Several Guernseys &c all new & unworn.
  ε. A Sheet at the bottom of the trunk, extensively stained & soiled, stains of a dark color, with others of a yellow tinge from mustard.— Used beyond doubt by a sick person.—

No 2. Large Leather portmanteau (locked)
  a. A Woollen shawl, old & unstained on top.
  β. Drawers, dirty & stained with mustard
  γ. Socks, pocket handkerchief, Coat & Trousers all worn & dirty & also a Guernsey
  δ. Sheet on bottom, stained all over, some dark, others of a lighter colour, also used in a sick chamber — mustard stains.—
  ε. Between these & the shawl on top were a quantity of Guernseys, shirts, flannel & cotton &c all new and two Yellow slips & a shirt all very dirty & stained, some of the stains as from port wine, all apparently having been used in a sick bed

No 3. Black Trunk (corded & locked)
  β. Shirt & Guernsey (flannel) perfectly new
  γ. Pocket handkerchief, stained & very dirty, stained all over with dark

10. The Second Shipment of Articles Contaminated 129

Opposite and above: Figure 15B. Pages from St. Georges Corporation Book, detailing the contents of the three trunks found in the house of Edward Swan after their removal to Nonsuch Island (St. Georges Corporation Minutes, Book 3, 1834–1870, unpaginated. Bermuda Archives, Hamilton, Bermuda).

and found to contain wearing apparel and bedding, made up in small packages, decently clean, with dirty flannel drawers and shirts on the outside, all evidently taken from a sick bed, intermixed with these packages were poultices, and many other things which could have been placed there for no legitimate purpose, were found; The whole of which were *burned* [emphasis the author's] by direction of the health officer." Only one sentence further, he said, "I shall use my utmost endeavors to have the contents of the trunks taken up at once and thoroughly destroyed...."[28] It appears that two independent transcriptions of Allen's handwritten letter came to different conclusions about a single word that changed the meaning of the action taken upon the contaminated articles. One source transcribed "burned," while another interpreted the word as "buried."[29] One letter of the alphabet was the difference. Likely the latter was correct. The original handwritten letter has not been preserved. It might seem today to make more sense to burn such material, but yellow fever in the 1860s was thought to be transmitted by "miasmas," or vapors, and the authorities perhaps reasoned that burning the contaminated articles might simply have hastened the distribution of such infectious materials into the air. If anything was actually burned immediately, it was a small fraction of the contents of the trunks, because extensive testimony later cited the health officer's return trip to Nonsuch Island, where the trunks had been buried.

Blackburn had employed Swan to keep and hide these trunks, and it was in Swan's house that they were found. Swan was arrested and charged with "keeping in his possession a nuisance prejudicial to the health of the community."[30] His bond was set at 50 pounds, with two additional sureties of 50 pounds apiece. Consul Allen also tried to obtain a warrant for the arrest of Blackburn, but the doctor had already gone back to Canada through Halifax.

Allen wrote a letter to Secretary of State William H. Seward on April 14, 1865, the day of Lincoln's assassination. Of course, Allen was unaware at the time of the writing that Lincoln had been murdered. He described to Seward what he knew about Blackburn's "diabolical scheme."[31] This time he described the fee paid to Swan in a slightly different way from other informants—$150 per month for keeping the trunks and $500 to take the trunks to New York. Some reports, including the testimony of George P. Black, cited the fee paid to Swan as a $250 "down payment" and another $250 after he had taken the trunks to New York.[32] In the same trial in Bermuda Frederick Buckstaff[33] testified that the fee was simply $150 per month that he held the goods.[34] Allen never named his informant, the Swiss ex-employee, although he referred to him as "a person intimate in the Office of N.S. Walker, Confederate agent here." Other details Allen relayed were similar to parallel versions of the story that witnesses would eventually report.

The first Bermuda Judicial Investigation about the yellow fever plot was held in the tiny police court in the town of St. Georges in late April 1865. Similar to a grand jury hearing, the proceedings were to determine if it was likely that a crime had been committed and if enough evidence existed to charge an accused party. Interest in the case was high, and space for observers was limited. Present were W.C.J. Hyland, the police magistrate; James H. Thies, the mayor; R. W. Outerbridge, John Fox, and W.S. Trott, aldermen; G. Wainwright, G.S. Rankin, Joseph M. Hayward, and W. Tudor Tucker, the magistrate. Hayward was again the secretary. Lawyers present were Seth Harvey, the solicitor general who represented George P. Black, and Richard D. Darrell, representing the board of health. During this trial both Blackburn and Hyams—the major players in the drama—would be absent.

The investigation began with a brief statement from James H. Thies, the mayor of St. Georges from 1862 to 1880 and president of the board of health. Thies testified that U.S. consul Charles Maxwell Allen had approached him on April 10 and told of three trunks secreted in the home of Edward C. Swan containing clothing infected with yellow fever intended for an "atrocious purpose." On April 12 Thies had convened a meeting of the board of health. Thies, two members of the board (Mr. John Fox and Nathaniel Jackson, the

10. The Second Shipment of Articles Contaminated

town's "nuisance inspector") had gone to Swan's home and searched for trunks potentially filled with clothing and bedding contaminated with yellow fever. A spy in that meeting had relayed word to a compatriot, who hurried to Swan's home to warn him, but the team arrived before Swan could do anything with the trunks. After discussion (including that statement of "some demur"), Swan admitted to keeping trunks for Blackburn but asserted that he didn't know anything about the contents except that they might contain some clothes. Swan turned the trunks over to the mayor and his committee, but Swan demanded a receipt for the trunks and requested that they be returned to him if nothing dangerous or adverse was found in them. Swan testified that he had been promised money for keeping the trunks, but that Blackburn thus far had paid him nothing. The team's nuisance inspector, Nathaniel Jackson, gave the trunks to the police, who waited for the health officer of the East End, Dr. Benjamin Burland, MB, and member of the Royal Artillery, who was out of town that day. The next day, April 13, police took the trunks to the quarantine station on Nonsuch Island, where the health officer examined them. Thies again noted for the record the following labels: on the leather "portmanteau" (the large leather suitcase) were two labels saying, "St. Louis Hotel, Upper Town, Quebec," and "Clifton House, Niagara Falls, Canada Side." The other two trunks (a black "shoe trunk lashed with rope" and a green "traveling trunk" with a broken lock) had no markings. The detailed reports of the entire contents of the trunks were entered into evidence.

As the proceedings against Swan developed and the connection with Blackburn became obvious, the U.S. State Department relayed the information to Judge Advocate General Joseph Holt, who arranged for the Bureau of Military Justice to issue a warrant for Blackburn's arrest in the United States. By then, Blackburn was back in Canada and outside the jurisdiction of U.S. authorities. Edward Swan then told members of the hearing that he indeed had kept three trunks for Dr. Blackburn but was unaware of the contents of the trunks, though he knew them to be of "great importance." He reported that Blackburn was pledged to pay him for his services, and that the Confederate Office would pay if for some reason Blackburn didn't return to claim the trunks. Swan identified Major Norman Walker as the person in charge of the Confederate Office, but since Walker was gone Swan had applied to Mr. George P. Black, who was temporarily in charge, for payment. Swan said that he had mentioned the trunks to his wife, to Frederick Buckstaff, and to a boarder of his, a Mr. Alexander, another clerk in the Confederate Office. Swan swore that he had never received any money from Blackburn, in spite of their agreement. He had not opened the trunks, but Blackburn had told him they contained clothes. Apparently Black had wanted the trunks to be transferred to the Confederate Office, but Swan refused and became nervous about the intense interest shown in the trunks and their contents. It might have seemed that the trunks contained something more valuable than clothing alone. The next witness was Matilda Swan, Edward Swan's wife, who concurred with her husband's testimony but added no new information.

Dr. Benjamin Burland, the health officer for the East End (St. Georges) and an assistant surgeon of the Royal Artillery, was then called to testify. He reported that he had been instructed by the president of the board of health to inspect the trunks on April 13 after they had been found in Swan's house and placed under custody. Burland rode from the police station to the Nonsuch Island Quarantine Station with the officer and the trunks. The men had been instructed to bury them on the island if the trunks contained any infectious material. His assistant in this inspection process was Nathaniel Jackson, the inspector of nuisances at St. Georges. On Nonsuch Island the inspectors opened the green trunk, the black trunk, and the portmanteau that had been removed from Swan's house. There they took an inventory of the contents, which included "shirts, blankets, pillow cases, drawers, pocket handkerchief, a bandage, &c., all more or less stained and soiled; the stains being partly similar to those made by black vomit [the characteristic of yellow fever]; partly of mustard, all evidently taken from sick persons. Intermingled with these were a quantity of clothing, as guernseys, shirts, flannel, and cotton, &c., quite new and still ticketed." Burland inventoried the suspicious items; Jackson listed the clean and unworn articles. Burland further described the stained articles in detail: "a white blanket, rather new, but covered with dark stains—they bore all the traces of having been used in a sick chambur [sic]— the stains resembled those from 'black vomit' ... a sheet very extensively stained ... a pair of drawers, very dirty, with yellow stains ... two pillowslips, very much soiled ... a white pocket-handkerchief, with dark colored stains, and a few dark spots such as would be produced by black vomit ... two pillow-slips on the bottom also stained as if from perspiration."[35] Finding this material to be suspicious, Burland concluded, "I considered them very prejudicial to the health of the community." The two inspectors ordered the trunks to be broken up, and both the trunks and the contents were buried. Mayor Thies at this point added that he had seen to it they were destroyed, probably meaning he had arranged for the combination of burial and subsequent application of sulfuric acid to them underground.

The next witness, George Hawthorn, a wharf worker denied knowledge of the trunks and their contents. Mayor James H. Thies reported the addresses listed on one of the trunks as hotels in Canada, but he had no further testimony. George Potts Black, the person in temporary charge of the Confederate Office in Bermuda, said that he had learned of rumors of the contents of the trunks only recently. Because he had heard his name mentioned in connection with the trunks he had written a letter to the mayor asking that the St. Georges

10. The Second Shipment of Articles Contaminated

Corporation Board of Health convene a meeting so he could dissociate his name from whatever the controversy might be. Black had retained a lawyer, Seth Harvey, for this hearing and submitted a statement that told of Blackburn's activities at the end of September 1864. Blackburn had told Black about some trunks he had left with Swan for safekeeping. Swan was reputed to be an honest man, although Black claimed to know little about him. Black said Blackburn had promised to pay Swan $250 initially and $250 later if Swan would store the trunks and take them to New York City in the spring of 1865. Blackburn had also intimated an alternate plan to transport the trunks if Swan's trustworthiness became suspect. Black went to Swan's house a few days later, and Swan showed Black the trunks that had been left for safekeeping. Black then forgot about the incident until March 31, 1865, when Swan sent a short note to Black asking about payment for Swan's services. On April 11, Swan sent that note to Black and said, in part, "I therefore deem it imperative to notify my intentions to you to see *undoubted* remuneration from another source should I not hear from you within the space of 24 hours." Black considered this letter to be a threat of blackmail or extortion. Black therefore notified the Mayor and requested a hearing of the Board of Health. Black still claimed ignorance of the contents of the trunks and reiterated that no money had changed hands between him and Swan. Court was then adjourned for the day.

Court reconvened on April 20, hearing U.S. consul Charles M. Allen. Allen offered no new evidence but submitted some names of possibly useful witnesses. Frederic Buckstaff was the next witness. He reinforced prior testimony and admitted that he had knowledge of the existence of the trunks for about three or four months; however, he had heard of the potential destructive nature of the contents only about one month earlier. Edward Swan, Mrs. Swan, and Mr. Alexander, a boarder at the Swans' house, had provided Buckstaff his knowledge. Buckstaff related that Blackburn was purported to be an agent of the Confederate government, and that "the object of his mission was the destruction of the Northern masses." The targets of the plot were New York and Philadelphia. Buckstaff testified that Blackburn had told Swan the payment would be $150 per month for each month that Swan kept and protected the trunks and the money would come from Major Norman Walker's office. Buckstaff implicated Black in a conversation between Black and Mrs. Swan in which Black encouraged Mrs. Swan to remove the trunks from the house, and Black told her that she could receive a lot of money for them.

The other Confederate in Walker's office, Mr. Alexander, appeared to know of the plot. Buckstaff alleged that Swan indeed knew of the contents and nature of the items in the trunks, as well as the purpose for them: "Mr. Swan told me that Mr. Blackburn had informed him that the intention of sending the clothing to New York was for the destruction of the masses there. Swan told me he knew the contents of the trunks from what Dr. Blackburn had told him; Mr. Swan also expressed his suspicion that other trunks taken by Dr. Blackburn were infected." Once again, testimony confirmed that no money had yet changed hands.

Buckstaff would suffer intense persecution after the trial from Southern sympathizers located in Bermuda. Assassins shot at him, wounding him under the right arm. In addition, he was ultimately threatened with death for his part in Swan's conviction. Consul Allen even recommended to Buckstaff that he leave Bermuda for a safer location. Buckstaff took the advice and went to New York City, where the local papers noted that he had lost two months' employment and wages for his honest testimony and that he deserved "some consideration at the hands of the city authorities in return for his valuable services" as the epidemic of yellow fever had been intended for New York City but was never successfully exported there.[36] Kit Swan testified next but claimed to know nothing useful to the court. Court was adjourned and reconvened on April 22.

Dinah Amery was a nurse in Bermuda who lived in Hamilton, Pembroke Parish, and worked intermittently with Dr. Blackburn at the Hamilton Hotel. She herself had contracted a mild case of yellow fever, but she recovered without severe complications. Unknown to her at the time, this mild case would give her immunity from future infection; thus, she was able to attend patients with yellow fever and not become sick again herself. She observed Blackburn attempting to cause patients to sweat profusely by covering them with multiple layers of clothing and blankets. She also helped Blackburn retrieve some additional heavy coverings from a trunk in his room, items he used to treat his patients. When she objected to this "treatment" of promoting excessive sweating, Blackburn seemed annoyed and objected to her interference in his care. Dr. Blackburn probably thought that the sweat contained the infectious agent of yellow fever, and more sweat would mean that the bedclothes would be more highly contagious. After he had left the room, Nurse Amery removed some of the heavy clothes and blankets from her patient. When he returned at 4:00 a.m. and discovered that she had removed the additional clothing and blankets, he was angry and scolded her. Blackburn took some of the used clothing items from the patient. "He then took all the things and placed them back in the Trunk, which witness [Nurse Dinah Amery] assisted him to carry back to his room." The garments were packed in the trunk unwashed.

William Blackman was the next witness. He was a carter, that is, he hauled belongings from place to place on a cart. He testified that he had taken trunks belonging to Blackburn from the Hamilton Hotel and Slater's Boarding House to Swan's house on Shinbone Alley at the foot of Barrack Hill in St. Georges. These hotels were the two sites where Blackburn treated patients.

10. The Second Shipment of Articles Contaminated

Frances (also alternatively spelled as "Francis") Cameron was another nurse who lived in Hamilton and worked with Blackburn. She had nursed one patient at the Hamilton Hotel and four at Slater's Boarding House. One of their patients was Captain John Wesley Galloway. Galloway, hailing from Smithfield, North Carolina, had organized ship pilots, fishermen, and sailors to form what was called Captain Galloway's Coast Guard Company. This organization served the Confederate navy by protecting Cape Fear near Wilmington, North Carolina, and Fort Fisher at the mouth of the Cape Fear River. They also provided skippers for many of the blockade-runners. Galloway had taken the ship *Mary Celestia*[37] to Bermuda as its pilot under the command of Captain Arthur Sinclair at the end of August 1864.

On August 24, 1864, Galloway had taken the *Mary Celestia* out of the Fort Caswell, North Carolina, harbor, bound for Bermuda under Captain Arthur Sinclair.[38] All arrived successfully, but Galloway soon came down with yellow fever while in Bermuda. Dr. Luke Blackburn attended him at Slater's Boarding House. Tragically, on September 6, just three weeks before Galloway's death on September 27 at age 52, Captain Arthur Sinclair, the mariner still in charge of the *Mary Celestia*, took her out of the Hamilton harbor, with John Virgin serving as the local pilot. The steamer was loaded with 125 boxes of bacon and 534 boxes of other merchandise—food, rifles, and ammunition—and was headed first for Nassau, then likely onward to Savannah, Georgia. They quickly passed at about 13 knots toward the South Shore of Bermuda, where the pilot and co-owner Colonel William Crenshaw, who was onboard, were planning to disembark near Gibb's Point Lighthouse, where both lived. As the steamer came close to shore, First Officer Stewart yelled a warning to Pilot John Virgin that he was too close to rocks on the shore. The pilot failed to heed the warnings of the first officer, claiming arrogantly, "I know every rock about here as well as I know my own house."[39] He was wrong. The *Mary Celestia* ran aground on a reef and sank within six to eight minutes in seven fathoms (about 42 feet) of water. The weather had been perfect; it was daylight. Many blamed the headstrong—though experienced—Bermudian pilot Captain John Virgin for causing the ship to sink because of his failing to listen to his first officer. One man onboard, the chief cook, died in the wreck as he tried to return to his stateroom to retrieve something valuable to him. As the vessel continued sinking, a door that wouldn't open trapped him. Divers retrieved much of the cargo, but the hull of the steamer itself remains on the floor of the ocean until this day, just beyond the sands of the southern tip of Bermuda off South Road. Officials speculated how the accident could have happened, and others later even suggested that John Virgin had taken a bribe from Union officials in Bermuda (maybe even from Consul Charles M. Allen himself) to sink the vessel purposely so the Confederates wouldn't have access to the valuable cargo onboard. Allen denied the charge.

The pilot commissioners suspended Pilot John Virgin from service for 18 months.

Galloway ultimately died of yellow fever on September 27 at age 52, his terminal event being a hemorrhage of the lungs. During this hemorrhage, he soiled many garments and a handkerchief with blood. After Galloway died, Blackburn sent everyone away on various errands, including making preparations for Galloway's burial. When Nurse Cameron returned about an hour later, Galloway was shrouded, but his clothing and those other garments had disappeared. Some of the soiled items Blackburn had thrown out the window of the hotel before Galloway died, and the proprietor of the hotel, Mrs. Catharine Slater, noted that many such items had disappeared similarly during Blackburn's treatment of patients.

Joseph Hayne Rainey was a barber and barkeeper at the Hamilton Hotel and was the next witness.[40] He coincidentally traveled once from Bermuda to Halifax with Blackburn, and Rainey noted that Blackburn had once come to the Hamilton Hotel with only one trunk but returned to Halifax with multiple trunks. A nurse had alerted Rainey to the fact that Blackburn covered his patients with heavy blankets to make them sweat, then packed the coverings in his personal trunk. Rainey observed that on Blackburn's second trip to Bermuda he had some baggage shipped from Hamilton to St. Georges, and Rainey later saw Blackburn's luggage at Swan's home. When Blackburn left Bermuda the second time he had only one trunk, and Rainey had overheard Blackburn tell Swan to take care of the remaining trunks. Though Blackburn filled multiple trunks with clothes during his stay at the Hamilton Hotel, Rainey never saw Blackburn buy or ship new or used clothing to the hotel from stores in town.

At this point, the court was recessed. Swan by now refused to post the bond (£50 and two sureties of £50 each), saying that he felt unsafe to remain free in town and requesting to be held in the "gaol," where his life would be in less danger. He had been threatened by some of the Southern blockade-runners, who told him that hundreds of men were out to kill him. Nor did Northern sympathizers likely think too much of a man helping to introduce pestilence into the North. Swan found himself in the unenviable position of being hated by men on both sides of the Civil War. The court granted his request and kept him in jail for his own protection. Swan thus chose "protective custody," which he thought was better than being killed on the streets. Swan was first incarcerated in the jail on April 22 and listed as a 28-year-old white Caucasian man from England. The St. Georges town constable, Robert Mageehan, took charge of him until the next day in court, which was to be April 25.[41] Court resumed on April 25, 1865.

Joseph Willington Stevens was the next witness. He was the son-in law of Mrs. Catharine Slater, owner and operator of Slater's Boarding House,

10. The Second Shipment of Articles Contaminated

where Blackburn had attended some yellow fever patients. Stevens was present when Captain John W. Galloway died, and Stevens watched Blackburn's behavior and the activity of Nurse Frances Cameron. Stevens was helping to care for Galloway, and he noted that just before Galloway died he coughed up some blood that Stevens caught in a handkerchief. Stevens threw the handkerchief on the floor but later remembered that the handkerchief had disappeared from the spot on the floor where he had discarded it. He noted that Blackburn removed Galloway's clothing—undershirt and drawers—and put them on the floor, but Stevens wasn't present when the clothing was removed from the room. Blackburn told Mrs. Slater not to destroy the soiled blankets but to "let them remain out in the dew for two or three nights and the infection would be removed."[42] Stevens also commented that Mrs. Slater had noticed quite a few clothing and bedding articles had disappeared from her hotel when Blackburn was there, and Blackburn would carry a "carpet bag" to the hotel when he came and went to Mrs. Slater's establishment.

Mrs. Catharine Slater was the next witness. She was the owner of Slater's Boarding House, in Hamilton (which would become the Victoria Hotel in 1866), located next to the Royal Bermuda Yacht Club on Front Street downtown, just down the hill toward the harbor and about three blocks from the new and elaborate Hamilton Hotel. The Bermuda Yacht Club had been established in 1844 and was then located east of its current location. The old yacht club was situated just opposite Pier 6 on Front Street. Slater's Boarding House was in one of the adjacent buildings.

Blackburn had attended six patients at Mrs. Slater's hotel, three of whom died, Captain Galloway being one of them. Mrs. Slater confirmed that Blackburn had thrown some soiled articles out the window during the course of his treatment of the patients. She didn't know what happened to Galloway's clothing. Blackburn had indeed told her to let soiled articles remain on the ground, the purpose being to let them become covered with dew. She never personally retrieved them from the ground, but they always mysteriously vanished. She testified that many articles of bed clothing had also disappeared when Blackburn was there (she had initially suspected that some of her employees had stolen them). She also confirmed her son-in-law's report that Blackburn carried a "carpet bag" with him when he came and went from her hotel.

George Potts Black was recalled as a witness to refute Buckstaff's story about the interactions between Mrs. Matilda Swan and himself. He denied that he had talked with Mrs. Swan about payment to retrieve the trunks. Black testified that Buckstaff had asked Black for help in procuring a job, which Black did, finding him a job as Purser on the ship *Stag*. When Buckstaff was fired from that job Black tried to help him find another job, but the war was coming to an end, and the decline of blockade-running made finding employment difficult. Black confirmed that he himself was a citizen of the Confederate States of America and a clerk in the office of Major Norman Walker, the Confederate States agent. Black was in charge of that office from June 1864 through February 1865 because Walker was absent from his post.

Nathaniel Jackson, as inspector of nuisances for St. Georges, testified about the removal of the trunks from Swan's house to Nonsuch Island. He swore that the items were as described—both soiled and clean clothing in the trunks. On April 19 he had gone back to Nonsuch Island to see if the trunks had been disturbed since they had been buried there. They had not. As an added measure of decontamination and security, he had personally "sunk several holes on the spot among the clothing and poured in Vitriol in sufficient quantities to destroy it."

John Fox was an alderman in St. Georges and a member of a committee from the board of health that had gone to Swan's home to inspect the trunks. He testified that Swan at first produced only two trunks but after some prodding revealed a third from another room. He stated that Swan was reluctant to part with the trunks unless he was paid what he had been promised by Blackburn. Mayor Thies reasoned with Swan that the trunks would be returned to Swan if nothing illegal or dangerous was found in them. Swan finally agreed, saying that Blackburn had given the trunks to him for safekeeping, and that Swan thought that they contained clothing but that he wanted to retain possession so he could be paid as promised.

Thus the hearing was completed on April 25. The magistrates decided that the case should go to the attorney general for trial in the Court of General Assize (the British court for the trial of both civil and criminal cases, held in Hamilton, Bermuda). Swan was again directed to post the equivalent of a bond in the amount of £50 and two sureties of £25 each or else he would be held in jail until the trial. He again chose to remain in the jail, as his life was still in danger.

Because the assize was held in Hamilton, Swan was transferred to the jail there on April 28, 1865, to await the Easter session of the general assize.[43] For some reason, the Hamilton Gaol Journal recorded his age as 36,[44] not 28 as listed at St. Georges. He was kept in the Hamilton jail for the time necessary for the assize to hold the trial, which began on May 5 and ended on May 8.[45] The Easter 1865 term of the Court of General Assize cited Edward Cork Swan, a "lodging house keeper," for harboring a "nuisance." He "did unlawfully and injuriously have and keep ... a great quantity of woollen [sic] and other clothing and of woollen blankets and cotton and other bed clothing impregnated and infected with certain deleterious and unwholesome matter or infection produced by a certain fatal and infectious disease called yellow fever." Swan was charged with keeping material that was "hurtful and dangerous to health and perilous and dangerous to the lives" of Bermudian residents. Confirming the theory of yellow fever propagation in the 1860s, the charge continued that Swan's actions produced the following nuisance: "The air there and then became and was greatly corrupted and infected to the great damage and common nuisance of all the liege subjects of our said Lady the Queen."[46]

No detailed records of testimony or deliberations of the assize remain today, only newspaper articles and the final rulings of the court. The assize trial of Edward Cork Swan was concluded on May 8, 1865. After having given explicit instructions to the jury, the Honorable Judge John Harvey Darrell, the chief justice of the assizes, sent them to their deliberations, which lasted only about 30 minutes. He instructed that there were only two issues necessary to consider: (1) whether Swan had indeed kept the infected clothing in his possession, and (2) whether the clothing was a threat to the local community's welfare. Swan was found guilty of the charge of harboring a nuisance, and he was sentenced to four months in the jail of the town of St. Georges.[47]

The jails in Bermuda (in St. Georges and Hamilton) in 1865 weren't comfortable. They were indeed punishment, and Swan's confinement for four months was harsh. The prisoner in the jail was given minimal bedding (a mattress, cot, or hammock), a canteen tin, a water pail, a urinal, and not much else. His clothing had a bold label visible from a distance: "Prison Dress." He was expected to clean his own cell, including disposal of his own human waste. One hour of exercise daily—by himself—was the prescribed amount, with no talking allowed if someone else happened to be nearby, although later regulations allowed more exercise "as deemed proper for the preservation of health." No "gaming" or liquor was allowed, and the penalties were harsh for infractions of this regulation. The prisoner's total subsistence for all necessary maintenance was sixpence per day. Fivepence of this amount per day was allocated for his meals—a pound and a half of bread and some milk. He was allowed a Bible and a prayer book.[48]

The prisoners had to clean their own cells at least weekly, and they had to report at muster daily in the morning and attend all parades and drills. The prisoners scraped, cleaned, and whitewashed the walls of the jail with lime at least yearly. Often prison labor was used for other projects thought to be appropriate for the improvement of the islands, including cutting lumber and quarrying stones. Hard labor was allowed—no more than 10 hours daily and not simultaneously with a bread-and-water punishment diet. The jail keeper had to inspect each cell daily. Leg irons and solitary confinement were liberally applied. The warden of the prison had a minor degree of latitude in the administration of punishments and labor duties. Occasionally the jail journal contained an entry like the following: "Prisoner was relieved of hard labor today, seeing that it was his birthday." Many prisoners were housed in ship hulks—decommissioned ships that were no longer seaworthy but were adequate for the confinement of prisoners. The worst risk, however, of being jailed was the threat of disease—yellow fever and dysentery being the most common ailments, many of the cases fatal.

While Swan was jailed, about 18 other prisoners were there with him, the number ranging from about 16–20 during his incarceration. Weekly attendants in the St. Georges jail were Dr. Frederick A.S. Hunter and the Reverend Doctor Tucker. The degree of medical or spiritual support given, however, was likely not extensive. Swan's tenure in the jail wasn't distinguished. Very little is recorded about his stay. His wife visited him in jail only three times, on April 29, May 6, and May 13 in the Hamilton gaol.[49] He had one other visitor, named Ann Hayward, on August 26.[50] Her exact relationship to Edward Swan and the purpose of the visit are unknown.

Matilda Swan couldn't bear the idea of waiting for her husband to be released, and she quickly retreated to New York, arriving on May 25 accompanied by Frederic Buckstaff. Matilda Swan and Frederic Buckstaff simply travelling together was considered scandalous, even though her son "Master Christopher Swan" had travelled to New York with them.[51] She would belatedly testify on May 29 before the Office of the Superintendent of the Metropolitan Police in New York that others were the principal parties involved in the shipping of the trunks. She was attempting to exonerate her husband, who by then was beginning his sentence of four months in jail. She implicated Joseph Hayne Rainey, the barber and bartender at the Hamilton Hotel, as the man who was actually supposed to transport the trunks to the United States. Rainey had been born a slave in Georgetown, South Carolina, and his father had purchased their freedom when the son was 14 years old. They had then moved to Charleston, where both worked as barbers.

Joseph Rainey and his wife Susan had moved to Bermuda in 1862. Susan, born a free black in Philadelphia, was a dressmaker. One of her clients was Mrs. Georgiana Walker, the wife of Confederate agent Norman Walker, who lived in St. Georges. When yellow fever decimated the shipping business in 1865 the Raineys moved to Hamilton, Bermuda, where Joseph worked in the Hamilton Hotel as a bartender and a barber. He would later return to the United States and become the first black member of the U.S. House of Representatives, elected from the State of South Carolina and serving from 1870 to 1879. The reports of the interrogation of Buckstaff and Mrs. Swan on May 29 discredited the stories they had fabricated since the trial in Bermuda, and their attempt to pin the blame for the storage and transport of the trunks on Joseph Rainey was unsuccessful.

District Attorney Gray said, in summary, "There is no truth in Matilda Swan's statement." Furthermore, regarding Rainey's involvement, Bermuda district attorney S. Brownlow Gray said that there was "no ground whatever for suspecting Rainey of complicity in this plot, much less for preferring any charge against him." Gray—in his letter of July 18, 1865, to Bermuda lieutenant

10. The Second Shipment of Articles Contaminated   141

governor and commander-in-chief Colonel William George Hamley—also expressed doubt about the veracity of Buckstaff's testimony. Gray questioned the propriety of the relationship between Buckstaff and Matilda Swan and said that "what was generally understood to be their relation the one to the other ... [shouldn't] command the respect or confidence of any Bermuda jury."[52]

Swan was finally released from the St. Georges jail on September 29, 1865.[53] He was reported to have "dieted" there for 123 days, a term used to denote the number of days the government had to furnish him with food and lodging. He had previously "dieted" in the St. Georges jail for 8 days (April 22–28) and 32 days (April 28–May 29) in the Hamilton jail.

11

Trials in Canada

Dr. Blackburn had fled back to Canada just in time to avoid being summoned to the trial of Edward Swan in Bermuda. He would face legal difficulties in both Canada and the United States, but his major risk was in the United States. So he remained in Canada.

After Blackburn returned to Canada, Sir James Hope, commander-in-chief of the North American and West Indies Station of the Royal British Navy, suggested that it would be appropriate to present the good Dr. Blackburn with a token of appreciation for his service to British subjects on the islands of Bermuda. The Lords of the Admiralty chose to bestow the Blackburns with two gifts—a gold watch for Dr. Blackburn and a gold bracelet for Mrs. Blackburn. Since the Blackburns were in Canada at the time, these testimonials were sent to the governor general of Canada, Viscount Charles Monck, who was to present the gifts at St. Lawrence Hall in Montreal, where the Blackburns were staying. But when the time came for awarding the watch and bracelet, stories began to circulate about the possible ulterior motives for Dr. Blackburn's generosity in Bermuda. Sir James Hope vacillated about presenting the gifts. Blackburn was feeling pressure about the accusations against him and wrote to officials in London asking for some support, at least some positive affirmation about his role in treating the yellow fever epidemic, as though he sensed an approaching need for witnesses and testimonials on his behalf. It is unclear if Dr. and Mrs. Blackburn ever received the watch and bracelet, but ultimately Queen Victoria of England gave him a humanitarian award, including a token gift of 100£ for his aid and assistance in fighting those yellow fever epidemics in Bermuda. But had his real motive been known, the queen might have thought twice about honoring this man who collected the clothing of dead and dying victims of the yellow fever epidemic in order to kill Northerners.[1] Blackburn's good luck would not last. Having fled Bermuda, he would soon be apprehended.

While Edward Swan's trial was being held in Bermuda, Blackburn was himself arrested in Montreal on May 19 (some sources say May 18).[2] His bail

11. Trials in Canada

was set on May 26, 1865, at $4,000, with two "sureties" of $2,000 each, and he was charged with violating Canada's neutrality laws. Coincidentally, he was received into the Catholic church and baptized at St. Lawrence Hall that week (having "abandoned [his] Protestant prejudices"), the reasons for his conversion to Catholicism from his Presbyterian roots being unclear.[3]

Detroit lawyer Halmer H. Emmons was working on retainer from the Union government "to assist in extradition cases" and trials involving international issues. He had been working with Godfrey Hyams, attempting to convince him to testify about the yellow fever plot. Emmons wrote to Judge Advocate General Joseph Holt in Washington, D.C., on April 28, saying that Blackburn would be detained in Canada for trial in the yellow fever plot. (Blackburn's associate Jacob Thompson had already escaped to England, where he remained until 1869.)[4]

Emmons reported to Holt on April 28: "Without efficient aid from our Government they [Blackburn and Thompson] cannot be convicted." He pleaded with Holt to cooperate with the lawyers in the Canadian trial, and to offer Hyams "an authoritative promise of protection." He mentioned needing for Hyams a "retainer for a few months ... [that would be] indispensable to success." Emmons wanted funding to pay for future transportation and support for Hyams, as well as repayment for what Emmons had already spent on the prosecution: "Is there no way in which I can be authorized to employ for a month or two one or two of these men [witnesses] at a moderate rate? I should like to realize too my advances." He wrote to Colonel La Fayette C. Baker, a Union spy, War Department official, and later general and chief of the National Detective Police, provost marshal of the War Department, and investigator of the Lincoln Assassination: "I have advanced some three or four hundred dollars in the matters in the belief that they were of such importance that Mr. Baker would deem it within his provinces." He also predicted that most suspects would be released after only a few days, like the St. Albans raiders, "because there was no proof of action in Canada," unless the United States government aided the investigation and the prosecution. "But without the immediate assistance the opportunity of securing the most important arrests will be lost. It is worse than useless to leave the matter simply to Canadian prosecution, as however well disposed, without our assistance they cannot succeed." He also suggested prosecuting Blackburn in Halifax, perhaps anticipating the jurisdictional disputes that eventually would result in Blackburn's acquittal and release: "I believe it will amply repay our Government in the end to promote their prosecution at Halifax. Unaided, however, the local authorities there can do nothing."[5]

Toronto police detective Francis McGarry had filed a complaint in Toronto on May 10, 1865, charging Blackburn and Hyams and "divers other persons unknown," beginning April 15, 1864, alleging:

[They did] combine, conspire, confederate and agree among themselves to commit the crime of murder in the United States of America, by importing and introducing from Her Majesty's dominions into certain cities of the said United States of America, to wit: the City of Washington, in the District of Columbia; the City of Norfolk, in the State of Virginia, one of the said United States of America; and the City of Newberne [sic], in the State of North Carolina, one of the said United States of America, and there disposing of, to and amongst the inhabitants of said cities, divers large quantities of shirts, blouses, coats, and other articles of clothing, infected with the virus of yellow fever and other deadly, poisonous and noxious substances, calculated and liable to produce said fever, for the purpose of creating and spreading the said fever amongst the said citizens, and of causing the death of the said citizens by means of said yellow fever and the poisonous, deadly and noxious substances aforesaid.[6] [Further] Luke P. Blackburn, to wit, the 1st day of June, 1864, did cause to be exported and sent from the said City of Halifax, in the Province of Nova Scotia, divers, to wit, tea-trunks containing such infected clothing into the said United States, and did cause the said infected clothing to be disposed of ... for the wicked and unlawful purpose, and with the wicked intent aforesaid; and that by means of the said infected clothing, so imported in and disposed of as aforesaid, in the said cities, in pursuance of said conspiracy, the death of divers persons in said cities, to the informant unknown, was caused and procured.[7]

McGarry charged that Blackburn shipped the clothing in trunks to the United States on June 1, 1864, and accused Blackburn of plotting to kill thousands of Northerners.

On May 19, 1865, officials in Montreal had arrested Blackburn and had him moved to Toronto. Just prior to his arrest as he left for Toronto, Dr. Blackburn said tearfully, "I am entirely innocent; but I have a secret presentiment that I am about to be delivered to the North, because I am being taken to Upper Canada."[8]

The magistrates court in Toronto was to hear the case. The star witnesses were to be Godfrey J. Hyams, William W. Cleary, and Edwin J. Hall. McGarry, the Toronto police detective, had located Blackburn at Montreal's St. Lawrence Hall, the fancy hotel where Confederate sympathizers and agents congregated. It was here and at other haunts in Montreal that Booth, Lawrence, Thompson, Clay, Blackburn, Sanders, and perhaps Kane had hatched many of their "black ops" schemes to destroy the North—fire-bombing cities, poisoning water supplies, kidnapping Lincoln, freeing Southern prisoners, destroying dams, and maybe even assassinating the president. The Canadian Rebel sympathizers wanted to remove the head from the body of the Union government. From there, events accelerated.

Blackburn's colleagues weighed in on the controversy. The *Medical and Surgical Reporter* of Philadelphia outlined the charges and concluded with these words about Blackburn: "A fiend, and he is a physician, in the employ of what professed to be 'a Government,' [the Confederacy] engaged in efforts to spread 'among the masses' in this country, a virulent and fatal disease, which, when it broke out in former years in Southern cities, enlisted the sympathies and cooperation of our profession in all parts of the country in behalf of those who ... were afflicted. It were too much to believe, if it had not the most convincing testimony to support it!"[9]

On May 23, 1865, following a warrant dated that same day, Blackburn was brought before the police court in Toronto on charges of violating Canada's neutrality laws by conspiring to overthrow the Northern government. Police magistrate Mr. Bloomer presided. Mr. James Paterson was the lawyer for the Crown, and Mr. M.C. Cameron and a Mr. Kerr appeared as lawyers for Blackburn. Paterson was a member of the law firm [James] Paterson, [James] Harrison, and [Robert A.] Paterson. Francis Henry Medcalf, the Toronto Mayor, Mr. Gilbert McMicken, the "Frontier Stipendiary Magistrate," and Mr. James Cahill, the police magistrate for Hamilton, Canada West, were also on the bench.[10]

Hyams testified first, swearing on a copy of the Old Testament (he was Jewish) that his testimony would be true. He was not charged with any infraction in this Canadian court, but essentially retold the entire story of the soiled clothing and Blackburn's plan to have Hyams distribute the contaminated articles in the Northern United States. Letters written in early 1865 and introduced in evidence at the Toronto trial stated Hyams' claims of Confederate military service. Hyams also told the court about his leg wound suffered at about the time Union general Samuel Ryan Curtis took possession of Helena, Arkansas.[11] Hyams told of his property that had been destroyed in Helena, Arkansas, by Union troops. He also told of being arrested and sent to St. Louis, where he remained for a total of 11 weeks, confined for being a Southern sympathizer. Other testimony described him as being "expelled" from Arkansas, so perhaps his arrest didn't occur until he resided a brief time in St. Louis. But records from Gratiot Street Prison and Alton Prison show that his imprisonment lasted only about one week, from August 27 through September 4, 1862, and then he lived in St. Louis for the next five months. He was indeed less than accurate in some of the details he would report.

The Rev. Dr. Stuart Robinson was the second witness at Blackburn's hearing. Both Hyams and Robinson testified orally. Robinson's testimony added little to Hyams' account, though Robinson claimed that the destitute Hyams frequently asked him for money. Robinson estimated that he gave Hyams about $20 three times over the course of their acquaintance, usually with Robinson thinking the money was going for supplies for Hyams' shoe repair business. Robinson again denied knowledge of the plot between Blackburn and Hyams to infect the North with yellow fever. His denial was likely a falsehood. He told the court he had introduced Hyams and Blackburn, establishing the personal connection between the two. Sworn documents from William W. Cleary, the Confederate Canadian secretary to Jacob

Thompson, and Edwin J. Hall, another Confederate operative, were also admitted into evidence in the Toronto hearing, though neither man appeared in person. Cleary was available to testify, but his personal appearance wasn't required. Cleary, Thompson, and Blackburn had all been rooming at St. Lawrence Hall in Montreal in January 1865. Cleary claimed that Blackburn first revealed the yellow fever plot to Thompson then. Blackburn, according to Cleary in his sworn deposition, believed Thompson would be funding the plot through Confederate sources. Thompson had refused to participate in the plot, claiming that he had a family and reputation to protect, and he "would not furnish a dollar for any such undertaking."[12] Cleary had no respect for Hyams' honesty, and Cleary claimed that Blackburn had paid Hyams to "distribute among the army of the United States clothing which he had prepared, I think he said, at Bermuda, infected with yellow fever."[13] Also through his sworn deposition Edwin J. Hall told of the $20 bribe Hyams had used to smuggle the trunks into Boston. However, Hall denied knowledge of the contents of the trunks, and he denied any understanding of a plot to infect the North.

To seek more expense money, Hyams had found it necessary to return from Baltimore to Canada and had briefly stored the trunks in Baltimore. He was penniless at the time and couldn't even raise money for his own transportation to the Clifton House, so Hall loaned him funds for this short trip. Watching his own expenses carefully, Hall had asked Blackburn for reimbursement. He reported that he received a telegram from some unnamed person at the Clifton House, asking him to tell Hyams to go meet with Blackburn at St. Catharines. Hall and Hyams traveled together on the ship *Silver Spray* to St. Catharines to meet with Blackburn. Hall said that on this trip Hyams vaguely related some outlines of the plot and told Hall he had encountered some difficulty at the Boston Customs House in obtaining passage for some trunks—that he had to pay some $20 gold pieces to bribe agents and personally traveled from Halifax to Boston, even though his mission wasn't completed yet. Hall denied knowledge even then of the purpose of the trip: "I had not the slightest idea of what his mission was or what enterprise he was engaged in until I heard it mentioned, by William L. McDonald, a few weeks since.... Mr. McDonald in speaking of Hyams' enterprise, said it was taking clothing infected with yellow fever into the United States to be introduced amongst the soldiers."[14] Blackburn's attorney was willing to admit— for the sake of argument—that the facts proposed by Hyams and Robinson might be correct. But he contended that technicalities of the case demanded that Blackburn be acquitted. Because Blackburn's lawyer didn't object to the facts presented, no other witnesses were called.

The trial in Canada relied heavily on Hyams' testimony. Hyams reported the promise of $100,000 from the Confederate coffers through Blackburn

11. Trials in Canada

and Thompson and revealed that they had actually given him only a paltry advance, not even sufficient to cover his travel expenses. While Hyams' statements implicated Jacob Thompson and even Jefferson Davis in the plot, William W. Cleary's affidavit stated that the plan was entirely Blackburn's brainchild, apparently cutting any link to Thompson, to the Confederate Secret Service's treasurer, and to any direct connection to Jefferson Davis. Since Hyams was clearly a man motivated by money and the need for immunity from prosecution, his testimony had to be viewed skeptically. Cleary's statements held more weight and seemed to be closer to the truth. Blackburn was unequivocally involved. Perhaps none of the others were conspirators in the scheme, and maybe Blackburn was acting purely on his own initiative. Most testimonies seemed to mesh.

Cameron, Blackburn's lawyer, proposed that "the evidence only disclosed a conspiracy to commit a crime abroad and beyond the jurisdiction of our Courts, and was consequently not triable here."[15] Blackburn didn't testify in Toronto, apparently because he was ill at the time. The police magistrate in the police court of Toronto ruled on May 25, 1865, that enough circumstantial evidence existed to proceed to a full trial. Blackburn would thus stand trial at the next assize (one of the Canadian courts). He was released on a $4,000 bail and two $2,000 sureties.[16] The trial was scheduled for October 1865. David Thurston, the U.S. consul in Toronto, wrote in May 1865 to Halmer H. Emmons, expressing his dismay at the matchup of Paterson for the prosecution against Cameron for the defense, because this case was the "most infamous scheme to injure our country." He followed by writing, "Paterson prosecuted, + it seemed to me a farce to pit him against M.C. Cameron. Paterson is so deaf he can't hear half that is said, + he is beside half dead with consumption. I protested against the suit being conducted without Harrison [Paterson's law partner] being present but to no effect. At any rate the trial is postponed to Oct."[17] On July 22, 1865, Edward Cardwell, secretary of state for the Canadian Colonies, wrote to Lord Monck stating that in his opinion Blackburn was indeed "triable in Canada for conspiracy to commit murder in the United States, though it is not apparent how he can be indicted upon the same facts for that which is termed a breach of the 'Neutrality Laws.'"[18]

As Blackburn awaited his trial in Toronto before the assize court, his public reputation deteriorated. He was described in newspapers as an "uneducated charlatan" who "knew even less than he supposed of the nature of the fearful epidemic, and expected contagious results that do not follow the latitude where he disposed of the infected goods." They called him a "large-bodied blusterer, who murdered his English and misspelled the simplest words." His plot was "regarded throughout Canada as one of the most diabolical crimes that a human being could possibly engage in, and Blackburn was designated as the yellow-fever fiend."[19] The *New York Times* wrote as follows:

> Such an act cannot be held to belong to civilized war. It is an outrage against humanity, calling for, and will receive, the universal execration of mankind. Civilized war implies an attempt to kill one's enemy while he stands up with arms in his hands, attempting on his side to kill; but it shrinks from seeking the lives of noncombatants and women and children by insidious sickness. No punishment can be too severe for such an offence. For the rest, it is an incident of human life to be most profoundly deplored that a man could fall from so high a position as that which Dr. BLACKBURN [emphasis in the original] held into so deep an abyss as this evidence seems to have placed him. It was an evil hour for him in which over-zeal for the cause of his country, or desire to take revenge for her injuries, or the temptation of the devil, led him to commit himself to so foul a crime. He had better himself have died.[20]

The *Philadelphia Inquirer* had this to say:

> Dr. Blackburn, of yellow fever notoriety, is there [at the Queen's Hotel] also, fat and pompous, but deploringly neglected, and wearing a worn and seedy appearance. He spends nearly all of his time in a saloon on King street, but is little noticed, even by the crowd that generally frequents a saloon. He denies that he is guilty of endeavoring to introduce the infected rags into New York and other Northern cities, but deems that it would have been quite a legitimate mode of warfare. He does not seem to entertain much hope of a pardon, or to fear that punishment will overtake him.[21]

The trial in October 1865 in Toronto was dependent upon a few technicalities (court records of this trial have disappeared, but newspaper accounts remain). The court ruled that since the trunks had been brought from Bermuda into Halifax—which then was not a part of Canada—the court in Toronto had no jurisdiction over the actual importation of the contaminated articles. The goods had never been on Canadian soil, nor did the prosecution purport that they had been there. And—though this was no technicality—since the trunks hadn't ever been recovered or taken to Canada as evidence, there was insufficient proof to convict Blackburn on the violation of neutrality laws. Much of the conspiracy to gather and distribute the trunks was directed from Halifax, Nova Scotia, although certainly many meetings dealing with the plot had taken place in Montreal and Toronto. However, the evidence for these meetings and their content were deemed to be too "circumstantial." Furthermore, Blackburn's lawyer, M.C. Cameron, successfully argued that even if the court had jurisdiction, the only relevant law on the books in Canada prohibited a citizen from plotting to kill a head of state. The court agreed that Blackburn, even if guilty, was not guilty of plotting to kill a head of state. Though the contaminated shirts to be sent to Lincoln certainly should have qualified as such a plot, this critical detail was not discussed. And "a conspiracy to commit a misdemeanor in a foreign country was not an offence against the law of this country," argued Blackburn's attorney, though he purported that the testimony presented wasn't even sufficient to prove such an alleged conspiracy. They were technicalities, most of them, for sure, though important ones.

The law officers of the Crown in Canada decided that the case against Blackburn was "by no means sufficient to enable the Crown to prosecute Blackburn with any chance of success, and there was no prospect of obtaining any further evidence." On October 16 the case was essentially dismissed, and the bail and sureties were refunded because the evidence was insufficient to make a conviction likely. The official letter confirming this judgment was penned on October 27, 1865. Blackburn wasn't completely released, however. He was admitted to bail on his own recognizance, and was "to appear whenever called upon,"[22] which turned out to be never. Blackburn was now a free man in Canada, but he still couldn't return to the United States.

Yet another detail inhibited Blackburn's prosecution. Even in the mid-19th century, a case was far more compelling if a party had actually been damaged by the accused's actions. Even though a huge outbreak of yellow fever had begun in New Bern, North Carolina, in 1864, the evidence connecting Blackburn to the epidemic was flimsy at best. No firm evidence existed that connected the trunks to any final destination in New Bern. The event also had occurred in another country—the United States. Had the connection between Blackburn's trunks and the outbreak in New Bern been more convincing, he might have been convicted, at least in a court in the United States. Since many doctors believed yellow fever could be transmitted from one person to the next by touching contaminated clothing, reliable medical testimony would certainly have implicated, if not directly connected, Blackburn to the 2,000–3,000 deaths in New Bern in 1864. But they didn't. So the Canadians ultimately dropped all of the charges against Blackburn. Of course, officials in the United States didn't look upon Blackburn so dispassionately.

New Bern, North Carolina, had indeed experienced a yellow fever epidemic in August 1864, near the time Blackburn's trunks were scheduled to be delivered there. As many as 2,000–3,000 people died—soldiers and civilians alike. Conditions in New Bern were ideal for the real terrorist responsible for the spread of yellow fever—the *Aedes aegypti* mosquito. New Bern lies about 170 miles to the south, and slightly east, of Richmond. In March 1862 the Union forces captured this low-lying region at the head of the Neuse River, a strategic location where railroad lines met water-shipping routes. Marshy lowlands, swamps, and poorly drained wetlands dominated the landscape. The town of New Bern itself was a typical Southern climate—hot, rainy, humid, and covered with mud. The unpaved streets provided ideal breeding grounds for the mosquito. Union forces held this region for the duration of the war, and it made an appealing target for recapture by the Confederate forces, hence Blackburn's goal of ridding this crucial port city of its Northern occupiers. When the yellow fever epidemic hit, panic followed.

All who could travel left the city. Since the mode of transmission of yellow fever was unknown, and the prevailing theory was that miasmas, or vapors, carried the disease, residents sought escape from the town where the stagnant air and smelly mud puddles dominated the environment. The Union military encampment added to the depressing scene. Sanitation was either horrific or nonexistent, and the troops would move from one site to a nearby new site whenever the stench of their own occupation became unbearable.

Yellow fever was a disease that spread rapidly and killed quickly. Mary Phinney von Olnhausen, an army nurse at the Morehead City Hospital, about 35 miles to the south of New Bern, wrote on September 30, 1864, "Till you are with it you can have no idea of this dreadful fever; nothing else approaches it except cholera. The effect upon the spirits would alone be distressing enough; but then the agony of the patient, and his consciousness of the danger add so much to the horror. No one expects to live, and when the black vomit comes that look of despair with the 'There is no show for me any longer' makes your heart just full."[23] It was a Confederate terrorist's dream of the ideal method to demoralize the Union army.

Even pro–Confederate Canadian newspapers reported that the yellow fever plot was a sinister deed falling outside the bounds of "gentlemanly warfare" or the morals of the routine conduct of hostilities. Of course, newspapers in areas targeted by the scheme were even more vehement in their denunciation of Blackburn: "This hideous and long studied plan to deliberately murder innocent men, women, and children, who had never wronged him in any manner, is regarded here as an act of cruelty without a parallel—a crime which can only be estimated and punished in the presence of his victims in another world."[24] The *Toronto Globe* said that Blackburn was "a criminal of the worst sort who should be deported under the Alien Act." Other reporters opined that Hyams should be hanged.[25] Later medical knowledge that the transmission of the disease required mosquitoes for the human-to-mosquito-to-human cycle would historically absolve Blackburn of his responsibility in causing yellow fever. While he could have been charged with conspiracy to murder thousands, he wasn't. Furthermore, charges could have been brought against Blackburn in Halifax, where the trunks were delivered en route to the North. Nova Scotia was a part of the British Empire, not yet a part of Canada, and officials there could have brought charges against Blackburn, as they had been in Montreal and Toronto. Detroit lawyer Halmer Emmons had even suggested prosecution in Halifax, but the government of Nova Scotia never took any action.

Research into even other means of killing people and spreading panic were underway in the Confederate laboratories, at least one of which was in Richmond. Richard Sears McCulloh was a chemistry professor from Columbia University in New York who had returned to his home in the South to support the Confederacy.²⁶ He developed a liquid in early 1865 that would both kill from the effects of its vapor and spontaneously combust. His invention was reported to Jefferson Davis on February 11, 1865, but the South lost the war before this weapon could be put to use.²⁷ Unlike Blackburn, McCulloh was apprehended off the coast off Florida, tried, and sentenced to serve two years in prison—solitary confinement in the Virginia State Penitentiary. But like Blackburn, he would return to polite society as a chemistry professor at Washington College (now Washington and Lee University) in Lexington, Virginia.²⁸

Godfrey Hyams not only gave evidence against Blackburn, he was also a witness in other trials of Confederate plotters, betraying their trust. He testified against William Lawrence McDonald in Toronto in April 1865. McDonald first resided with his sister on Adelaide Street in Toronto, the same street where Dr. Blackburn had initially established a medical practice in Canada. In October 1864 he moved to Agnes Street, where he labored for the Southern cause, allegedly under the order and financing of Jacob Thompson. There McDonald made "torpedoes, hand shells, Greek fire and other explosive missiles." He was accused of manufacturing those bombs to be used against Union targets, and his trial began on April 26 in the Toronto Police Court. Hyams had been McDonald's friend (and Hyams was involved in the making of bombs, or at least he was intimately aware of the activity and its purpose). Hyams as a witness said, "I have been engaged in some of the raids and occupations above mentioned, and by these means became informed of and intimate with the action of McDonald and others." Officials found the bombs in the house Hyams had identified, so at least part of his testimony was accurate. Hyams had knowledge that could have been obtained only through close association with McDonald. He knew not only the location of the munitions factory, but he was also able to lead authorities to the residence and expose the cache of explosives under a small trap door on the ground floor of the building. Police Sergeant Major Hastings testified that he went to the Agnes Street residence, where Hyams descended through the trap door and retrieved 26 "torpedoes." Hyams' friend J.A. Posey testified to similar details, and the case was referred by the grand jury for trial as a "true bill," meaning that the evidence seemed to indicate enough proof to hold a formal legal hearing.²⁹

Hyams also testified against the St. Albans conspirators, specifically Bennett H. Young. In fact, Hyams' testimony against McDonald had to be delayed because he was simultaneously giving evidence against Young in the trial of those charged in the St. Albans raid. Hyams was indeed probably the least reliable witness against Blackburn, though his story fits well with the known facts, dates, and movements of the Confederate agents and corresponds well with independent testimony of other witnesses. But Southern-leaning newspapers gave Dr. Blackburn the benefit of the doubt, based on Blackburn's prior reputation as a compassionate physician and Hyams' history of being a traitor.[30]

Conflicting views of all of these persons were numerous, however. The Confederate blockade-runner Thomas Taylor recorded, speaking of Blackburn, that an "eminent Confederate military doctor proposed to me during the prevalence of the yellow fever epidemic that he should ship by our boats to Nassau and Bermuda sundry cases of infected clothing, which were to be sent to the North with the idea of spreading the disease there. This was too much, and I shouted to him, not in the choicest language, to leave the office. It is difficult to conceive of such a diabolical idea, not only to spread havoc among combatants, but among innocent women and children, being present in an educated man's mind"[31]

12

Trials in the United States

The trial of the Lincoln assassination conspirators would be held in Washington, D.C., beginning in May 1865. Even the venue raised serious questions. In fact, the opening dispute of the trial centered on which court—military or civilian—should try the case. The first ruling dealt with this jurisdiction, and the military option would win: "That the persons implicated in the murder of the late President, Abraham Lincoln, and the attempted assassination of the Honorable William H. Seward, Secretary of State, and in an alleged conspiracy to assassinate other officers of the Federal Government at Washington City, and their aiders and abettors, are subject to the jurisdiction of, and lawfully triable before, a Military Commission...."[1] Even today many constitutional scholars believe it should have been held in civilian courts.

This Military Commission comprised nine military officers who would be chosen by the assistant adjutant general and approved by President Andrew Johnson, with the judge advocate general of the army and recorder of the commission being Brigadier-General Joseph Holt. The assistant judge advocates would be Honorable John A. Bingham and Brevet Colonel H.L. Burnett. The trial was convened on May 8, 1865, with preliminary statements before the nine-person Military Commission; the first witness was heard May 12. The document initially stated the following:

> CHARGE.—For maliciously, unlawfully, and traitorously, and in aid of the the [sic] existing armed rebellion against the United States of America, in or before the 6th day of March, A.D. 1865, and on divers other days between that day and the 15th day of April, A.D. 1865, combining, confederating, and conspiring together with one John H. Surratt, John Wilkes Booth, Jefferson Davis, George N. Sanders, Beverly Tucker, Jacob Thompson, William C. Cleary, Clement C. Clay, George Harper, George Young, and others unknown, to kill and murder, within the Military Department of Washington, and within the fortified and intrenched lines thereof, Abraham Lincoln, late, and at the time of said combining, confederating, and conspiring, President of the United States of America, and Commander-in-Chief of the Army and Navy thereof; Andrew Johnson, now Vice-President of the United States aforesaid; William H. Seward, Secretary of State of the United States aforesaid; and

Ulysses S. Grant, Lieutenant-General of the Army of the United States aforesaid, then in command of the Armies of the United States, under the direction of the said Abraham Lincoln....[2]

The Military Commission carefully allowed itself latitude to add later to the charges the names of any other suspects who might be implicated by testimony during the trial:

A Military Commission is hereby appointed to meet at Washington, District of Columbia, on Monday, the 8th day of May, 1865, at 9 o'clock a.m., or as soon thereafter as practicable, for the trial of David E. Herold, George A. Atzerodt, Lewis Payne, Michael O'Laughlin, Edward Spangler, Samuel Arnold, Mary E. Surratt, Samuel A. Mudd, and such other prisoners as may be brought before it, implicated in the murder of the late President, Abraham Lincoln, and the attempted assassination of the Honorable William H. Seward, Secretary of State, and in an alleged conspiracy to assassinate other officers of the Federal Government at Washington City, and their aiders and abettors.[3]

Only the eight primary defendants were ultimately tried in these proceedings.[4] Blackburn, whose efforts attempting to import yellow fever to the North were mentioned at the outset of the trial, would be the subject of some of the testimony. One of the official records of the trial begins with a summary of the various aspects of the proceedings:

Containing the Orders convening the Commission; Rules for its guidance; Pleas of the accused to the Jurisdiction of the Commission, and for Severance of Trial; Testimony in full concerning the Assassination, and attending circumstances; Flight, pursuit and capture of John Wilkes Booth; Attempted Assassination of Hon. W.H. Seward, Secretary of State. Official Documents and Testimony relating to the following plots: The Abduction of the President and Cabinet, and carrying them to Richmond; The Assassination of the President and Cabinet; The Murder of President Lincoln by presents of infected clothing; The introduction of pestilence into Northern cities by clothing infected with Yellow Fever and Small Pox; Starvation and murder of Union prisoners in Southern prisons; Attempted burning of New York and other Northern cities; Poisoning the water of the Croton Reservoir, New York; Raid on St. Albans; Contemplated raids on Buffalo, Ogdensburg, etc.; Burning of Steamboats on Western rivers, Government "Warehouses," Hospitals, etc.; Complicity of Jefferson Davis, Judah P. Benjamin, Jacob Thompson, George N. Sanders, Beverley Tucker, C.C. Clay, etc.; Jacob Thompson's banking account in Canada; The mining of Libby Prison, and preparations to blow it up; The "disorganization of the North" by a system of terrorism and infernal plots; Arguments of Counsel for the Accused; Reply of Hon. J.A. Bingham, Special Judge Advocate; Findings and Sentences of the Accused, etc.[5]

Blackburn was involved in some of the deeds listed. Initially, prosecutors thought the assassination of President Lincoln was closely connected to the Canadian Confederates, based in part upon a bank receipt found on John Wilkes Booth's body. This receipt for 61 pounds, six shillings, 10 pence was

12. Trials in the United States

dated October 27, 1864, and was signed by 'H. Stanus, Manager, Royal Ontario Bank in Montreal," where Booth and Thompson both had accounts. Booth was known to have gone at least twice to Canada in the months immediately prior to Lincoln's murder. Prosecutors would try to connect the other Canadian conspirators to the assassination.

The United States government tried to have Blackburn arrested and extradited to Washington, D.C., for the conspirators' trial because it believed he held some information that would link Jefferson Davis and the Confederate government to the plot to assassinate Lincoln. Though Davis had sent his commissioners to Canada and had provided them with funds, the directions for their activity were both vague and verbal. The United States needed a witness who could provide evidence against Davis. Blackburn was at this very time being tried in Canada, and efforts to extradite him might have been delayed for that reason.

Consul Charles M. Allen in Bermuda had relayed his information about Dr. Blackburn and Edward Swan to Judge Advocate General Joseph Holt. Holt was beginning the proceedings headed toward a trial against the Lincoln conspirators in Washington, D.C. The U.S. Bureau of Military Justice recognized that Blackburn might be an important suspect in the trial. Blackburn's yellow fever plot had included the gift of the fancy valise with the elegant but contaminated shirts to be given to Lincoln to infect him with yellow fever. Since Blackburn was connected with a scheme to kill Lincoln, Holt directed the Bureau of Military Justice to investigate how he might have been involved in Booth's actions.

By now Hyams had discovered that his financial plight had worsened, if that were even possible. When he started his odyssey, he at least had a shoe repair business. Now he had nothing, as his wife had been forced to sell everything to buy food. Given the turn of events, Hyams couldn't have had anything but contempt for Blackburn and his entire scheme. He had been promised a minimum of $100,000; he had received a meager $520, which barely covered his expenses for travel, food, and lodging. Had Blackburn ever intended to pay him? Was Hyams just a tool for someone else to achieve a goal? Hyams was livid. He had been languishing in poverty for months, and now it was time to strike back. He was finally convinced that he'd never be paid the $100,000 for his dangerous work, so he gave up the idea of riches coming from the Confederates. Tired of being used and not being paid by the Confederate operatives in Canada, he decided to expose the plot and "turn state's evidence." Maybe the Union would reward him.

On April 5, 1865, Hyams went into the office of David Thurston, the U.S. consular agent in Toronto and told him he had valuable information he would give in exchange for money and a pardon for his parts in the Confederate schemes. (Hyams may first have given some information to Robert Harrison,

Toronto's Crown attorney, a position similar to a district attorney in the United States.) Hyams offered to testify about many of the Confederate schemes, not only the biologic warfare but others as well. He needed money, and he needed protection from prosecution. Thurston held out the possibility of the former, and perhaps he would be able to secure the latter. Thurston wrote to Secretary of State William H. Seward on April 7:

> [A] person by name of Hyams, resident in this city + who has been intimately associated with the rebels here, called on me + stated that he was in possession of important information in relation to the plans of the Rebels.... He had been connected with the Rebels for several years—+ that all their schemes and plots were well known to him—which he was desirous of communicating to me if I would remunerate him for so doing. I said to him that I would be glad to receive any communications of the kind which he had to make, but I wished him to understand that the information he gave me would be submitted to the Gov't of the U.S + if it was considered of value a proper remuneration would be made, but that the Gov't of the U.S. would be the judge whether it was or was not of any value, or if any use could be made of the information given—but under no circumstances would I guarantee any return for his communication, if he gave it on these conditions he might do so. He replied he was willing to accept those terms.[6]

While Hyams has been censured by the press as a poor witness—he was popularly known as a perjurer-for-hire—many others corroborated his testimony. He has been described frequently in derogatory terms—penniless, willing to do anything for money, fearful for his role in Blackburn's plot, and wanting immunity for his own crimes. He was poor and low-class, a Southerner who had defected twice. Starting as a Union supporter, he converted to being a Southern sympathizer when Union troops attacked his house. In addition, he wanted money from the United States government for his testimony. Blackburn's biographer called Hyams "an inglorious turncoat whose loyalties responded to money rather than to a cause."[7] Not considering further how his testimony might tarnish his reputation and the subsequent effect it would have on his monetary value as a witness, Hyams described his view of the Blackburn plot as the importation of clothing "carefully infected in Bermuda with yellow fever, smallpox, and other contagious diseases."[8] On April 12, 1865, three days after Robert E. Lee surrendered at Appomattox and two days before Lincoln was shot, Hyams revealed his knowledge of Blackburn's scheme to Union authorities.

Detroit lawyer Halmer Hull Emmons had heard similar rumors from other informants even before Hyams had offered to provide testimony about the yellow fever plot. On March 3, 1865, an acquaintance of Godfrey Hyams named Samuel Lewis wrote to Emmons offering information about "affairs that may be of some importance to you."[9] Lewis alluded to a prior meeting he had conducted with Emmons, though the date wasn't recorded. Lewis lived on the same block as Hyams on York Street in Toronto, Hyams being at 120 York Street and Lewis at 177 York Street. Lewis's information was second-hand at best. He and another friend, John Alexander Posey, would try to report what they had overheard about Confederate schemes—for money, of course—but their information was neither new nor extensive. Lewis was a "colored whitewasher," according to the 1866 Toronto directory,[10] and Posey initially advertised himself as a carpenter.[11] Emmons described Posey as "a tall young man, smooth face, stout."[12] They were friends and tag-alongs with Hyams, likely seeking money wherever they detected a possible source. Posey, at a point in time before Hyams defected to the North to deliver his evidence against Blackburn, was a spy within the cabal of Confederate conspirators, seeking information while trying to gain the confidence of those Confederates plotting against the North.[13] Of course, Emmons wouldn't know the extent of Posey and Lewis's first-hand knowledge (or lack of it) until he could question them.

The first note extant between Lewis and Emmons was dictated by Lewis but penned by Posey (he often went by the name "Alexander"). Perhaps Lewis had experienced some hand injury that briefly prevented his writing himself. Lewis later proved that he was literate and could write by composing his letters in his own handwriting. Lewis referenced Godfrey Hyams and some communication regarding information Lewis had about the Confederate Lake Erie Raid and the *Georgian* affair. Lewis promised to "bee [sic] faithful and do all that I can to help the Federal Government."[14] Lewis also dictated the next letter—put to paper by "J.A.P.," presumably Posey again—on March 11, 1865. It conveyed no useful information, but he asked for money: "If you can send me some money I would like it very much for I would like to stay in Chatham [a city near Toronto] five or six days that I may get on the trace [trail] of some things that is [sic] very important."[15] Lewis and Posey seemed to have identified the lawyer Emmons as a potential source of money in exchange for information.

Emmons, at about this time but after the revelation of the yellow fever plot, made notes about Posey and his connection with Hyams. Emmons was just beginning to piece together the story of Blackburn's trips to Bermuda, but he noted that Blackburn, "who was out of money + who had quarrelled with some of the leaders because his services had not been sufficiently requested would not be able to proceed with it."[16] On May 1, 1865, Posey wrote to Emmons, also revealing no useful information but again asking for money: "As I have no means to stay here on, will you send me some [money] and I will come to Detroit and you can then send me from there home.... I will do all I can against all of these raiders.... I hope that we bee [sic] able to get them.... Mr. Emmons I am owing some money hire [sic] for board and will you please send me eneouf [sic] to pay off here and pay my way to Detroit and from there you can send me home. I owe about twelve or fifteen dollars in Canadian money."[17] Posey appended a note on the back of the letter saying, "Mr. Hyams wrote you a letter to day but I thought that I had better write to you myself and let you know the exact condition that I am in."[18]

The trio on that block on York Street in Toronto—Hyams, Lewis, and Posey—had to have known what the others were doing, and all were trying to extract money from Emmons. The letter to Emmons from Hyams, written on May 1, said, in part, "I this day saw Mr. Patterson [sic] who told me he thought the trials of those men would not come off this court setting. I therefore would like to come to Detroit with my family.... Posey wishes to come allso [sic]. I should like you to send me some funds. I have paid off my debts. I am short now."[19] Both Posey and Lewis maintained contact with Emmons over the next few months. On June 19, 1865, Posey wrote to Emmons from Henderson, Kentucky, where he had gone home to live with his family and where he once again had become a farmer. He spoke of his rather dismal financial state, the need to pay former slaves $30–35 and board per month, and the scarcity of both male and female workers.[20]

On July 1, 1865, Lewis wrote to Emmons inquiring about his son, whom Emmons had given employment on the Emmons' farm near Detroit at the junction of the Escorse River and the Detroit River.[21] A final note from Posey to Emmons was dated January 23, 1866, also from Henderson, Kentucky. It said, "I shall never forget the kindness that you and your family showed to me while I lived with you."[22] Clearly, Emmons had befriended the Canadian informants. Posey had actually lived with Emmons for a time.

Emmons, a lawyer and not a physician, immediately sought help from a physician friend regarding the probability that Blackburn's plot could actually produce yellow fever. Dr. E.M. Clark wrote to Emmons on April 15, 1865: "I find that medical writers differ in opinion as to the contagiousness or noncontagiousness of yellow fever. The evidence seems rather to preponderate in favor of noncontagiousness. My own opinion is that fomites will under favorable circumstances convey yellow fever. I know that smallpox is very frequently so transmitted."[23]

• • •

The first "depositions" for hearings in the United States were taken in Toronto and Detroit. On April 5, 1865, Hyams told his story to the U.S. consul to Canada. He was directed to give a more complete and formal accounting to attorney Halmer H. Emmons in Detroit on April 12. Emmons was primarily a lawyer in private practice, his specialty being railroad law. Beset by chronically bad health, he also ran a farm in Ecorse, Michigan, about seven miles southwest of his office at 15 Bank Block in downtown Detroit. Emmons sent Hyams' story to United States attorney general James Speed in Washington,

12. Trials in the United States 159

D.C., on April 22. It would soon prompt a request for Hyams to testify in the Lincoln assassination trial, which would be held between May 9 and June 30 in Washington, D.C. Hyams would appear before this military tribunal on May 29, 1865.

He had much information to reveal and first disclosed details about the plot to free Confederate prisoners on Johnson's Island on Lake Erie.[24] After exposing his knowledge of this Confederate scheme he then proceeded to tell about a munitions factory in a house in Toronto where torpedoes, hand grenades, and "Greek fire" were being produced. Ultimately, his story proved to be true. He also claimed knowledge of the inner workings of the St. Albans Raid, the Confederate foray into St. Albans, Vermont, during which three people were killed, three banks were robbed, and other citizens were injured. Authorities willingly thrust Hyams into the witness chair at the trial of the St. Albans conspirators on April 10, even before he had outlined the Blackburn yellow fever plot for Emmons on April 12. Defendants in the St. Albans trial, including the leader of the St. Albans raid, Bennett Young, were quite unprepared to see Hyams perform as a surprise (and only) witness. Hyams further proved his knowledge by revealing the plan to disrupt fishing in the Atlantic. All of this information suddenly made him appear to be a valuable witness. It was then suggested that Hyams might be offered a pardon for his part in the yellow fever plot if he would disclose the details, and he subsequently gave the entire story as he knew it. His "confession" was tendered on April 12, 1865, just two days before Lincoln was shot. After giving the equivalent of a deposition in Toronto, he then repeated the information before attorney Emmons.

Details regarding the delivery of this testimony are conflicting. One report has Emmons traveling to Hamilton, Ontario, to meet Hyams and take his deposition.[25] Other reports say the testimony was proffered in Detroit. Likely it was given in Canada, as the original handwritten verbatim deposition document was dated by Emmons as "Hamilton April 12th, 1865," though the cover note has Emmons' Detroit address.[26] Hamilton is located between Detroit and Toronto, only about 40 miles from Toronto and 200 miles from Detroit. Alfred Russell, the district attorney for the Eastern District of Michigan, was in Chicago at this time, so Emmons took charge of the questioning and the communications about the matter. Emmons was both chronically ill and acutely sick around the time of all of these transactions, at times being "confined to my bed."[27]

Emmons had initially written to Attorney General James Speed "a few days" before April 17, the day he told Speed of the plot of "spreading infectious diseases" in the United States (his note arrived in Washington, D. C., on April 21). He alluded to Hyams' testimony, which he had in hand, and asked for assistance in his investigation by receiving a promise of pardons in return for the testimony of his informants. On April 18 Emmons affixed a P.S. to his note, saying that he would forward the necessary documents as soon as they had been copied. (Hyams' testimony was 19 handwritten pages long. Emmons needed to produce multiple copies and did most of the transcription by hand himself.) Nevertheless, he transmitted Hyams' testimony to Attorney General James Speed on April 22, adding that Blackburn and Thompson would likely have warrants issued soon for their arrests in Canada. In a telegram on April 19 and a letter on April 21, Attorney General Speed in Washington, D.C., quickly granted Assistant District Attorney Alfred Russell in Detroit the discretionary powers to offer pardons "in certain cases" in return for cooperation in the prosecution of higher-level conspirators. Russell replied on April 24: "I appreciate the responsibility involved [sic] upon me and shall endeavor to act discreetly and usefully to the Government in the matter. I have had occasion to promise fully but one pardon altho' I have held out hopes to others." It's unclear if he is referring to Hyams when mentioning the "one pardon," but certainly "others" would have included Hyams if Russell had not already proffered it.[28]

Alfred Russell, the assistant U.S. district attorney for the Eastern District, Detroit, Michigan, wrote to Brigadier General Joseph Holt, the judge advocate general, in Washington, D.C., on May 11, 1865, saying, "The Atty. Gen. [James Speed] of the U.S. has directed me to forward to you any information I might gather respecting the assassination and I accordingly enclose the affidavit of one Hyams, whom I have induced to come to this city from Canada, under promise of a pardon, which promise the Atty. Gen. empowered me to make. If you should deem the oral testimony of Hyams important, I can send him to Washington."[29] On May 19 Emmons and Russell sent a telegram to Speed informing him of Blackburn's arrest in Canada and again requesting assistance and financial support ("several thousand dollars") in the prosecution of the case.[30]

• • •

Securing Hyams' cooperation would indeed require funding. Hyams had experienced major financial difficulty in pursuing Dr. Blackburn's plot. The grand total of the payments to him from Blackburn and his associates had been only $520. On multiple occasions Hyams had sought small amounts of money from the Canadian Confederate agents simply for travel, housing, family support, and food expenses—$10 here, $20 there. So the $520 from the Canadian Confederates for all of his work and travels, hardly enough to cover his expenses, was becoming a major source of his anger. He had even found it necessary in the middle of his delivery of the contaminated trunks in the North to return to Canada from Baltimore to obtain more money to fund his travels and the distribution of the contents of the trunks. Hyams lived on a shoestring from day to day, and his testimony, particularly if he would need to travel to Washington, D. C., meant that he needed money. While making a large profit on his testimony was likely Hyams' goal, he certainly couldn't travel without at least having his expenses provided. He would testify at the Lincoln assassination trial in Washington on May 29, 1865. So his goal of making a fortune *from* the Confederates changed to at least making a reasonable sum *from testifying against* the Confederates.

Records show that Emmons was reimbursed $4,452.04 during the years 1864–1865 for "services and expenses in sundry extradition cases, and other business in Canada, during two years—1864 and 1865."[31] These monies were payment for *all* of Emmons' work during these two years, only a small fraction of which went for Hyams' pay and reimbursement of expenses incurred by Hyams and Emmons in the investigation of the many schemes reported to have been hatched by the Canadian Confederates.[32]

Another ledger entry in Washington reported monies paid to Emmons that included $1,000 "in the matter of the extradition of prisoners, the St. Albans raiders, &c." and $3,052.04 "for services in extradition cases, &c., in the British provinces." These two entries likely represented the same payment, considering that the amounts were nearly identical, and noting the correspondence of the terminal "52.04." Emmons commented in a letter to George E. Baker at the State Department that he [Emmons] might have already been reimbursed "$400 or $500" and that Baker was supposed to revise upward the sum requiring payment if Emmons had not been sent the $400, based on Baker's records. Adding $1,000, $3,052.04, and $400, the sum is $4,452.04, accounting for all of the money that flowed through Emmons' accounts.[33] Buried within this diplomatic and legal correspondence is proof of what the Union did indeed pay Hyams to secure his testimony. The sums Emmons and Russell paid him are documented by Emmons' ledger and an invoice he submitted to the U.S. government for payment. Probably the money initially given to Hyams was only slightly more than the expenses he incurred going to Washington, D.C., and subsequently to Boston.

Hyams was first given $39 on April 13, just one day after he began his discussions with Emmons. Hyams wrote, "Hamilton Apl. 13, 1865. Rec'd of H.H. Emmons thirty nine —— dollars U.S. currency compensation for my services for him in matters for the U. States. Godfrey J. Hyams."[34] In a telegram dated April 21, James Speed, the attorney general, wrote to Emmons: "Authorized [Alfred] Russell to promise pardons[.] Act with him."[35] On the same day, Speed wrote to Emmons in a letter confirming his message by telegram: "Night before last I telegraphed the District Attorney [Russell] to promise pardons as liberally as in his discretion, the exigency of the case demanded. It is horrible to think that such monsters [those charged with Lincoln's assassination] live in this age and that they are of this nation. Their conduct however, is an apt sequel to the rebellion.... I have written to day [sic] to Mr. Russell confiding [sic] all the power of this Department to his discretion."[36] Also, Hyams wrote a telegram to Emmons on the same day, April 21: "I will be on the first train [to Detroit;] meet me."[37] On May 6, 1865, he penned to Emmons, who was then staying at the Queen's Hotel in Toronto, "I have been waiting ... thinking I was to be paid witness fees, but he [James Paterson, the Canadian lawyer working with Emmons] refused to pay them on the grounds that the U. S. Government has given me some employment.... My rent is due on Monday morning the 8th, I shall sell out on Monday and go to the states."[38] It's unclear if Hyams was actually employed doing menial jobs for Russell and Emmons, if he was hired for other tasks, or if this statement simply reflected the "reasonable" payment for his time necessary to give his testimony, as opposed to "witness fees," which Hyams felt should have been much higher. Nevertheless, he wasn't handsomely rewarded as he wished and expected.

Negotiators wrote back and forth rapidly and furiously as discussions progressed. David Thurston, the U.S. consul in Toronto, wrote to Alfred Russell twice on May 20. Initially he said, "Consul General directs me to say pay Hyams['] passage and expenses both ways [to testify in Toronto]. [Pay him a] reasonable allowance for time—and draw on him for the amount."[39] Adding a paragraph, also dated the 20th, on the same page, Thurston then expressed some hesitation in paying Hyams in advance for his job: "Perhaps better pay Hyams['] expenses to Toronto only, assure him his time + expenses back [to Detroit] will be paid here by me."[40] Russell forwarded these two notes to Emmons on the same day and added a note on the same page with yet an additional paragraph, saying that he [Russell] hadn't been able to pay Hyams, but that he had sent him on to Toronto.[41] La Fayette C. Baker, the official at the War Department, on June 15, 1865, instructed Emmons by telegram: "Advance Hyams one hundred and fifty (*150*) dollars and draw on me at eighty for the amount."[42] Emmons wrote to George E. Baker at the State Department on June 16, summarizing his fees and expenses and asking for reimbursement for work between December 1864 and June 1865. He spoke of "the prosecution of conspirators in Canada," of expenses for travel "from March 20 to April 14—25 days in reference to matters of introducing yellow fever by Doctor Blackburn + his + others [sic] attempts to take the life of President and Members of Cabinet by infection." His ledger listed "Paid Godfrey G. [sic] Hyams who aided in obtaining details of Blackburn's scheme $2. gold. $40. Currency. Ck. $100. Currency 10. Currency." The sum was $155, though his subheadings of payment methods totaled only $152. A later entry for June 14 said, "Paid note for G. J. Hyams *35.75*."[43] The total for Emmons' invoice to the U.S. government for all of his services corresponded to the amount on Washington's records of what Emmons was paid; the rest of Emmons' ledger reports all of

12. Trials in the United States 163

the expenditures, none of which went to Hyams. Hyams thus received only a paltry sum from Emmons or Emmons' government connections totaling just $379.75. Hyams wrote to Halmer Emmons on May 30, 1865, after he had arrived in Washington, D.C., where he had gone to testify in the trial of the Lincoln assassination conspirators:

> "I write to inform you I arrived on Saturday Night. I reported at the War Department on Sunday morning to Gen'l Fay. He sent me [to] Col Burnett Judge Advocate. I meet him Sunday morning[;] he told me to report at the War Department at 1/2, 8 oclock at night. I did so he keep [sic] me there till near 10 oclock that night told me to report next morning at 9 oclock. Told me then to go to the Hotel and lay there subject to orders. If I had means I should come home at once and attend to my work. I am here without a cent to my name [and] had to beg this paper stamp and envelope. Cannot buy paper to do what I promised. Trusting you still keep well. I am sir your humble servant Godfrey J. Hyams.[44]

He was offended that he wasn't greeted as an important part of the trial hearings, and he was annoyed at repeated delays in his appearance at the Military Tribunal. After this letter, La Fayette C. Baker in the War Department telegraphed Emmons for that $150 to sustain him during the hearings. Baker's instruction to "draw on me at eighty for the amount" is a perplexing request; whether he meant to take $80 out of some account for which Baker was responsible or whether this was an additional $80 is unclear.

John Potts, the disbursing clerk for the War Department, reported total Union Secret Service payments for the quarter ending June 30, 1865, to be $39,966.52.[45] Hyams' share of that amount was only $10. The government also used other sources of funds to pay informants and witnesses, and the sums seemed to be allocated according to the perceived value of the information and testimony. Payments of $50–100 for expenses were common, while witnesses perceived to be important, such as J.B. Merritt and Sanford Conover, commanded payments in the thousands.[46] J.B. Merritt's ledger showed payments of at least $6,768 by July 7, 1865.[47] Hyams had written to the government, on May 30, 1865, a letter that was subsequently lost, but letterbook ledger entries remain: "States he was the means of having numerous rebels in Canada arrested and asks that he be furnished money so that he can [give] testimony against them."[48] It was a long shot, but Hyams needed to keep pleading for money.

The Confederate government lavished huge sums of money on the conspirators in Canada, requiring little to no accountability for the outlays. However, the Union government clearly wasn't generous with its expense money, but it wasn't sure that Hyams would be worth much as a witness, either. Hyams had a high estimation of himself, and he thought he would be a crucial witness in the Lincoln trial. Indeed, he had given sworn testimony about John Wilkes Booth earlier, on May 11, 1865, to Alfred Russell, the United

States district attorney in Detroit.[49] In this testimony Hyams claimed knowledge of Booth's movements and meetings in Canada. He even claimed to have seen Booth perform on the stage in Philadelphia, New York, Baltimore, New Orleans, and St. Louis, an unlikely assertion, given Hyams' known residences and chronic poverty.

Hyams had first gone to Washington, D.C., to testify at the trial of the Lincoln assassins. His financial straits remained severe, even as he resided at the posh Kirkwood Hotel in Washington. While in Washington he petitioned the government for more money, knowing that he needed to travel to Boston for yet another trial. He found himself again begging for tiny sums of money. The paperwork for such requests was almost ludicrous. Hyams applied for additional money; Charles A. Dana, assistant secretary of war, wrote a note to John Potts granting Hyams ten dollars. Hyams had to sign a receipt for even that pittance. Government officials finally relinquished the $10 on June 22, 1865,[50] bringing his payments to $389.75. In Washington Hyams had been summoned to Boston to testify at the trial of Bryan O'Brien, the boat captain who had smuggled the trunks into the United States in July 1864. Little did he know that his appearance in the Boston trial might actually incriminate himself rather than simply be an opportunity to testify against a lowly boat captain accused of smuggling. Hyams wrote from Boston on June 26, 1865,

> When I arrived at Washington I reported to Mr. Baker, who ordered me then to report to the Judge Adv Gen'l Holt, he then ordered me to report at once to the Hon. J.Z. Goodrich Collector of Customs at Boston not telling me what for[.] [H]ere I learned that Capt Obrien [sic] had been arrested for smuggling infected clothing into the States and I have to appear as witness for the United States against him, who's [sic] trial comes off on the 29 inst. When I was in Washington I saw the Attorney Gen'l who told me I must lay the whole matter before the Sec'y of State, who will not return to Washington for two weeks yet, Dear Sir when I get home I shall give up having anything more to do with those cases. Trusting this will reach you in good health. I am sir your humble servant Godfrey J. Hyams.[51]

Clearly Hyams wasn't becoming rich from his testimony, and he was ready to abandon his role as informant.

In Boston, Hyams was scheduled to testify in the U.S. Commissioner's Court at the trial of Bryan O'Brien, the captain of the barque *Halifax* accused of smuggling Hyams' trunks, as well as the goods contained therein. (Hyams always incorrectly referred to the Halifax, Nova Scotia, captain of the *Halifax* as "John O'Brien," and some newspaper articles referred to him as "John" O'Brien or "Brian" O'Brien.) The Indictment was titled, *The United States versus Bryan O'Brien et al.* The big surprise was the "et al." William Patterson was another mariner charged in the same documents in the case of defrauding the government of tax revenues, but there would be another surprise defendant. O'Brien's first hearing was on June 3 before Henry L. Hallet, counselor

12. Trials in the United States 165

and U.S. commissioner, charged with smuggling by Assistant District Attorney Thornton K. Lothrop. O'Brien had Charles R. Train as his attorney.[52] The issue was initially scheduled for a hearing before Commissioner Hallett on Monday, June 12. Hyams thought he himself was to be the primary witness (though initially authorities referred to him by his alias, "J.W. Harris"), but he was still in Washington, D.C., testifying at the Lincoln assassination trial, so the hearing in Boston was postponed. O'Brien argued that he needed to continue his job as a ship's captain and that it would take two weeks for him to sail to Halifax and return to Boston, so the trial was postponed until June 29 at 10:00 a.m. in the U.S. District Court before Judge John Lowell. O'Brien's bail was set at $2,000 (some newspapers incorrectly reported it to be $1,000). Newspapers also reported that the charges would likely be dropped against O'Brien if Hyams couldn't or wouldn't testify. On June 26 Hyams was present in Boston, where he wrote to Halmer H. Emmons in Detroit that he was awaiting the trial to begin on June 29. He had been ordered to report to the Honorable John Zaccheus Goodrich, the collector of customs in Boston, which he had done. Hyams' letter was written on the stationery of the United States Hotel in Boston, proving his presence there. The grand jury indictment against O'Brien was dated June 27, 1865, and read in part as follows:

> Bryan O'Brien, master mariner, and William Patterson, mariner ... on the twenty fourth day of July in the year of Our Lord one thousand eight hundred and sixty four, at Boston ... knowingly and wilfully and with the intent ... to defraud the revenue of the United States did then and there smuggle and clandestinely introduce into the said United States certain goods, wares and merchandize, to wit, one hundred woolen shirts and thirty woolen blouses ... subject to duty by law, and ... without their ... paying or accounting for the said duty on the said goods, wares and merchandize as aforesaid.... And the Jurors aforesaid, upon their oaths aforesaid do further present that Godfrey Joseph Hyams late of Detroit in the State of Michigan, trader, at Boston in the District of Massachusetts on the twenty fourth day of July ... did then and there knowingly and wilfully smuggle ... certain goods, wares and merchandize, to wit, one hundred woolen shirts and thirty woolen blouses ... subject to duty ... without ... paying or accounting for the said duty thereon as required by law....[53]

Hyams thus found himself indicted with O'Brien and Patterson. All were charged with the crimes of smuggling and tax evasion. Hyams wasn't just a witness, as he had originally believed. He was a defendant.

Hyams' and O'Brien's versions of the story were quite different. Hyams claimed that O'Brien had helped him smuggle the trunks from Halifax to Boston, but O'Brien obviously denied this assertion. Part of Hyams' physical description of the *Halifax*—sliding panels in the porter's quarters behind which the trunks were hidden—didn't exist, according to Captain O'Brien. O'Brien also disputed Hyams' report of the location of the *Halifax* on the dates in question, saying that the ship wasn't in the Boston port on the day

Hyams claimed the smuggled goods were unloaded from the barque.[54] But the barque was indeed in Boston around this time and Hyams didn't have intimate knowledge of the interior of the *Halifax*, so most of his story could have been true.

Hyams was justifiably fearful of testifying and hesitant to appear. He didn't show for court on the 29th. Perhaps he was concerned not just about being named in the indictment; perhaps he also feared for his own safety. In the mid–1800s the stereotype of a sailor was that of a person who could be rough and who could extract vengeance by physical means; testifying against Captain O'Brien might be dangerous. For certain, Hyams worried about his own legal prosecution. He had gone to Boston thinking that he was to be a witness in O'Brien's trial, maybe even receiving payment for his testimony, but he found himself named in the indictment. The trial was again postponed ("continued") until September 12 in the U.S. district court of Judge John Lowell, with Ellis W. Morton acting as the assistant district attorney for the government. However, the trial never materialized, likely because Hyams was no longer in Boston and he had no intention of returning.[55] Even if his presence was to be as a witness only and not a defendant, he had declared that he was finished with testifying in matters concerning Blackburn: "[W]hen I get home I shall give up having anything more to do with those cases."[56]

Hyams' detailed expenses for the Washington and Boston trips are unrecorded. He had stayed in Washington at the Kirkwood House and in Boston at the United States Hotel. Both establishments were rather exclusive places of lodging. In fact, Vice President Andrew Johnson had rented a two-room suite in the Kirkwood House on the day of Lincoln's assassination and actually took the presidential oath of office there on April 15, 1865. Each hotel in Washington and Boston where Hyams stayed cost about $1–2 per day for lodging and about $2.50–3.50 for both room and board. An individual meal cost about $0.75. Menus from 1865 list chicken stew and dumplings for $0.30, veal pot pie for $0.25, beef soup for $0.15, and beef roast for $0.30.[57] Hyams could have found much more modest accommodations. It's not certain whether his rooms had been arranged by the government or by Hyams himself. The train travel from Toronto to Washington was $22.70 and from Washington to Boston $14.35.[58] He was away from home for at least four weeks and likely closer to six. The total of all his railway fares would have been about $74.10; his room (assuming he was gone six weeks) would have been about $63.00, and his food also somewhere near $63.00. So his total expenses would have been a minimum of about $200, while he received only about $389.75 from the U.S. government through Emmons and the small payment from the government while he was in Washington in June. Therefore, Hyams likely cleared no more than about $190 on the trip, certainly nothing like he

12. Trials in the United States

had originally expected to earn from his involvement in the entire affair. Remember that an average sailor in 1865 was paid about $500 per year. Hyams' profit from his "witness fees" to this time was hardly enough to maintain his family for more than a few months. This monetary gain could hardly be called exorbitant. He wanted more. His original expectation through Southern sources, based on his discussions with Blackburn 18 months earlier, had been at least $60,000–100,000. The North was not making him rich, either. If Hyams' past behavior were any prediction of the future, he might soon be defecting back to the South. He needed to make another pitch for money for his testimony. Having returned to Washington from Boston, he again petitioned the government for payment for his role as a witness. He wrote to Edwin M. Stanton, the secretary of war, on July 6, 1865:

> I submitt [sic] to your kind consideration. Compensation for time and expenceses [sic], Since the 20th of February last I have been taking a considerable ... time to Bring to Justice, Clearry [sic], Young, Blackburn, McDonald, and also in laying up of the Steamer Georgian in Canada since them [sic]. I appeared before the Military Commission and have been to Boston in the case U.S. vs Obrien for smuggling. I have been the means of getting them all committed for trial. My traveling and board ... cost me nearly $800 Eight hundred dollars. And my time should be worth according to my Business about $25.00 [sic] two hundred and fifty dollars per month, making about—$1,800 dollars One thousand eight hundred dollars. I was promised by the Consul Gen'l in Canada I should be paid something in addition, I pray payment will be made as I wish to go home, I have received about two hundred and fifty dollars. I shall have some great work yet in attending to the convicting of the above named parties in October next which I promise to do faithfully. Hoping I shall recive [sic] pay I remain your humble servant Godfrey J. Hyams.[59]

In partial support for his requests and claims, Hyams submitted two receipts from the United States Hotel in Boston dated June 30 for one week ($24.50), and July 5 for 4¾ days ($17.00).[60]

On the same day, July 6, 1865, Judge Advocate General Joseph Holt in the Bureau of Military Justice wrote to Edwin M. Stanton, the Secretary of War:

> Respectfully submitted for the consideration of the Secretary of War. This witness has rendered important services for the government, + in traveling + for board has no doubt incurred—for him—heavy expenses. He should be indemnified by an allowance sufficient to compensate him for his time + reimburse him all that he has paid out. The sum demanded strikes me as large + might probably be reduced without injustice. He is now in the city, + is, I presume, little able to bear the expense of remaining.[61]

Stanton replied on July 8: "Referred back to the Judge Advocate General for input as to what sum would in his opinion would be just and reasonable."[62] Holt responded, also on July 8: "Respectfully returned from a conversation with this man. I am satisfied that $1200 besides what he has received would not more than indemnify him. It is recommended that this sum be paid."[63] Stanton approved.

Hyams was paid $1,200 on July 8 "for services + expenses in cases of Young, Cleary, Blackburn + McDonald." The payment was listed as an "Appropriation" for "Army Contingencies."[64] So his total compensation for his work in 1864 and 1865 was $520 for expenses delivering the trunks, $389.75 for his subsistence during the trials, and $1,200 as a witness fee. Though he didn't get fabulously rich from his testimony, the additional $1,200 dollars went a long way to keeping Hyams' family solvent for a couple of years.[65] He was still playing in a different league from high-priced witnesses like Dr. James B. Merritt and Charles A. Dunham, but $1,200 over expenses was the best that he could do. Such an amount might even be considered prejudicial to an honest testimony or bribery for Hyams to tell a good story. Nevertheless, the general scope of what he reported to authorities correlated well with evidence obtained from more reliable sources. Some of the details may have been questionable, but the themes were accurate.

Hyams was also pardoned as part of the deal, his amnesty papers being completed on June 22, 1865. Amnesty is actually the correct term because a pardon is granted for a convicted offence; amnesty is a proclamation that a person will not be prosecuted for an alleged or suspected crime. Even though he was named as a defendant in the Boston smuggling indictment, Hyams was never formally charged, tried, or convicted in either Canada or the United States for the yellow fever plot itself.

• • •

Overall, Godfrey Hyams performed as a rather inconsistent and contradictory witness. He told his story about Dr. Blackburn at least four times (excluding the trial in Boston, at which he never actually testified), and the details changed slightly with each telling. The first was the preliminary accounting given in Toronto; then he told his entire, more detailed, story to Halmer H. Emmons on April 12; next he testified at Blackburn's first hearing in Canada; and finally he testified before the military tribunal for the Lincoln assassination conspirators in Washington, D.C., on May 29. While the general story was the same, certain details—such as the number of trunks and the amount of money he was paid to participate in the plot—were slightly different. But his testimony corroborated the others' stories. Dr. Luke Blackburn was guilty.

• • •

The trial of the eight Lincoln assassination conspirators—Herold, Powell, Atzerodt, Surratt, Mudd, Spangler, Arnold, and O'Laughlin—concluded on June 30. The jurors reached a guilty verdict for all. The verdict and sentences were transmitted to President Andrew Johnson, who approved them on July 5. The four most seriously involved in Booth's murder scheme—David Herold, Lewis Powell, George Atzerodt, and Mary Surratt—were hung on July 7, 1865.

13

Jefferson Davis
His Involvement in the Plots and the Consequences

President Jefferson Davis was implicated in the conspiracy to assassinate Abraham Lincoln and in the plots emanating from Canada, but what is the evidence of it?

Testimony in the trial of the Lincoln conspirators in Washington, D.C., confirmed that $1,000,000 had been earmarked for clandestine projects emanating from Confederates living in Canada. Though this exact dollar amount can't be found in Canadian Confederate bank records, during the Lincoln conspiracy trial Robert Anson Campbell, the chief teller at the Ontario Bank at Montreal, testified that Jacob Thompson's account, opened on May 30, 1864 (and closed on April 11, 1865—three days *before* Lincoln was assassinated), at one time had a balance of $649,873.28.[1] Many of his deposits were monetary instruments that seemed to have originated in the South—Southern sterling exchange bills, gold, and bills of exchange from the Confederacy passing through Liverpool, England, a known Confederate banking route.

In other testimony at the conspiracy trial, Sanford Conover (aka James Watson Wallace), whose real name was Charles Dunham, testified that Jacob Thompson, the head of the Canadian Confederate Secret Service, said that the goal of the "black ops" was to "leave the government entirely without a head."[2] This meant killing President Lincoln, Vice President Johnson, Secretary of State William H. Seward, General Ulysses S. Grant, and perhaps Secretary of War Edwin M. Stanton. The Constitution of the United States at that time didn't specify a chain of succession of the presidency any further down the ranks of the political or military spectrum. That being said, Conover/Wallace/Dunham was not considered to be a reliable witness, so the veracity of the testimony was questioned. Another witness, Henry Von Steinacker, testified that he had been present in the summer of 1863 close to Swift Run Gap near Harrisonburg when Booth had this to say: "If we only act our part, the Confederacy will gain its independence. Old Abe Lincoln must go up the spout, and the Confederacy will gain its independence any how." Von Steinacker continued his testimony:

> By this expression I understood he meant the President must be killed. He said that as soon as the Confederacy was nearly giving out, or as soon as they were nearly whipped, that this would be their final resource to gain their independence.... [Conspirators would] send certain officers on "detached service" to Canada and the "borders" to release rebel prisoners, to lay Northern cities in ashes, and finally to get possession of the members of the Cabinet and kill the President. This "detached service" was a nickname in the Confederate army for this sort of warfare.[3]

Of course, the testimony was disputed. Steinacker was first a member of the Union army, from which he became a deserter. He then became a member of the Confederate military, the 2nd Virginia Infantry, Stonewall Brigade. A fellow soldier from the same brigade, H.K. Douglas, testified that no such statements as alleged by Steinacker had been made, that the fellow soldiers of that brigade were honorable and that any consideration of assassination was an "unrighteous act."[4]

Samuel Chester testified that Booth had originally developed the plan to kidnap Lincoln and take him to Richmond. The initial plan wasn't received well in Richmond, though. Richard Montgomery testified that another conspirator, Beverly Tucker, had said it was "too bad that the boys had not been allowed to act when they wanted to." Richard Montgomery was a double agent Union spy in Canada who said Jacob Thompson verbalized that it would be a blessing to rid the world of Lincoln, Johnson, and Grant. The conspirators in Canada expressed their belief that the killing of a tyrant should not be considered a murder but a duty. Yet another testimony, from Henry Finegan, revealed that he had overheard a conversation between George Sanders and William Cleary in Montreal, in which Sanders had said, "If only the boys have luck, Lincoln won't trouble us much longer." Leary queried, "Is everything going well?" Sanders retorted, "Oh, yes. Booth is bossing the job."[5]

Louis Weichmann testified at the Lincoln conspirators' trial that on March 27, 1865, about three weeks before the assassination, John Surratt went to Richmond and visited with Attorney General Judah Benjamin and President Jefferson Davis. Surratt appeared in Montreal, Canada, on April 6, just a week before Lincoln was killed, and reported that the assassins had the approval of Davis and the Confederate government. On that same day, Jacob Thompson withdrew $184,000 (some sources say $186,000) from his Montreal bank account, which had over $600,000 in it at the time, the magnitude of which could not have come from Thompson's personal income. This information is quite circumstantial, and the communication—allegedly written in a secret cipher—was never preserved. If true, it would strongly implicate high-level Confederate complicity in the plan. Charles Dunham also testified that he was present at that meeting with John Surratt and Jacob Thompson and that Thompson read the messages from Davis and said, "This makes the thing [presumably the kidnapping or assassination] all right." It's another obscure reference, perhaps, but seems to support the theory that Davis was onboard with at least some kind of black flag warfare. Dunham, however, was later proved to be an unreliable witness, a perjurer, in fact. Though trained as a lawyer, it's unclear if he ever passed the bar or practiced law.[6] He was a fraud, a liar, a confabulator, and an inventor of self-aggrandizing tales. However, all of his stories and lies contained just enough truth and detail to make them seem convincing. He impersonated both Union and Confederate supporters, and his list of aliases was almost endless. Taken as a sole witness, his testimony was useless, but when correlated with other accounts it occasionally provided some useful details. Although multiple other witnesses in this escapade corroborated his stories, Dunham was eventually found guilty of perjury and sent to prison.[7]

Ultimately, evidence would surface that seemed to connect Jefferson Davis even more closely to Dr. Blackburn. One of the Confederate agents who worked in Canada was Episcopal minister Kensey Johns Stewart. Stewart originally served in St. Paul's Episcopal Church in Alexandria, Virginia. In 1861 he went to Richmond in response to being arrested for refusing to offer a special prayer for the Union. There he became a chaplain in the Sixth North Carolina Infantry and then briefly served the Union prisoners in Richmond hospitals. He subsequently went to England, where he worked for one year on a prayer book, returning to Richmond in 1864. He then went to Canada as a Confederate agent. His assessment of the efforts of the other Canadian agents was less than complimentary. He attacked the effectiveness of these other agents, calling them "useless annoyances" and "miserable failures," and he thought that some of their techniques were less than honorable. Stewart wrote to Jefferson Davis about some "inhumane and cruel" plans that the others in Canada were attempting. He spoke to Davis in humanitarian and moral terms:

> I cannot regard you [Davis] as capable of expecting the blessing of God upon ... plans such as I describe below. As our country has been and is entirely dependent upon God, we cannot afford to displease him. Therefore, it cannot be our policy to employ wicked men to destroy the persons & property of private citizens, by inhumane and cruel acts. I name only one. $100.00 of public money has been paid here to one "Hyams" a shoemaker, for services rendered by conveying and causing to be sold in the city of Washington at auction, boxes of small-pox clothing.... It is only a matter of surprise, that God does not forsake us and our cause when we are associated with such misguided friends.[8]

This letter confirmed Hyams' testimony, regardless of his motives or unsavory character. It would add strong weight to the story that would be told about

Blackburn in Bermuda, in Canada, and at the conspirators' trial in Washington. If Jefferson Davis didn't know about Blackburn's scheme before then, he knew it after he received Stewart's letter, written on December 12, 1864. Stewart was a moral man, and he couldn't countenance such activity. Many witnesses would ultimately testify to the existence of the yellow fever plot, but Stewart's admission that Hyams was paid from Confederate funds would add conclusive proof that the entire story was true. The later testimony and depositions of all of the other witnesses were confirmed, at least the substance if not the fine details. But Davis didn't order a stop to this activity. Even in April 1865 the trunks with the contaminated articles sat in Edward C. Swan's house in Bermuda awaiting shipment.

When Booth was caught and killed, William Eaton was instructed by the War Department to go to the National Hotel in Washington to search Booth's belongings. (Eaton was the same official who arrested Edmond Spangler, the carpenter and stagehand employed at Ford's Theatre who was accused of aiding John Wilkes Booth.) Eaton took the contents of a trunk found in Booth's room and turned them over to the provost marshal's office, and in turn they were given to Lieutenant William H. Terry. One of the papers found there was a ciphered letter marked "Important." Cipher communication was common during the Civil War. A cipher was a mechanical gadget, either utilizing concentric circles or rotating cylinders. The cylinder type used for the letter in question measured about six inches long by two-three inches in diameter. This "machine" functioned by simple letter/number substitution and wasn't very elaborate or secure. One such machine was found in Booth's belongings. A ciphered letter, dated October 13, 1864, and delivered to Richmond from the Confederate Rebels in Canada by Richard Montgomery, said, "We again urge the immense necessity of our gaining immediate advantages. Strain every nerve for victory. We now look on the re-election of Lincoln in November as almost certain, and we need to whip his hirelings to prevent it.... Our friends shall be immediately set to work as you direct." This text, of course, is a vague reference, but evidence showed that it had been written with the same cipher used in the State Department in Richmond—in Confederate President Jefferson Davis's office. The implication was that the phrase "as you direct" meant that Jefferson Davis was involved in the planning and direction of the assassination. A ciphered reply went back to the Canadian Southerners on October 19 urging them to continue to recruit voters against Lincoln's reelection bid and to be patient for a turning tide: "A blow will shortly be stricken here. It is not quite time."[9] During the conspirators' trial, the validity of this ciphered letter was disputed, and the defense sought to have it expunged from the admissible exhibits of evidence. The defense argued that the ciphered letter was actually fictitious and inadmissible because it was not signed. There was no proof of any connection between the cipher and the accused on trial; it was not taken from the possession of anyone currently on trial; and there was no handwriting connecting the cipher and the accused. The judge rejected these objections, and the cipher was kept as evidence (Exhibit #7).

Final evidence of Davis's sentiments, if not his foreknowledge, about the assassination plot was his reaction to the news that Lincoln had been killed. Davis was staying at the house of a friend, Mr. Louis F. Bates, in Charlotte, North Carolina, when he received a telegram from John C. Breckinridge, the Confederate secretary of war, which said, "His Excellency, President Davis: President Lincoln was assassinated in the theater in Washington on the night of the 14th inst. Seward's house was entered on the same night and he was repeatedly stabbed, and is probably mortally wounded." Davis then said, "If it were to be done, it were better it were well done." Later that same day, Breckinridge expressed distress that the assassination had occurred because it came at a time when it could have been a detriment to the terms and conditions imposed on the South after losing the war. Davis again said, using many of the same words, "Well, General, I don't know; if it were to be done at all, it were better that it were well done; and if the same had been done to Andy Johnson, the beast, and to Secretary Stanton, the job would then be complete."[10] Much interpretation can surround these statements, but none of it is good. Judge Advocate General Joseph Holt summarized his view of them by concluding that Davis should be tried as the other conspirators were and that hanging was the appropriate end for the Confederate president. "The blood of the President [Lincoln] is still calling to us from the ground, not for vengeance, for that his nature was incapable, but for justice—that justice without which no nation can long live in honor or peace or happiness."[11]

The judge in the trial of the Lincoln conspirators, Special Judge Advocate John Bingham, summing his opinion of the results of the evidence and testimony presented at the trial, said, "What more is wanting? Surely no word further need be spoken to show that John Wilkes Booth was in this conspiracy; that John Surratt was in this conspiracy; and that Jefferson Davis and his several agents named, in Canada, were in this conspiracy.... Whatever may be the conviction of others, my own conviction is that Jefferson Davis is as clearly proven guilty of this conspiracy as John Wilkes Booth, by whose hand Jefferson Davis inflicted the mortal wound on Abraham Lincoln."[12]

The first indictment against Jefferson Davis was dated May 2, 1865, presented by Judge Advocate General Joseph Holt to Secretary of War Edwin M. Stanton in a cabinet meeting. It charged Davis and others who had been based in Canada (including Jacob Thompson, William Cleary, Beverly Tucker, George Sanders, Clement Clay, and others) with conspiring to murder President Lincoln. Davis wasn't cited in this indictment for treason emanating from his Southern rebellion, but only for his alleged role in the murder of the president. The charge also placed a $100,000 bounty on Davis's head. This indictment would ultimately never make its way to a trial.

Lieutenant-Colonel Benjamin Pritchard of the 4th Michigan Cavalry arrested Davis on May 10, 1865, in Irwinsville, Georgia, and took him from Irwinsville to Savannah, Georgia, and then to Hilton Head, South Carolina, before transporting him to prison at Fortress Monroe.[13] Davis, Clement Clay, Vice President Alexander H. Stephens, Postmaster-General John H. Regan, General Joseph Wheeler, and other Confederate prisoners arrived at Fortress Monroe in Hampton Roads from Port Royal, South Carolina, on May 19 aboard the Steamship *William. P. Clyde*, accompanied by the steamship USS *Tuscarora*. Aboard the *Clyde* they waited in the harbor for their imprisonment. Davis and Clay were incarcerated at Fortress Monroe in Virginia on May 22, 1865, both under solitary confinement. They couldn't even communicate with their wives and children. The other prisoners were conveyed to Fort Warren (Boston), Fort Delaware (Delaware City, Delaware), or Fort McHenry (Baltimore).[14]

At Fortress Monroe Davis and Clay were housed under extremely strict security in the casemate cells, rooms carved out of the walls of the fort. Davis was in #2, Clay in #4. Soldiers were stationed in #1, #3, and #5, separating Davis and Clay and providing additional security for the prisoners. Barred doors and windows separated them from any hint of freedom. Initially, a lamp burned in each cell continuously, and guards checked the prisoners every 15 minutes. Guards walking in the hallways provided yet more observation of Davis and Clay, making it extremely difficult for the prisoners to sleep. Their rooms were furnished with a stark hospital bed, a metal bedstead, a stool, a table, and a small closet. In their early confinement, they were allowed only a Bible; no other reading material was approved (Davis would later be allowed a prayer book). Letters—even from family—were forbidden.

On the first day of Davis's confinement, guards didn't use iron shackles, but on May 23 shackles were forcibly placed on his ankles. He fought the guards trying to attach them, later recounting that he had hoped the guards would shoot or bayonet him to end his humiliating ordeal. Dr. J.J. Craven would later recount, "These fetters were of heavy iron, probably five-eighths of an inch in thickness, and connected together by a chain of like weight."[15] Davis protested: "'I tell you the world will ring with this disgrace. The war is over; the South is conquered; I have no longer any country but America, and it is for the honor of America, as for my own honor and life, that I plead against this degradation. Kill me! Kill me!' he cried passionately, throwing his arms open wide and exposing his breast, 'rather than inflict on me, and on my People through me, this insult worse than death.'"[16] The fetters remained for five days, though Davis's hands were free. The directors of the prisoners' confinement, Assistant Secretary of War Charles Anderson Dana and Major General Nelson A. Miles (the commander of the fort was Major General H.W. Halleck), were later accused of abusing Davis and Clay, and many (including Union sympathizers) believed that the confinement and treatment of the two men were imposed simply to humiliate them—and the South in general.

Davis began his incarceration in failing health, which further deteriorated rapidly, though some reports may have been exaggerated to encourage more lenient treatment from his jailers. Brevet Lieutenant Colonel Dr. John J. Craven (the chief medical officer of Fortress Monroe) was assigned to monitor Davis and Clay's health, and he first saw them on May 24. Craven quickly recommended an additional mattress and a pillow and that Davis be allowed to have some tobacco (the only personal item Davis had been allowed to bring into the cell was his meerschaum pipe). Dr. Craven made all of these requests allegedly to help Davis sleep. The doctor also requested on May 25 that the ankle irons be removed because they were irritating Davis's skin. These irons were removed on May 28. Guards remained physically present in Davis's cell until June 23, continuing to make his sleep difficult. On June 24 he was allowed some newspapers, books, and magazines, and he was given the freedom to walk one hour each day on the ramparts of Fortress Monroe. On June 25, 1865, Brevet Major General Nelson A. Miles wrote to Assistant Adjutant General E.D. Townsend: "I think him [Davis] to be as strong now as he was on the day he entered the fort. The statement in the papers that his health is declining under his imprisonment are utterly false and in my opinion are intended to excite sympathy in the North."[17]

Dr. Craven found Davis more debilitated on July 20, 1865: "Found Mr. Davis in a very critical state; his nervous debility extreme; his mind more despondent than ever heretofore; his appetite gone; complexion livid, and pulse denoting deep prostration of all the physical energies."[18] Later he said, "Mr. Davis said when he had last been out on the ramparts he had met Mr. C.C. Clay, similarly walking under guard. Clay was looking wretchedly, and seeing him made Mr. Davis realize more acutely his own humiliating position."[19] Secretary of War Edwin M. Stanton was concerned. He wrote to Major General Miles on July 22, 1865, outlining a six-point plan to insure Davis's health and to allay the fears of the public that his troops were mistreating the former president of the Confederacy. Stanton said,

> [I]t has been determined:
> 1st—That you may remove the guards and lights from Mr. Davis' room if they are inconvenient to him, taking such precautionary measures as you may think adequate for his security.
> 2nd—That you may allow him to take such exercise in the open air, under your own immediate supervision, as the Surgeon in charge may deem essential to his health, but allowing no other person to hold communication with him.

3rd—You may allow him such books and papers as he may desire to read.

4th—*You should see him personally every day* and if any other relaxation consistent with his secure detention is deemed beneficial to his health by yourself or his Surgeon, you will report it to this Department.

5th—*You will make daily reports of your visits to him*, and the state of his health— and oftener if his health changes for the worse.

6th—You will continue every vigilance and precaution against efforts to escape by surprise, strategem or other means, but it is not the desire of the Government to subject him to any hardships not essential to his secure detention[20] [emphases added].

It would not serve any worthwhile purpose for Davis's heath to worsen or to have him die. On the contrary, there was much to lose if he were to die in custody. Both sides of the conflict would be upset with such an outcome. Many Northerners wanted a trial and severe punishment (even execution) for a man they deemed to be a traitor; Southerners would see it as unjust punishment of their hero president. Death would elevate Davis to the status of a martyr. In addition both sides would see it as an impediment to Reconstruction. It was unprecedented to ask a major general to visit a prisoner and to write a report daily to the secretary of war, but on July 24 there began months of close observation of this very important prisoner and daily reports from Miles to Stanton.

Davis rallied slowly over the next few days, but on August 14 he again worsened, with high fever and facial swelling that later erupted in erysipelas, a skin infection and inflammation often caused by the bacterium streptococcus. He progressively worsened through August 20. Dr. Craven reported to General Miles on August 20, 1865, that Davis's general condition was deteriorating, that he was losing weight, and that his mental state was bad, in addition to the erysipelas. Davis began improving on about August 25, only to worsen again on September 1. His condition thus waxed and waned continuously, though from a baseline of extreme weakness and debility. On October 2 (some sources say October 5) he was finally moved to Carroll Hall on the south end of the second floor. This building was a structure used for officers' quarters. Both Grant and Sherman had quartered in the very room to which Davis was assigned, although it had been converted to a prison cell for the Confederate president.

Dr. Craven was transferred in December 1865 and replaced by surgeon Dr. George E. Cooper. Dr. Cooper relayed on January 21, 1866, that "both of the state prisoners are men of delicate appetites."[21] They both received their food from Fortress Monroe's hospital. "Jefferson Davis is much troubled with dyspepsia, and cannot eat the food furnished in the soldiers' rations, without having the same aggravated and with an exacerbation of the dyspeptic symptoms comes severe neuralgia of the face and head."[22] In addition, Dr. Cooper found that Dr. Craven had actually been feeding Davis from his own table. Craven's young daughter Anna often brought Davis's food to him, and Davis thanked her by giving her one of his prayer books that had been a gift from his wife. Cooper commented upon Clay's severe asthma only parenthetically and ended by recommending that money from the hospital fund (which had excess money at the time) be used to provide "proper food for the state prisoners." That amount was $15 per month per prisoner.[23]

Davis's health improved and worsened cyclically over the months. On March 21, 1866, Edward D. Townsend, assistant adjutant general, described Davis as being "in a state of high nervous excitability [and] is complaining of fullness of the head and a tendency to vertigo. He seems to be wasting away gradually + loosing [sic] flesh. This is scarcely perceptible to one who sees him day by day—but is nevertheless certain." On April 18 Townsend reported, "His appetite seems to be diminishing. Complains of muscular weakness."[24] Davis's wife, Varina, monitored her husband's health from reports she received at her residence in Montreal, Canada East. Worried, she wrote a telegram to President Andrew Johnson from Montreal on April 25: "I hear my husband is failing rapidly. Can I come to him? Can you refuse me! Answer."[25] In another communication, this one an undated letter to the president, she said, "May I hope once more to sit near my sick husband. I cannot do anything for him in his great peril and agony but speak to him of my love.... Will you not let me do this? ... I will take any parole." As a postscript, she added, "Mr. President *please decide* this matter *yourself*. For the love of God, and his merciful Son, do not refuse me. Let me go to him, and admire and bless your name every hour of my life" (emphasis in the original).[26] Varina received permission to visit her husband on April 26, and on May 3 she took an oath of parole:

> I, Varina Davis, wife of Jefferson Davis, for the privilege of being permitted to see my husband, do hereby give my Parole of Honor, that I will engage in, or assent to no measures which shall lead to any attempt to escape from confinement on the part of my husband, or to his being rescued, or released from imprisonment, without the sanction, and order of the President of the United States, nor will I be the means of conveying to my husband any deadly weapons of any kind [emphasis in the original].[27]

Varina and Jefferson Davis met, and his health improved. Townsend reported on May 10, "Since his wife has been here he seems to be in better spirits."[28]

Almost simultaneously, President Andrew Johnson received additional information about Davis's failing health from sources other than the letter and telegram from Varina Davis. On May 9, 1866, President Johnson directed that Secretary of War Edwin Stanton order Dr. G.E. Cooper to file a report about how Davis was faring under arrest. Cooper reported as follows:

13. Jefferson Davis

He is considerably emaciated, the fatty tissue having almost disappeared, leaving his skin much shriveled. His muscles are small, flaccid and very soft, and he has but little muscular strength. He is quite weak and debilitated; consequently his gait is becoming uneven and irregular. His digestive organs at present are in comparatively good condition, but become quickly deranged under anything but the most carefully prepared food. With a diet disagreeing with him, dyspeptic symptoms promptly make their appearance, soon followed by vertigo, severe facial and cranial neuralgia, an erysipelatous inflammation of the posterior scalp and right side of the nose, which quickly affects the right eye (the only sound one he has) and extends through the nasal duct into the interior nose. His nervous system is greatly deranged, being prostrated and excessively irritable. Slight noises, which are scarcely perceptible to a man in robust health, cause him much pain.... Want of sleep has been a great and almost the principal cause of his nervous excitability. This has been produced by the tramp of the creaking boots of the sentinels on post round the prison room, and the relieval of the guard at the expiration of every two hours, which almost invariably awakens him.[29]

General Miles objected to this description, saying that he felt that both President Davis and Davis's wife had unduly influenced the doctor. Dr. Cooper's wife and Varina were friends. Newspaper reporters and the public at large (even those who were North-leaning) seemed to believe Dr. Cooper's report, however. Officers at Fortress Monroe relaxed the conditions under which Davis and Clay were held. On May 25, 1866, Davis swore that he would not attempt to escape, and he was allowed intermittent access to the interior grounds of Fortress Monroe.

• • •

The stories of Davis's trials are complex. The first indictment for conspiracy to assassinate Lincoln never came to trial because it appeared the evidence for such a charge wasn't strong enough for a conviction. The logistic impediments to Davis's trial greatly lengthened the judicial process. Lincoln's assassination occurred in Washington, D.C. Had that trial been held, as it was for the trial of the other conspirators, opinion was divided whether a military or civil court should be the venue. For the other defendants, the military option had been chosen, though not without fierce opposition. Davis would likely have faced the same military tribunal, but the charge of conspiracy to murder was never pursued either in a military or a civilian court.

The saga of the many other (at least four) indictments for treason is likewise convoluted. The proceedings were repeatedly interrupted, in part by the fear that an impartial jury couldn't be found either in the North or the South. Since it would ultimately be declared to be a civil trial rather than a military one, it would fall within the jurisdiction of Virginia. During the attempts to begin the trial, the Fourteenth Amendment to the Constitution was being debated and ratified, and it would ultimately be pivotal in Davis's fate.

The crime of treason—or at least secession, if that constituted treason—had occurred primarily in Virginia. Civilian courts in Virginia were open and functioning, and any trial of Davis for treason would probably have been held there. However, Davis was incarcerated in a military prison. Military jurisdiction needed to be abandoned for a civil trial to occur. Revocation of military control was needed to convert to a civilian venue. This transfer never occurred.

Political considerations also came into play often. Many hearings and court dates were postponed, often simply because one or the other parties claimed to need more time; occasionally key members of the process simply didn't appear at appointed court dates. Key government officials came and went as their jobs and job descriptions changed; people were hired; people were fired or resigned; and others simply moved to different positions.

Before his death, Lincoln had favored leniency for the leaders, officers, and soldiers of the South. President Andrew Johnson wasn't as sanguine in his mercy toward the South, and ill will still existed between Johnson and Davis. Supreme Court Chief Justice Salmon Portland Chase played a prominent role in the judicial proceedings against Davis. Chase was an ardent abolitionist, but after the war he favored leniency and reconciliation for the perpetrators of the rebellion. He had actually helped to author some of the antislavery legislation, but he had little desire to wreak vengeance on Davis and the other secessionists. Indeed, almost all of the Confederates would ultimately be pardoned; however, many Northern sympathizers wanted to see Davis punished.

Some of Chase's hesitations were more legal or logistic considerations than expressions of mercy. He foresaw the difficulties in prosecuting Davis, and he knew what consequences would follow from either acquittal or conviction, if indeed the trial could ever be held, considering the impossibility of finding an unbiased jury. An acquittal of Davis would tend to negate the outcome of the war, including the seeming trivialization of the loss of over 600,000 lives during the conflict. A conviction, on the other hand, might cause further retaliations against the South. Perhaps simply not holding the trial would be the best plan. Furthermore, Chase thought like a politician, as he had harbored thoughts himself of being president of the United States. He didn't want to anger either block of voters, the north or the south. He had been a potential candidate both in 1860 and 1864; 1868 might be his golden opportunity to become president.[30]

Chase's counterpart in the judicial process in the Virginia Judicial District was Federal District judge John Curtiss Underwood.[31] Underwood was known to display "temperamental partisanship,"[32] and even his competency was questioned. Initially Underwood thought that Davis shouldn't even be prosecuted. A guilty verdict and an execution would possibly make a martyr of the Confederate leader. However, after meeting with President Andrew Johnson in August 1865, Underwood proceeded to begin preparation of an indictment against Davis, without naming any other Confederates in the charges.

Congress had passed a law on July 31, 1861, stating that "conspiracy to overthrow the government or to interfere with the operation of its laws was guilty of 'a high crime.'"[33] This offense was punishable by a fine of $500-$5,000 and a prison sentence of not more than six years. These penalties were significantly less severe than capital punishment for treason. This law was intended to punish crimes against the government that were not as serious or that were deemed to justify leniency. Another law passed on July 17, 1862 (part of the "Second Confiscation Act"), provided that a conviction for treason could result in a sentence of a prison term of up to five years and a fine of not less than $10,000. This law also allowed the courts to sentence more leniently someone convicted of treason, avoiding the penalty of execution.

To avoid the possibility of execution should Davis be found guilty, Underwood's team used this "Second Confiscation Act" as the basis for the charges; this act provided the opportunity to seek only fines and a prison sentence as punishment, not the execution that would have been possible under alternative forms of indictment. Connally points out that the most ardent supporters for punishing Davis were Secretary of War Edwin Stanton and Judge Advocate General Joseph Holt.[34] (Holt has been criticized for his vigor and aggressiveness in pursuing many alleged conspirators in the assassination of Lincoln.)[35] Davis was charged in the United States District Court of Virginia with treason under this latter law in June 1865, shortly after his arrest in May. Another indictment for treason would be filed in the District of Columbia later in 1865.

President Johnson had made a Proclamation of Peace on April 2, 1866, trying to calm emotions over the Civil War and its aftermath. Though perhaps offering a means to an end to the military aspect of Davis's imprisonment, it wasn't sufficiently clear to Judge Chase that it was yet appropriate to proceed with the trial. Johnson wanted Davis kept under military control, and though the accusation against Davis for participating in the assassination plot was never rescinded, President Johnson wanted to proceed instead with the trial for treason.

While all of these legal wranglings continued, Davis was released on $100,000 bail on May 13, 1867. Many friends, including Commodore Cornelius Vanderbilt, Horace Greeley, Gerritt Smith (all Northern sympathizers), and ten Richmond businessmen, paid his bail. Davis, now freed, retreated to Canada, traveling through Washington, New York, and Montreal and arriving at Milloy's Wharf at the foot of Yonge Street on Lake Ontario in Toronto on the steamer *Champion* on May 30, 1867. He appeared quite ill upon arrival.

George T. Denison, a Canadian Southern supporter present at the dock, said in horror, "They have killed him."[36]

Davis had gone to Canada in part to join his family, in part for sanctuary, and in part because he had given his secret papers to his sister-in-law. She had taken them to a vault in the Bank of Montreal in Place d'Armes, and he needed to retrieve them. He first went by the boat *Rothesay Castle* to Niagara-on-the-Lake, about 30 miles south of Toronto, where he remained until June 3. From there, he traveled to Montreal with part of his family.[37] A depressed recluse during the early part of his time in Montreal, thin, gaunt, limping, and using a cane, Davis was finally persuaded to attend a play—*The Rivals*—at the Royal Theatre in the back of St. Lawrence Hall on July 18, 1867. The play was a benefit for the Southern Relief Association, an organization raising funds to reconstruct portions of the South after the war. The crowd recognized him and cheered, demanding that the band play "Dixie," which it did, but even the cheers and song didn't elicit a smile from the depressed former president of the Confederacy.[38] Davis remained in Montreal for about two years, where he slowly wrote his manuscript *The Rise and Fall of the Confederate Government*.

Perhaps surprisingly to observers of today, Davis reportedly actually wanted to go to trial. He felt that he would be vindicated, both on the charges of treason and of complicity in the assassination of Lincoln. Davis eagerly sought a hearing, and his lawyers claimed that he was being denied an appropriately speedy trial. Further delays pushed the process into October 1866. All this time, the 14th Amendment was gaining momentum as the trial was repeatedly delayed. The trial was eventually scheduled as *United States v. Jefferson Davis* in the United States District Circuit Court in Richmond, Virginia, in the spring of 1867. However, the trial was postponed twice, in part due to the impeachment trial of Andrew Johnson, brought against Johnson for firing Edwin M. Stanton from his office of secretary of war. Johnson's opponents believed that the Tenure of Office Act had protected Stanton from being fired.

The timing for Davis's trial was crucial. The statute of limitations for the original indictment was three years from the alleged crime. The date of the crime specified on the indictment was June 1864 (paperwork from a previous indictment had been "lost"). A grand jury in the United States District Circuit Court in Virginia handed down another indictment for treason on May 8, 1866. Underwood's grand jury charged Davis with a crime under that statute that held only fines and imprisonment as punishment.

President Johnson's impeachment consumed March-May 1868. He was impeached but not convicted (conviction failed by one vote). Underwood and a grand jury in Richmond, on March 26, 1868, issued yet a new and more complete indictment against Davis, this being the fourth indictment for the charge of treason. The charge was based on the old 1790 law that demanded execution upon a guilty verdict. Again, the trial was repeatedly delayed. Months elapsed, and the 14th Amendment to the Constitution was passed and finally ratified on July 9, 1868. The crucial portion of this amendment addressed the ability of an insurrectionist to hold a government office in the future:

> **Section 3.** No person shall be a Senator or Representative in Congress, or elector of President and Vice President, or hold any office, civil or military, under the United States, or under any State, who, having previously taken an oath, as a member of Congress, or as an officer of the United States, or as a member of any State legislature, or as an executive or judicial officer of any State, to support the Constitution of the United States, shall have engaged in insurrection or rebellion against the same, or given aid or comfort to the enemies thereof. But Congress may by a vote of two-thirds of each House, remove such disability.

Underwood released other prisoners on the strength of his own interpretation of this amendment. Underwood and Chase disagreed on the propriety of Underwood's rulings. Here the question of Section 3 of the 14th Amendment came into play. Judge Chase favored dropping the charges against Davis because of a "technicality," and it would save the country from a treason trial that might invoke the death penalty. It was still unclear in many judicial minds whether secession constituted an act of treason. Furthermore, if disqualification from holding future political office was really a "punishment," then Davis had already been punished and he couldn't stand trial for a second "punishment" for the same crime. When interpreted with the understanding of the issues boiling at the time of its writing, the 14th Amendment to the Constitution assumes a more poignant meaning. The Civil War had just ended, and some politicians/statesmen wanted to punish the rebellious Southerners. They believed that those who had participated in the secession should never hold elected office again. This amendment was a means of assuring that those who had committed treason would be so limited.

Section 3 was the crucial passage. Did it mean that Davis and others would simply be *disqualified* from holding future office, or was it an actual *punishment*? The distinction was important, for disqualification was a mild rebuke, while punishment meant that Davis could not be tried for his "crimes" otherwise—additional punishment would violate the section of the Constitution prohibiting double jeopardy for an offense. The initial interpretations of Section 3 of the 14th Amendment called it a criminal sanction, which meant that Davis might be protected from further prosecution, an effect likely not predicted by those who had drafted and voted upon this amendment.

The adoption of the 14th Amendment to the Constitution meant that

Davis could never again hold public office (unless ⅔ of both the Senate and the House of Representatives voted to allow the restoration of his office-holding rights). Some of Davis's supporters claimed that such a punishment was sufficient and that no harsher sentence was needed. Restoration of the union would be promoted by such leniency, they argued. However, the District Court (which included Supreme Court chief justice Salmon Chase, in his role as circuit court judge, who wanted to dismiss the treason charges, and Underwood, the district judge in Virginia, who wanted further punishment for Davis) was thus split in its decision to dismiss the charges against Davis. The case eventually moved up to the Supreme Court, of which Chase was the chief justice. Then President Johnson issued his Christmas Day 1868 Proclamation of General Amnesty for former Confederates. That proclamation required application for amnesty, but such amnesty was almost certain to be granted. It included all Confederates, whereas the previous amnesty proclamations had excluded various classes of Southerners or specifically excluded certain high Confederate officers. That amnesty restored any Confederate's civil and property rights and protected the person from charges of treason. However, the amnesty didn't confer rights to vote or to hold office, as outlined in the newly passed 14th Amendment. The amnesty made moot any future criminal prosecution of Davis, and the Supreme Court recommended abandonment of charges against him. So in February 1869 Davis was a free man again. This interpretation of Section 3 of the 14th Amendment meant that any future legal wrangling over the Civil War wouldn't ever happen. The Constitution had been (and remains) silent on whether secession is treason.

Though the Supreme Court under Chief Justice Salmon Chase ultimately rescinded the treason indictment against Davis in February 1869, Davis still wasn't included in the provisions of the Amnesty Proclamations of 1872 and 1876, which restored to some Confederates the rights of citizenship, including the right to vote and to hold office. Davis never asked for a pardon. He said in 1881, "It has been said that I should apply to the United States for a pardon, but repentance must precede the right of pardon, and I have not repented."[39] For all of the legal wrangling over nearly four years, Davis appeared in court for only portions of two days. He was never tried or convicted; on the other hand, he was never completely exonerated during his lifetime. Davis died in 1889. Senate Joint Resolution 16, Public Law 95–466, signed by President Jimmy Carter on October 17, 1978, posthumously restored Davis's citizenship and full rights.[40]

14

The Fate of the Co-Conspirators

Jacob Thompson

Sometime toward the end of the war Jacob Thompson's wife Catherine was told incorrectly that her husband was dead. Fortunately, at about the same time, Thompson had sent a messenger—a Canadian girl—with a letter to Catherine telling her to come to Canada and to bring the receipts for $200,000 he had invested in stocks in England. Catherine needed to use forged identity papers to make the journey, and on two occasions (in Memphis, Tennessee, and in Cairo, Illinois) the illegality of her travel documents was almost discovered, but she eventually successfully joined Jacob in Canada.

Money would become a crucial issue for the Thompsons as the war drew to an end. Judah Benjamin and Thompson had begun communications in December 1864 regarding Thompson's inability to function effectively as the Canadian Confederate commissioner. Union spies knew everyone in Thompson's camp. Furthermore, virtually all of Thompson's schemes had failed—from Blackburn's yellow fever plot to the burning of New York City to the St. Alban's raid. Nothing the Confederates had planned ultimately succeeded. Benjamin wrote to Thompson on December 6, 1864, telling him that General Edwin Gray Lee, a second cousin to Robert E. Lee, would replace him. Another letter from Benjamin to Thompson on December 30 said, "We are satisfied that so close espionage is kept upon you that your services have been deprived of value which is attached to your further residence in Canada. The President thinks, therefore, that as soon as the gentleman [General Lee] arrives who bears this letter … that you transfer to him, as quietly as possible, all the information that you have obtained and the release of funds in your hands and then return to the Confederacy."[1]

Benjamin subsequently ordered Thompson back to Richmond on March 2. In so doing, he told Thompson to keep sufficient money to cover his personal travel expenses back to the South but to deposit the rest of the Confederate money in Liverpool, England, with Fraser, Trenholm and Company, one of the financial institutions there that held Confederate assets. General Edwin Gray Lee delivered this message personally to Thompson in Montreal. In addition, Lee directed Thompson to give him $20,000 before the transfer of funds to Liverpool, probably for Lee's personal and travel expenses. The original infusion of cash into the Canadian accounts in 1864 had been close to $1,000,000 of the $5,000,000 allocated for the Confederate Secret Service. Benjamin estimated that about $400,000 should have been remaining in the account, and he instructed Thompson about a secret code he should use to tell Benjamin how much money would be transferred. Thompson was to place an advertisement in the *New York Herald* stating that a piece of land was for sale—the price being the amount Thompson would transfer to Liverpool. Thompson gave Lee only $10,000 and apparently kept most—if not all—of the remainder for himself. These funds would allow Thompson and his wife to live lavishly in Europe for the next few years. It's uncertain how much money he brought back to the States when he ultimately returned in 1869.[2]

Jacob and Catherine Thompson left Montreal on their journey to Halifax on April 14, the day Lincoln was shot. Thompson traveled by land through Quebec, and during his trip he discovered that Lincoln had been assassinated and that he himself was listed as one of the co-conspirators. He composed a lengthy denial of the charges, which was published in the *New York Tribune* on May 22. In it he claimed to be the object of "unjust persecution," and he feared that his "silence might be construed into an admission of the justness of the attacks" (on Thompson's character and accusations of his role in the assassination). Thompson expounded upon the legality and propriety of the Southern states in seceding from the Union on the basis of states' rights. He told of his work in the Canadian Confederacy as a "duty" and a "service." Speaking of President Andrew Johnson, Thompson said, "He [Johnson] took sides with power; I took sides with weakness." He further denied that he had been involved in the plot to burn New York City and said that any implication made by Captain Robert Kennedy about Thompson's role in the arson was made under the duress of Kennedy's death sentence, Kennedy's presumed intoxication at the time of the accusation and initial interrogation, and Kennedy's coercion by the authorities. Thompson called President Johnson's proclamation implicating him in the killing of Lincoln false and claimed the "Bureau of Military Justice" was a trumped-up court that deserved only shame: "I aver upon honor that I have never known, or conversed, or held communication, either directly or indirectly, with Booth ... or with any one of his associates."

Such a denial was clearly untrue. Boldly he proclaimed, "I know there is not half the ground to suspect me that there is to suspect President Johnson himself." Then he proceeded to list some reasons why Johnson might have

14. The Fate of the Co-Conspirators

actually wanted to see Lincoln dead. He lamented that Lincoln's killing "at the time it was done, was most unfortunate both for me and for the people of the South." He claimed, "President Johnson was to acquire a dazzling power in the event of Lincoln's death." Thompson suspected some kind of acquaintance—even friendship—between Booth and Johnson. Thompson called Lincoln's death Johnson's "great good fortune" and decried the public's need to demand a victim. He finished his diatribe as follows: "I am denounced as a traitor and rebel in this [presidential] Proclamation [naming Thompson as a co-conspirator]. Let the world judge between President Johnson and myself, not according to the law of *might*, but according to the law of *right*" (emphasis Thompson's). Then Thompson protested: "Now, mark me, I do not say that all this creates a suspicion in my mind of the complicity of President Johnson in the foul work upon President Lincoln." Finally, he penned, "There was no need of offering $25,000 reward for my arrest. If I felt the least assurance of being tried according to the recognized principles of law, without a prejudgment, without the arbitrariness of a Court acting under the instructions of this 'Bureau of *Military Justice*,' [emphasis Thompson's] and without contumely, I would go in person and deliver myself up to the proper judicial authorities. Until I have such an assurance, I think I ought to keep out of the way, which no doubt will gratify my enemies."[3] Since Thompson had just accused—or at the very least, libeled—President Johnson, perhaps exile was a reasonable course for him to take.

Thompson and his wife thus fled to Europe. During this time, the legislature of Mississippi claimed in a petition on Thompson's behalf on December 8, 1865 (received and filed on December 26), that Thompson didn't actually flee to avoid laws or prosecution, but that his trip was performed as a part of his "duty"—he "obeyed the call that told him a duty was to be performed," a "duty to the state where he had a home." Further, the Mississippi legislature and senate argued to President Johnson that Thompson had been "debarred from the benefits of your amnesty proclamation by its exceptional clauses, a reward offered for his arrest should he return—he necessarily remains an exile from this state he loves, and the country he once so honorably and faithfully served." They pleaded, "We ask that he may be permitted to return and to remain unmolested by your authority, that the provisions of amnesty may be extended to him, and that his once happy home may be again enlivened by his presence."[4] Sent on behalf of the Mississippi legislature, this petition was signed by S.J. Gholson, the Speaker of the House of Representatives, John M. Simonton, the president of the Senate, and Benjamin G. Humphreys, the governor of Mississippi. Thompson would later write to his supporters: "Your petition is well intended, I am thankful to each and every one who signed it. I regard it as friendship's offering; but I fear it will be unavailing."[5] It was indeed unavailing.

Jacob and Catherine traveled throughout Europe extensively. They hardly led a Spartan existence, and many Confederates believed Thompson had embezzled or transferred additional large hoards of Confederate money from the Canadian banks prior to his departure to Europe. Jacob and Catherine toured Paris, Switzerland, Rome, Naples, Egypt, Palestine, the Greek Isles, up the Adriatic to Venice, Vienna, Munich, Frankfort, Cologne, Brussels, Scotland, the Lakes of Killarney, and then back to Halifax and Canada. Catherine eventually returned to Mississippi, while Jacob went to Canada, where he remained for two more years, after which she joined him there. He returned to the United States in May 1869. Catherine and Jacob still had substantial resources upon their return to the United States, despite losing much property in Oxford, Mississippi, during the war. They finally settled in Memphis, Tennessee, where he died on March 24, 1885.[6]

Clement C. Clay

Toward the end of 1864, it seemed clear that the Canadian Confederates weren't accomplishing much to help the war effort. Confederate communications often took the form of advertisements or personal notices in newspapers. In November 1864 Clement C. Clay suffered yet another setback in his health, even as a personal notice in the *New York News* informed him that he was to leave Canada.[7] He departed Canada on either December 1, 1864,[8] or January 13, 1865,[9] and relinquished his remaining funds (about $32,000) to Jacob Thompson before he left. Clay's difficult journey took him from St. Catharines to Halifax, then on the steamer *Old Dominion* to Bermuda, where he arrived January 17. He then took the blockade-runner *Rattlesnake* from Bermuda to Nassau, departing Bermuda on January 18.[10] His original destination had been Wilmington, North Carolina, but the Northern blockade of the Wilmington port was complete and total. Fifty-nine ships enclosed the harbor at Wilmington, so trying to go there would have been futile.[11] Charleston was the only remaining port where he could go. He arrived safely in Nassau, and on January 31 he steamed from Nassau to Charleston. The *Rattlesnake* ran aground as it approached the Charleston port, and Clay was forced to board a lifeboat that took him close enough to shore for him to wade the remaining distance to land. In the process, he lost many of his possessions.

The *Rattlesnake* burned when it grounded near Charleston. The attrition rate of ships during the Civil War was extremely high. Any commercial company in modern days would never survive the loss or capture of so many vessels. At the beginning of the war, about 10 percent of each Confederate blockade run was captured or sunk by the Union navy, but by the end of the

14. The Fate of the Co-Conspirators

war fully 50 percent of blockade-running attempts were captured or sunk. Blockade-runners were to a certain extent expendable. Losing a ship was simply the cost of doing business. Couriers of supplies viewed the initial limited attrition as acceptable; however, as it approached 100 percent, the Confederates could no longer maintain this activity.

Clay then worked his way slowly homeward to his family. First he went from Charleston to Columbia, South Carolina, then to Augusta, Georgia (where he destroyed some of his papers that had survived the shipwreck).[12] He finally arrived at Macon, Georgia, on February 10, 1865, where he stayed with a friend until he was reunited with his wife.

Clay met with Secretary of State Judah P. Benjamin and President Jefferson Davis on April 2, 1865, as the war was about to end. He started a trip toward Mexico to join Confederate forces in exile there, but upon hearing that President Lincoln had been assassinated and that President Andrew Johnson had issued orders for Clay's arrest, along with other alleged co-conspirators, he changed his plans. All conspirators had rewards posted on their heads: Davis, $100,000; Clay, $25,000; Thompson, $25,000; George Sanders, $25,000; Beverly Tucker, $25,000; and Cleary, $10,000, again incorrectly identified as William C. Cleary[13] (offers of rewards for capture of Cleary, Tucker, Sanders, and Thompson were revoked on November 24, 1865).[14] Clay surrendered to General James H. Wilson, in Macon, Georgia, where he was arrested for the suspicion that he was involved in the plot to assassinate President Lincoln. He was imprisoned at Fortress Monroe, Hampton, Virginia, where Jefferson Davis was kept (they were housed in cells near each other). Clay spent 11 months in prison, from May 1865 to April 1866, but was never tried.

During the trial of Lincoln's assassins, Clay's sentiments and his role in the conspiracy achieved center stage. Not only did he have close personal attachments to many of those charged with conspiring to kill Lincoln, the government also had both physical evidence and testimony that implicated Clay in the plans to assassinate the president. Witnesses swore that Clay had access to the secret cipher device used to transmit messages to and from the conspirators in Canada, and John McGill testified that Clay had dealings with Robert C. Kennedy, the mastermind of the attempt to set New York on fire. Kennedy allegedly involved Clay in the discussions about killing Lincoln. The witness—John McGill—told of a meeting among McGill, Kennedy, Clay, McDonald, Cleary, and another unnamed friend. Four of them (Clay, Kennedy, Cleary, and McDonald) came out of a private meeting, and Kennedy said:

> He (alluding to me [McGill]) is the man to lay Stanton out [kill him]. Clay said, "Boys, it is a very risky job, and furthermore, if you undertake to do it you must take your lives in your own hands." He said to me (calling me by name): "Mr. Stan-

> ton is a very big man and if you cannot undertake to do the job you had better not try it." I told him I thought I could do anything in that way I was called upon to do. He said: "If you get back to Canada after the job is completed you will be a rich man. If you happen to fail in the attempt you will swing [be hung]." Captain Kennedy had previously stated to us in the conversation that we should have $5,000 apiece if we got back from Washington, and that the Confederate Government would give us a good deal more.[15]

Kennedy would later tell McGill that other men had been chosen to do the killing, men more competent for the job, and McGill was removed from the assassination team. But it seemed clear that Clay was part of the plan and that he approved of this approach. He had responded to the suggestion of killing Lincoln, expressing the idea that nothing was a crime if it advanced the cause of the Confederacy: "That is so; we are all devoted to our cause, and ready to go to any lengths, to do anything under the sun to serve our cause."[16]

Supporting these schemes of burning towns, killing presidents, and importing pestilence was partially the responsibility of Thompson and Clay as the designated keepers of the purse strings of the Confederate coffers in Canada. Large quantities of money passed through various Canadian banks. Movements of $50,000–100,000 were commonplace. The Lincoln trial testimony heard one Robert Anson Campbell, a teller at the Ontario Bank of Montreal, who told of such transfers in 1864 and 1865. Thompson and Clay managed these accounts, and Campbell would later identify John Wilkes Booth as another depositor.[17]

Clay was also closely associated with Blackburn and the latter's plan to import disease into the North. Hyams connected the two as well: "On disposing of the trunks I immediately left Washington and went straight through until I got to Hamilton, Canada. In the waiting room there I met Mr. Holcombe and Mr. Clement C. Clay. They both rose, shook hands with me, and congratulated me on my safe return and upon my making a fortune. They told me I should be a gentleman for the future, instead of a workingman and a mechanic. They seemed perfectly to understand the business in which I had been engaged." That Clay was aware of the diabolical schemes seemed obvious, and that he was concerned about the devious and unethical nature of the jobs he approved and funded is suggested by the fact that Clay used many aliases: Mr. Hope, Mr. Lacey, Mr. Tracey.[18] Valiant and honorable jobs rarely require aliases. Judge Advocate General Joseph Holt summarized his investigation by saying, "It is therefore advised by this bureau that as soon as such preparations shall be completed this party [Clay] be brought before a military commission upon charges, not only of complicity in the plot of assassination, but also of violation of the laws of war, in authorizing and directing guerilla raids and the burning of cities, and in promoting the introduction of pestilence into our territory."[19]

Clay's order for release from incarceration was sent to Fortress Monroe on April 17, 1866. The conditions were "that he takes the oath of allegiance to the United States and gives his parole of honor to conduct himself as a loyal citizen of the same and to report himself in person at any time and place to answer any charges that may hereafter be prepared against him by the United States."[20] On April 18, 1866, he was released, and he returned to his old home in Huntsville, Alabama. The July 4, 1868, Third Presidential Proclamation of Amnesty to Southern Civil War Participants did not include those charged with treason or a felony, so Clay wasn't pardoned (proclamations occurred on May 29, 1865; September 7, 1867; July 4, 1868, and December 25, 1868). However, on December 25, 1868, when President Johnson extended his Christmas Amnesty Proclamation, he gave universal amnesty to Confederate Civil War participants, and Clay was included in this order, making his pardon official. He died on January 3, 1882, and was buried in Frankfort, Kentucky.

James Philemon Holcombe

Professor Holcombe returned to the United States in September 1864 on a blockade-runner bound for Wilmington, North Carolina, from Halifax. His ship, the *Condor*, left Halifax on September 24, and the U.S. consul sent a message to the Navy Department in Washington, D.C., warning them of Holcombe's presence on the ship. The blockading squadron was alerted, and they were ready to intercept the *Condor* to arrest Holcombe when it came to Cape Fear on October 1. The *Condor* was a three-funneled steamer, piloted by a veteran British admiral on a one-year's leave. He was blockade-running for adventure and some extra cash, and the *Condor* was on its maiden voyage as a blockade-runner. The captain was named Augustus Charles Hobart-Hampden, the Eighth Earl of Buckinghamshire, also known by the aliases Captain Roberts, Captain Hewett, and Captain Gulick.[21] However, a storm intervened and the *Condor* escaped past the blockade, only to falter as it approached New Inlet, one of the two entries to the Cape Fear River.

The Union blockade ship *Niphon* pursued the *Condor*, firing guns as the race toward the inlet continued. The *Condor*'s captain steered his ship away from what he thought was another Union vessel, but the object he had spotted was the blockade-runner *Night Hawk* from Bermuda, a vessel that had been sunk just hours earlier and was burning on the rocks of the New Inlet Bar outside Wilmington, near Fort Fisher. Missing the *Night Hawk*, the *Condor* ran aground on a sand bar. Holcombe boarded a lifeboat and began rowing toward shore with three others: Captain Hobart-Hampden, Rose O'Neal Greenhow—a Confederate spy and famed author of the book *My Imprisonment and the First Year of Abolition Rule in Washington*, from which she had earned nearly $2,000—and a Lieutenant Wilson, a recently paroled Confederate prisoner of war. A wave capsized the rowboat, and Holcombe and two others survived by clinging to the overturned rowboat. Passenger Rose O'Neal Greenhow never surfaced after the rowboat capsized. Her money from the book profits went with her to the bottom of the bay. Holcombe then left Wilmington on October 2 to travel to Richmond, where he reported to Jefferson Davis. Holcombe didn't give a detailed account of his finances and completed duties until mid–November, at which time he stated he had successfully repatriated 55–60 Confederate soldiers during his seven months in Canada. He then traveled to his home in Bellevue, Bedford County, Virginia, arriving in October 1864.[22]

Judge Advocate General Joseph Holt, at the request of Secretary of War Edwin M. Stanton, reviewed Professor James P. Holcombe's case at the end of December 1865. Holt completed his review on December 29, 1865, and gave a scathing summation regarding Holcombe's involvement in the assassination of Lincoln and Blackburn's yellow fever plot. Holt based much of his opinion on the testimony given at the trial of the accomplices of Lincoln's assassination. Holt called them the "well known rebel agents and conspirators through whom was executed the assassination of President Lincoln."[23] Holt further said, "Associated as he [Holcombe] was with these men, it is not possible that he should not have been cognizant of their detestable schemes, and ... it can hardly be doubted that he cooperated in the plot of assassination."[24] Specifically to the question of Holcombe's involvement with Blackburn and Hyams, Holt commented that the attempt to introduce yellow fever into the North was "perhaps the most fiendish devised in the history of the war."[25] Holt believed Hyams' account and those of the other witnesses: "Not only is it full and frank and consistent throughout, but it is in its most material particulars corroborated by the depositions of various other witnesses entirely unconnected with the scheme in question or with the rebel interests."[26] He continued: "The guilt which must be attached to one of his intelligence and position must be deemed far more flagrant than any which can be imputed to the subordinates who executed the deeds of infamy which he and his confederates inspired and controlled."[27] He then concluded: "The offence of this man is unique in its character, and has about it features of foulness and barbarism more revolting than those which characterize any of the horrible crimes to which the rebellion has given birth. This monstrous attempt to poison whole communities and armies—undertaken as it was by high officials and traitors engaged in war upon the Government, and indeed resorted to as a mode of prosecuting that war—is not only a dishonor to our own country and people but a stain upon the very civilization of the age."[28]

However, Holt's protestations that Holcombe needed to go to trial came to naught. At the same time, Holcombe's request for pardon was being reviewed and considered at another level. In an undated letter to President

Andrew Johnson, probably written about June 28, 1865 (the filing date listed on a covering paper), Holcombe had asked for clemency. He signed a certificate of allegiance to the United States (called by some the "Oath of Allegiance," and by others the "Oath of Amnesty") on June 21, 1865, in Lynchburg, Virginia. His letter probably accompanied that oath, and they were transmitted in response to the Proclamation of Amnesty by President Johnson on May 29, 1865. Holcombe's letter said that he went to the "British Province" (Canada) in the spring of 1864, "not as a general agent of the Confederate States but upon a clearly defined and limited mission."[29] He alleged that he went to Canada only to investigate the "*Chesapeake* Affair," to determine the legality of the capture of that ship. He concluded that the Confederate States had no title to this vessel, and Holcombe asserted that he had conducted no other business in Canada except to furnish escaped Confederate prisoners with transportation back to the South via Halifax and Bermuda. He denied any connection with Clay and Thompson, stating that they had been sent to Canada for a different purpose. (Holcombe conveniently avoided any description of his unquestioned meetings with Clay, Thompson, Sanders, Blackburn, and others, and he even neglected to mention his participation in the attempt to negotiate peace through Horace Greeley's connections—meetings that President Lincoln himself had approved and had granted special passage through Union lines to conduct.) Holcombe said that he had left Canada on about the 22nd of August, 1864, "before most if not all of the detestable transactions which have since shocked the country."[30] He further denied being involved in any plots to perform raids into the North from Canada, any plans to burn Northern cities, any schemes of murder or arson, or the "introduction of pestilence."[31] As proof, he offered not only his oath of allegiance but also all of his public papers and his private diary. The attorney general of the United States and Judge Noah Haynes Swayne recommended approval of Holcombe's request for pardon. Apparently no one acted immediately on his petition, but Holcombe was finally granted a special pardon on December 28, 1865, only one day before Holt recommended the opposite. Time and logistics had been on Holcombe's side for the late arrival of Holt's scathing description of Holcombe's activities. Holcombe received his pardon and went on to live in Virginia, although he didn't return to his law professorship at the University of Virginia. He established a high school for boys near his home in Bellevue, Bedford County, Virginia. James Philemon Holcombe died on August 22, 1873.

William Walter Cleary

The press ultimately didn't treat William Walter Cleary with much respect, either. Soon after hearings and trials had begun, Cleary was described as a man who "sneaks round in a very subdued manner, and if he is seen in the bar of the Queen's [Hotel] it is only when he hopes to receive an invitation to drink."[32] Cleary initially had a bounty price of $10,000 on his head, but he never faced trial. He did not apply individually for a pardon, but the Presidential Proclamation of General Amnesty ultimately covered him. He finally returned to Cynthiana, Kentucky, where he continued to practice law and was later elected county judge. In 1873 he was elected to be the Twelfth Judicial District commonwealth's attorney. He died in Covington, Kentucky, on March 16, 1897, at age 66, of Bright's disease.

Edward Cork Swan

Edward Cork Swan disappeared from history after he was released from the Bermuda jail. There is no record of his having children born in the Parish of St. Georges in Bermuda, nor is his death recorded there or elsewhere in the country of Bermuda. Perhaps after he was released from the jail he decided that Bermudian life was less glamorous than had been advertised. He disappeared completely.

Bermuda, of course, survived its involvement in the Civil War. It returned to its more sleepy island identity after Confederate blockade-running rather abruptly disappeared, robbing the islands of the economic boom it had brought to the country. The environmental and sanitary conditions that promoted yellow fever persisted, though they gradually moderated with improvement in the overall health of the islands. Because the epidemics had largely been brought by ships and their occupants, the exposure to contagion decreased with the decline in shipping. Over decades, yellow fever completely disappeared as the mosquito responsible for the disease, the *Aedes aegypti*, was eliminated from the islands. In modern times yellow fever has been a disease unknown to the inhabitants of Bermuda.[33]

15

Godfrey Joseph Hyams
The Aftermath

The facts of the yellow fever plot seem rather indisputable. Although the prime witness, Godfrey Joseph Hyams, was disreputable and had turned from being a supporter of the North to a tool for the South and then back to an informant for the North, his descriptions of the events surrounding the plot are mostly true. While he had demanded immunity from prosecution for his testimony and had received payment for his testimony and for the expenses incurred for his travel and attendance at the many trials, his profit wasn't the riches he had desired. But the other witnesses and evidence firmly testify to Dr. Blackburn's intentions to spread an epidemic throughout the North. Few original documents exist today in the records of the Civil War dealing with this episode, except for those cited in the trials. Of course, no physical evidence remains. But Dr. Blackburn's legacy is tarnished because both the circumstances and the trial testimony are compelling.

• • •

Hyams seemed to disappear from sight after giving his testimony at the various trials. The United States government granted him a pardon on June 22, 1865. On January 19, 1866, he requested the paperwork concerning his pardon through Alfred Russell, the United States district attorney for the Eastern District of Michigan in Detroit. At this time, Hyams was living in Detroit at 116 6th Street between Abbott and Porter streets, near the Detroit River. Russell transmitted Hyams' request to Washington, D.C., and the attorney general of the United States in Washington confirmed on June 26, 1866, that the pardon had been completed almost a year earlier, on June 22, 1865.[1]

Hyams had a wife and children (at least two) in Toronto in the early-mid 1860s, according to the Rev. Dr. Stuart Robinson. Robinson called Hyams a "scoundrel" for failing to provide for his wife and children. He also referred to Hyams' spouse as a "half crazed wife."[2] Hyams' first child was Jefferson

Davis "Jeffrey" Hyams; the second was Thomas Francis Stonewall Jackson Hyams, who died at just over one year of age in Toronto in March 1865. The next was Joseph Godfrey Hyams, who was being carried by Hyams' pregnant wife in Toronto in early 1865, but he was born soon after the Hyams moved to Detroit.

From Detroit, after the trials in Toronto, Washington, D.C., and Boston, Hyams' precise travels are unclear. In 1866 or 1867[5] he moved to Charleston, South Carolina, where he had relatives at that time. Perhaps a fourth child named Mary Jane Hyams was born in Charleston. Charleston was a chaotic city during the early years of Civil War Reconstruction. Many Southerners didn't want to accept the abolition of slavery, and political parties were exceedingly polarized. Democrats (of which Hyams was one) clung to the idea that Lincoln had been an oppressor; Republicans (many of whom were black) resisted any thought of minimizing the freedoms of the newly emancipated slaves.[3]

The center of political expression in Charleston's historic peninsula was the corner of Broad and Meeting streets. At this intersection were the federal courthouse and post office, Charleston City Hall, the county courthouse and guardhouse, and St. Michael's Episcopal Church. Severely damaged by the war, many buildings in this area were simply carcasses of their past incarnations. Streets were cobblestone mixed with dirt, and near Broad and Meeting streets many of the buildings had vanished, remnants of Southern society with entry steps leading nowhere. Heavy metal and wrought iron fences remained, but flames and missiles had destroyed the parlors and bedrooms.

In subsequent years, this street corner in Charleston would be called the "Four Corners of Law" because of the concentration of legal activity at this site. There, as in Hyde Park in London, advocates of all political stripes would stand on the street corners and shout their beliefs. It was the proverbial soapbox of Charleston. Altercations were common, and the rhetoric often degenerated into physical battles resembling gang warfare. Newspapers referred to the groups participating in these spirited debates as "the Broad Street corner belligerents."[4] Here Godfrey Hyams once again would find an opportunity for the expression of his frustration with the broken promises he had experienced from both the South and the North. However, he remained a Southern supporter in spite of never receiving his promised fortune for the transportation of the trunks filled with garments and bedding from the yellow fever victims. Many Southerners viewed Hyams as a traitor to the Southern cause; he had revealed mountains of evidence and had testified against famous Southern operatives. Many thought that he deserved to be killed. He was "Public Enemy #1" to many of those who knew his history.

Hyams lived at least briefly in Charleston at 120 King Street, a scant one block from the intersection of Meeting and Broad.[5] Residing at this address, he had ample opportunity to engage his political opponents. (His residence today, after successive renumberings of the Charleston streets, likely would be at 132 King Street, the southern extent of a new Charleston parking garage.)[6] There Hyams was listed in the 1869 South Carolina census as living with five other persons, but their identity and exact ages were not recorded.[7] This census cataloged only the name of the head of the household, the number of males over the age of 21 in the home, the number of children between ages 6 and 16, and the total number of males and females of all ages. Hyams is listed as the only male in his living group over the age of 21. There were no children between the ages of 6 and 16, and the household had 4 males and 2 females. One can only speculate who the other 5 persons were, but perhaps it was the family associated with Bridget Hyams detailed below.

Hyams registered, as required by law, in the Charleston County Militia in 1869.[8] All males in South Carolina between the ages of 18 and 45 were compelled to enroll, much as the Selective Service required males to register later in our country's history. Exempted from this registration were government officials, clergymen, firemen, practicing physicians, professors, teachers, and students in colleges, academies, and common schools, soldiers and sailors, "idiots, lunatics, paupers, and persons convicted of infamous crimes."[9] Arguably, Hyams didn't fall within any of these categories, although he approached the "pauper" and the "infamous crimes" designations, notwithstanding the fact that he had never been tried or convicted in the yellow fever plot. He never performed any duties for this militia, however. Others clearly knew Hyams was residing in Charleston in the 1860s. "Dead letter" files in Charleston list him as a recipient of letters in December 1866 and January 1867.[10]

Hyams soon ran afoul of the law in Charleston, as he had elsewhere. He was charged with assault and battery sometime before 18 July 1867.[11] However, those detailed court records with repeated "continuances"[12] and police arrest documents have been lost. He was also charged on November 24, 1869, with assault and battery in an altercation. Falling back into his old ways, he had found assimilation into polite Southern society to be difficult. He was arrested for engaging in a fight that began at about 3:30 p.m. on November 23, 1869, at the corner of Meeting and Broad streets, involving one Lafayette I. Woolf. Woolf lived at 114 St. Philip (about 10 blocks from Hyams' house).[13] Arrest records have been lost, but the court documents have survived.[14] Hyams was charged with assault and battery, bludgeoning Woolf "without cause or provocation" about the face and then beating him as he lay on the ground. Perhaps the incident wasn't exactly "without provocation," as the victim was a member of the Republican party and first vice president of the Republican Party in Ward No. 4 in the Charleston area (Hyams, as noted, was a Democrat). The same Lafayette I. Woolf was prone to disputes and infractions of the law himself, based on other newspaper reports and court documents in Charleston.[15]

Hyams and Woolf filed competing charges against each other. They both accused the other of assault with intent to kill. A warrant for Hyams' arrest was issued on November 24. Hyams was apprehended and released on $100 bail. The trial began on February 7, 1870, but was continued until June 1870 and again until September 1870. He was found guilty (therefore Woolf was found not guilty), and on October 13, 1870, Hyams was fined $15 and court costs, or two months in the county jail if he failed to pay the fine. Positive confirmation that this Godfrey J. Hyams was the same Hyams of the Blackburn plot was provided by Hyams' signature on the court documents in Charleston, a signature identical to at least seven other signatures on documents extant from 1862–1866.[16] However, Lafayette I. Woolf would later find himself again on the wrong side of the law. He was fond of disputes and confrontations, and he repeatedly appeared on the front page of the *Charleston Daily News* for various infractions—assault and battery, assault with intent to kill, and murder. So Hyams' victim in 1869 wasn't exactly an innocent or upright citizen.[17] Hyams habitually seemed to run afoul of the law. Hyams was again charged with assault and battery in Charleston in June 1870 and was found guilty in September 1870. Detailed court records of this trial have also been lost.[18]

One Bridget Hyams also lived in Charleston during this time,[19] and she most certainly was Godfrey Hyams' wife (she would have been his second wife; his first was Hannah Martin in England in 1854). Likely this was the same Bridget Sheehan Hyams who was born in Ireland on November 16, 1850. However, the only documentation that her birth year was 1850 is her death certificate, listing January 17, 1903, as the date of her death from "Apoplexy" and the age as 50.[20] The Charleston, Irish Bridget was listed as an illiterate laundress who lived at 20 Broad Street and who later resided at the corner of Tradd and Southeast Legare streets, both sites just one and two blocks, respectively, from the reported address for Godfrey Hyams in 1869. Three of her children, Jefferson Davis "Jeffrey," age seven, Henry Michael, age five, and Joseph Godfrey, age three, were admitted to the Charleston Orphan House on June 16, 1870.

Located at 160 Calhoun Street, the site of old Revolutionary War barracks just about eight blocks from the area where Godfrey and Bridget lived, the Charleston Orphan House was established in 1790 for the "purpose of supporting and educating poor and orphan children and those of poor and disabled parents who are unable to support and maintain them." It was the first municipal orphanage in the United States.[21] While it accepted children whose parents had died, it also housed the poor. The Hyams children, listed in the 1870 census as being "Charleston Orphan House Children," were incorrectly reported in that census as having the last name "Haines." Another possible child of Godfrey and Bridget listed in the records of the Charleston Orphan House was Mary Jane Hyams, but details of her subsequent life are unknown.

Life in the Orphan House was secure, though not lavish by any means. Children were actually called "inmates," a term with derogatory connotations in the 1860s, as it is today. Education, segregated by gender, was delivered within the Orphan House. Classes included reading, writing, mathematics, literature, geography, and "elocution." Girls learned sewing and provided many of the articles of clothing needed by the children, as well as other items such as sheets and blankets. Boys participated in agricultural projects that helped put food on the table, tended a vegetable garden, chopped wood, and milked cows. Bright girls helped with the education of the younger children. Inmates were not allowed to leave the Orphan House grounds for any reason, even to visit family if they had one. Boys were kept until age 21, girls until age 18. All children, after arriving at the appropriate age, were subject to indenture and apprenticeship with a sponsor. For boys that age was 14, and the common training was as cobblers, shoemakers, tinsmiths, carpenters, mariners, sailmakers, ship chandlers, metal workers, clerks, farmers, and blacksmiths. Girls, who could be indentured at age 13, had only the career paths of seamstress and domestic helper. On one occasion a generous donor offered to provide dresses for the girls, but the Orphan House officials rejected the notion of the girls wearing anything but the standard homespun school uniform, as they wanted the girls to be "reminded ... of their place in society." Life as an indentured apprentice was often quite harsh, usually worse than living in the Orphan House itself.

It's not absolutely certain that Bridget Hyams was Godfrey's wife, although the ages of her children (approximately 7, 5, 3—or 5, 3, 1, and newborn at the time of the 1869 census) would correspond roughly to the ages of children known to have been born to Godfrey and his second wife. Furthermore, the four males and two females listed in that 1869 census would correspond to this family group. Jeffrey was later indentured to a carpenter named Ed O'Brien, in July 1877. Bridget reclaimed Mary, Henry, and Joseph in 1879 (Jeffrey would likely still have been indentured at this time), about eight years after Godfrey had left Charleston. Bridget told the Orphan House officials that she was moving to St. Louis to join her husband, perhaps a new husband. She signed the legal documents for this transfer with an "X" since she was illiterate. Perhaps she told the story of "joining her husband" because divorce or abandonment then was socially very unacceptable. She said she was going to St. Louis with her five children—likely Jeffrey, Henry, Joseph, Mary, and Mamie, born September 16, 1870. Jefferson Davis "Jeffrey" Hyams would subsequently die at age 19 on February 10, 1884, in a St. Louis smallpox hospital. (Thomas Francis Stonewall Jackson Hyams, another child of Godfrey and Bridget, had died in Canada in 1865.) In both the Charleston and the St. Louis directories beginning in 1881, Bridget claimed to be the "widow" of Godfrey J. Hyams, not his wife nor the wife of another husband. Perhaps Godfrey had even feigned his own death in Charleston to escape his destitute family and his many enemies in Charleston. This family likely was Godfrey Hyams' second wife and children. Bridget Sheehan Hyams died in St. Louis in 1903.

Hyams' exact whereabouts and activities around 1870 are obscure. However, one Godfrey J. Hyams married Eliza Miller Nichols Childress on March 1, 1871, in Union Schoolhouse District, Christian County, Kentucky.[22] Godfrey and Eliza had acquired their marriage license the previous day, February 28, 1861, in West Christian County for the exorbitant price of one hundred dollars. That amount would be roughly the equivalent of two thousand dollars today. Marriage was indeed a costly venture in the mid–19th century. The signature on the marriage certificate again matched other known signatures from Godfrey Joseph Hyams. They were married by the Reverend E.N. Dicken of the local Baptist church (current-day descendants say that it was the Mt. Zion Baptist Church), somewhat of an anomaly for Hyams, who was Jewish.

Born on March 9, 1848, Eliza was the daughter of Jesse Nichols and Kate Childress Nichols. She first married a widower named William T. Childress on August 26, 1866. His last name was the same as her mother's maiden name, confusing the heritage somewhat. So her last name was Nichols, and then Childress following her first marriage. Likely her first husband died before 1871, though his death is not recorded, and they had a son named John Childress. The Godfrey J. Hyams of her second marriage was the same Godfrey J. Hyams of the Blackburn plot. This Godfrey Hyams was listed as a boot and shoemaker born in London in 1822 (the year and city where our protagonist was born and the same occupation of the Godfrey Hyams of the Blackburn conspiracy). Hyams appeared in the June 12, 1880, federal census of Union Schoolhouse District in Christian County, Kentucky.[23] His wife Eliza was listed as having been born in Virginia, and that 1880 census reported that they had four children: John, 15 (likely the child of Eliza's from her previous marriage to William Childress, since Godfrey and Eliza had been married only 9 years at the time of the census); Robert Lee, 8; Louisa, 6; and Irene (Rena), 3. It's unclear how Hyams had been able to remarry in 1871. Probably he neglected to tell authorities in Kentucky that he was already married but had abandoned Bridget and the children in Charleston (in addition to his first marriage to Hannah Martin).

In 1876 Hyams was incorrectly reported to have died. The *Cincinnati Commercial Tribune* recounted rather indecisively, "It is said that Hyams after this [the yellow fever plot] came to Louisville, but learning of an indictment against himself for forgery fled to Charleston, South Carolina, where he was killed in an attempt to rob. Such is the account of persons who pretend to be familiar with the circumstances."[24] A letter from Hyams signed by him was published in the *Cincinnati Daily Gazette* in 1879, proving that he was still alive. In this letter, Hyams again defended himself against the charges leveled by Dr. Stuart Robinson, who had called Hyams "a lying tool, Hyams, who would swear to any falsehood for $5." Hyams retorted by saying, "It is not quite evident why he (Dr. Robinson) should *manifest a personal interest in discrediting me before the public, unless he imagines that I may know something that would inculpate him* [italics in the original].... Mr. Editor, this communication is written as a public protest against Dr. Robinson's treatment of me."[25] Furthermore, Hyams appeared with his family in the 1880 U.S. census, living in Christian County, Kentucky. So the 1876 report of Hyams' demise was premature.

Godfrey never achieved the riches he sought so tenaciously. In the tax records of Christian County, Kentucky, in the 1870s each adult male citizen was listed with the taxable items in his possession. These items included lots, land, homes, stores, cows, horses, mares, donkeys, jennys (called "jennets" in the tax records), buggies, carriages, wagons, gold, silver, clocks, and watches. In 1875 Hyams (incorrectly spelled "Hymes" on the tax records in that year) had no possessions; he was listed as the sole male over age 21 in the household, with only one child age 6–20.[26] He reported that he was a member of the Kentucky militia, which still existed even after the Civil War, reported to have been 195,881 strong in 1873.[27] In 1879 Hyams (this year spelled "Hyam" in the tax records) had blanks in every column reporting his possessions except for a mule valued at $20. His good fortune since the Civil War had produced an accumulation of only this single item of value for taxation. But by then he had two children ages 6–20.[28] When 1880 rolled around, however, even the mule was gone.[29] At least in 1862 in Helena, Arkansas, he had four mules. In 1880 he had none.

But, astoundingly, in 1880, even after the Civil War, Godfrey and his wife had servants. Charlatt Wallace and Sallie Roach lived with the Hyams in Union Schoolhouse District, each with a son, James Wallace (age 12) and Sam Roach (age 2). How Hyams had managed to achieve sufficient financial status to allow him to have servants is unknown. It is of interest that many of Hyams' neighbors also had servants. Not listing them as "slaves" but calling them "servants" was the Southern "politically correct" response to the outcome of the Civil War.

Godfrey J. Hyams had some additional run-ins with the law in Hopkinsville, Kentucky, in March 1885. The charge this time was "false swearing," an infraction akin to perjury, so he must have been involved in some other legal issues at the time.[30] Arrest documents and court records for these events have been lost.

The family subsequently moved to Trenton, Kentucky. Godfrey Hyams' family doesn't appear in the 1890 U.S. census, but in 1900 his wife Eliza is listed as a widow living with Robert Lee Hyams and Joe Hyams in Trenton, Todd County, Kentucky. Mary Mae (Jane) Hyams had been born on March 1, 1880, and Joe (Joseph Godfrey) Hyams was the 16-year-old "baby" in that 1900 census, born in Kentucky on March 1, 1883.[31] (Godfrey had named a son of his second marriage "Joseph Godfrey"—his first and second names reversed—and repeated that name in his third family.) Irene "Rena" Hyams had married Robert Davenport and lived nearby.

Godfrey was said to have died in November 1886 in Todd County, Kentucky. This region was Jefferson Davis country (Davis had been born in Fairview, Kentucky, on the border between Christian and Todd counties). Hyams' family today tells the story that Hyams was never accepted in this intensely Southern community. He had turned on the South when he repeatedly testified against Blackburn, and the Southerners in Kentucky could hold a grudge for decades. Hyams was a traitor in their eyes.[32]

Early November 1866 saw Godfrey beginning to exhibit rather strange and perplexing behavior. He seemed agitated and nervous and was even more detached than usual. One day he gave Eliza some money and said that he might be gone for a few days. The next day he returned and gave her some additional money, very unusual behavior in the Hyams household. Then he disappeared. A few days later a local herbal doctor named John Ware (often called "Uncle John" or "Doctor John" and described in his obituary after he died at age 110 or 112 as "part Indian and part Negro") told the Hyams family that he had found Godfrey lying dead in a sinkhole on the family property. Sinkholes and caves were common in this part of Kentucky. Uncle John reported that Godfrey had been murdered, although he didn't describe the methods that had been employed by the assassins. However, when the family went to the site, the body was gone. In a strange twist, near the sinkhole they discovered his gold wedding ring and his "artist's case," perhaps his shoemaker's tools, as the word "artist" as used in the 1860s included the activities of skilled laborers, not just those dealing in the fine arts. A wedding ring doesn't accidentally fall off a man's hand, nor is it likely to drop spontaneously next to a dead body. The murderers probably wanted the family to know Godfrey was dead but didn't want them to have the body available for evidence when the police became involved. As there was never any body found, the Commonwealth of Kentucky never issued a death certificate. Some of the family suspected that he had feigned his death to avoid yet another hostile encounter with the Todd County Southerners and escaped to begin a new life yet again, perhaps this time with a different name. He had a history of such behavior. Whether this story is true will never be determined. Uncle John, however, never changed his story about the murdered body in the sinkhole.[33]

15. *Godfrey Joseph Hyams*

Some Hyams' family members today believe that Godfrey was the victim of an even more sinister plot.[34] Godfrey Hyams couldn't escape the reputation of his repeated public testimonies against Dr. Luke Blackburn and other Canadian Confederates. Hyams disappeared in November 1886. Coincidentally, that was the same month Jefferson Davis returned to Fairview, Kentucky, to dedicate the Bethel Baptist Church of Fairview at the site of Davis's birthplace, just a few miles from Hyams' home in Trenton.

Davis had been born there on June 3, 1808, on land owned by his father, Samuel Davis. His birth home had long since been dismantled and removed from the site, but a committee headed by Captain Lewis Clark, a local tobacco broker, had purchased a nine-acre portion of the property on which the old log cabin had sat. The committee in turn had donated the small plot to Davis with the agreement that Davis would pass it along to the church. On March 10, 1886, Davis donated the land to the church for construction of the new sanctuary. He had come for the dedication of the completed building in Fairview on November 19, 1886.[35] To the chagrin of many, Robert W. Downer, one of the dedication committee members, asked Davis to give "a little address for which we can charge admission to help pay for furniture &c." Davis was offered $100 for this appearance, but he denounced it as "degrading.... The proposition has shocked me but will not prevent my attendance if I am physically able to go."[36]

Weather that day was gloomy, with a temperature of 58 degrees and a "cold disagreeable rain." Davis was feeble, and he required physical support to stand, though he gave a brief address to the congregation in which he thanked them for "[commemorating] the spot of my nativity." Davis was the honored guest, but Blackburn didn't attend that ceremony. Hyams family members today suspect that either Davis's or Blackburn's henchmen or both kidnapped and killed Hyams. Alternatively, men not associated with Davis or Blackburn but men simply loyal to the Southern cause who had been reminded of Hyams' treachery by the return of Jefferson Davis to the area might have been inspired to act against Hyams, a symbol of the lost Southern cause. These men could have given Hyams his death as his last—though delayed—payment for the treachery he had inflicted upon the South. The truth will never be known.

Godfrey Hyams' pardon for his Civil War crimes had allowed him to live reasonably peacefully in the United States after 1865, continuing his employment as a shoemaker, though still frequently running afoul of the law as he tried to reenter Southern society. His periodic indiscretions revealed his true character, and his life had been characterized by lying and perjury. A man without scruples, he followed his love of money rather than a love for the South. He and Dr. Luke Blackburn shared guilt equally but with different motives. A reed in the wind, Hyams bent in whatever direction might be advantageous for accumulating material wealth. A man without a cause other than his own survival and advancement, he abandoned his family—at least twice, maybe three times—to make a new start, and he sold out friend and foe alike for money. Granted, he was a pawn, a man manipulated by others more powerful than he, but he was guilty nevertheless. He had been driven by profit, not principle, but he didn't repeat any attempts to poison the populace—at least as far as we know.

16

Dr. Luke Pryor Blackburn
Ghoul or Governor?
Is This the Same Man?

Dr. Blackburn returned to Canada after he had made his second trip to Bermuda in the fall of 1864. His activities there were little recorded until his arrest in the spring of 1865. Initial interrogations and a preliminary hearing suggested a basis for his prosecution, but he was spared from undergoing a trial on the technicality that he had done nothing illegal within the borders of Canada as they then existed. He wanted to return to the United States, but he feared the liability of arrest and trials there. So he languished in Canada.

Blackburn's status in Canada gradually improved thereafter. The *Philadelphia Inquirer* had previously described him as "fat and pompous, but deploringly neglected, and wearing a worn and seedy appearance."[1] In late December 1865 Blackburn was "practicing medicine in the city [of Toronto] with much success. He is boarding with his wife, who occupies the splendid mansion of the late Mr. [Henry] Eccles, who was the most talented lawyer in Canada West.... [They live in] a suite of rooms most elaborately and extravagantly furnished, [with a] greenhouse, which is connected with a richly furnished sitting room." Dr. Blackburn there was "engaged in writing a 'treatise on cholera and how to repel its attacks,' which he intends publishing gratuitously, as he said, for the benefit and good of his poor, deluded Yankee countrymen. The Doctor is looking wonderfully fine, and seems to be enjoying himself like an English nobleman."[2] Blackburn's dignity had improved, but he still longed to return to his home in the South.

The trial of Lincoln's assassins had concluded, and evidence of Blackburn's plot had been discussed as a part of the proceedings, but he had not been charged with the other conspirators, nor had he been extradited. Judge Advocate John A. Bingham didn't even have much of the incriminating testimony (it came mostly from the Bermuda trial), but he declared,

205

> It may be said, and doubtless will be said, by the pensioned advocates of this rebellion, that Hyams, being infamous, is not to be believed. It is admitted that he is infamous, as it must be conceded that any man is infamous who either participates in such a crime or attempts in anywise to extenuate it. But it will be observed that Hyams is supported by the testimony of Mr. Sanford Conover, who heard Blackburn and the other rebel agents in Canada speak of this infernal project, and by the testimony of Mr. Wall, ... the well-known auctioneer of this city, whose character is unquestioned ... that Hyams consigned the goods to him in the name of J.W. Harris, a fact in itself an acknowledgment of guilt.... The very transaction shows that Hyams' statement is truthful. He gives the names of the parties connected with this infamy (Clement C. Clay, Dr. Blackburn, Rev. Dr. Stuart Robinson, J.C. Holcombe, all refugees from the Confederacy in Canada) ... in none of which facts is there an attempt to discredit him.... It is a matter of notoriety that a part of his statement is verified by the results at Newbern [sic], North Carolina, to which point, he says, a portion of the infected goods were shipped, through a sutler, the result of which was that nearly two thousand citizens and soldiers died there, about that time, with yellow fever.[3]

This judge believed the evidence against Blackburn, even though Blackburn ultimately was never tried in the United States. Such was the cloud under which Blackburn functioned while remaining in Canada.

President Lincoln had previously issued two proclamations granting amnesty to the Confederates if they would vow allegiance to the United States, one on December 8, 1863, and another on March 26, 1864. These proclamations did little to stem the tide of Southern Rebels. President Andrew Johnson likewise first issued a proclamation on May 29, 1865, granting amnesty to participants in the rebellion. This proclamation granted blanket amnesty and pardon to all who had fought against the Union, with the goal of inducing "all persons to return to their loyalty, and to restore the authority of the United States." This first proclamation from President Andrew Johnson excluded 14 categories of Confederates, mostly those in positions of high leadership. Those claiming the amnesty and pardon had to swear an oath to the United States and promise to abide by all laws and proclamations of the government, including those proclamations that freed the slaves. Persons in the excluded classes had to petition the president individually for a pardon. The government issued many pardons to the Confederate Rebels for varied offences against the Union.

In the spring of 1866 a friend pleaded for amnesty for Blackburn, that he be allowed to return to the United States from Canada. On April 28, 1866, Ms. C.C. Leathers wrote to Brevet Major General James Bowen asking for mercy for her "old friend exiled to Canada." She cited Dr. Blackburn's medical care of her family in Natchez, Mississippi: "I do not believe that Doctor Blackburn did any more harm during the late rebellion than a little talking that might have been left unsaid.... His trying to run the blockade with a few bales of cotton for the support of his family gave rise to the evil reports against him. I believe Dr. Blackburn to be perfectly innocent." She asked General Bowen to intercede through General Ulysses S. Grant and the president to obtain permission for Blackburn to return to the States. Her opinion was that Blackburn, "instead of aiding in the introduction of disease … would have tended friend and foe alike."[4] Bowen sent the letter to the president. The request was denied. Blackburn was never individually granted pardon for his role in the attempt to spread pestilence across the North.

George W. Gayle, of Dallas County, Alabama, was the lawyer who had published an advertisement in the *Selma (AL) Dispatch* on December 1, 1864, which said, "If the citizens of the southern confederacy will furnish me with the cash or good securities for the sum of $1,000,000, I will cause the lives of Abraham Lincoln, William H. Seward, and Andrew Johnson to be taken by the 1st of March next. This will give us peace, and satisfy the world that cruel tyrants cannot live in a land of liberty."[5] Even Gayle was individually pardoned on April 27, 1867.

On September 7, 1867, a second presidential proclamation reduced the number of excluded classes from fourteen to three. By late in 1867 over 13,000 individual pardons had been approved. A third proclamation came on July 4, 1868. On December 25, 1868, President Johnson issued a decree that advanced pardon to everyone. The Christmas Day Proclamation brought an end to the exile of many Confederates still hiding in the United States or foreign countries.

On May 1, 1867, Blackburn had personally petitioned the attorney general of the United States to allow him to return to Kentucky from Canada.[6] This request was unsuccessful. From Toronto on September 4, 1867, Blackburn again wrote letters to both President Andrew Johnson and the American consul in Canada (David Thurston in Toronto), volunteering to go to New Orleans and Galveston "without compensation" to aid in the treatment of patients during the yellow fever epidemic rampant at the time. He said to Johnson, "I have had much experience in the treatment of this disease, and feel confident I could render essential service to my suffering and dying Countrymen. If you can Mr. President consistently with your duty accept my offer, my conduct shall be such as to meet and merit your approbation."[7] David Thurston sent a dispatch to Secretary of State William H. Seward on September 17, 1867, including Blackburn's oath of allegiance to the United States and asking for a pardon for Blackburn, based upon the most recent Presidential Proclamation of Amnesty on September 7.[8] Seward recommended against a pardon for Blackburn. Blackburn's offer to help yellow fever victims in Louisiana and Texas was never answered formally by President Johnson himself, although William H. Seward wrote to Consul David Thurston on September 25, 1867, stating that Blackburn's case had not fallen under any of the blanket pardons that had been issued by the president, specifically the pardon of September 7, 1867. Seward said that Blackburn was "under one of the classes excepted":

> All that is known is that he lies under the charge of felony in this, that he conceived and put into execution, within a foreign dominion a plot to disseminate contagion and pestilence in this and other cities of the United States by clandestinely transmitting, for an unsuspicious market here, masses of infected clothing taken from the corpses of persons who had died of yellow fever in the tropics. It is not easy to understand how an offense of that character, which is a detestable crime against mankind, can be supposed, even by the felon himself, to be entitled to be regarded as an act of insurrection, rebellion or civil war [the classifications of crime pardoned by the proclamation]. The President's proclamation offers no amnesty in this case.[9]

Blackburn, though, acted as though the pardon for his crimes and permission to travel back to the United States would be forthcoming. He went to Louisville, arriving on September 25, 1867. Border crossings then were easy, and he was not detained as he tried to reenter the United States. From there he went to New Orleans and participated in the treatment of patients with yellow fever. After the epidemic had subsided he traveled back to Helena, Arkansas, where both his and his wife's families had farms. There he remained for about six years, farming cotton and practicing medicine. Tax records in Pine Bluff, Arkansas, place Luke Blackburn there as early as 1869, and an article in the *Little Rock Arkansas Gazette* on July 24, 1869,[10] spoke of Dr. Blackburn's presence on the streets of Little Rock and of his farming activities below Pine Bluff, Arkansas. The Civil War effort had produced serious needs for revenue, and Blackburn, now living in Arkansas, was taxed $1 on a gold watch he possessed.[11] Other tax documents list Pine Bluff as the residence of a Dr. Luke Blackburn, physician.

The government never formally prosecuted Blackburn in the United States for his Confederate allegiance or his diabolical plots. His story simply disappeared quietly. Likewise, Hyams wasn't prosecuted. Hyams, of course, had a lower profile as a shoemaker than Blackburn as a physician. While Blackburn's later history is well documented, Hyams officially received his pardon and then disappeared into relative obscurity.

Blackburn moved back to Kentucky in early 1873, living initially in Louisville. Soon after arriving, an outbreak of yellow fever drew him to Memphis, Tennessee. There newspaper headlines heralded the arrival of the expert in that disease: "Dr. Blackburn Comes to Our Relief and Takes Charge of a Hospital." The text of the article read as follows: "Dr. Luke P. Blackburn arrived last night from Louisville, and this morning tendered to the Mayor his services [having been asked by a citizen committee who wrote to Blackburn,] 'As the yellow fever is now prevailing to an alarming extent in the South, with a certainty of its increasing for several weeks to come, and from your long experience in the treatment of the disease, we would respectfully ask and beg that you go at once to our afflicted friends of the South and render such aid to such portions of the afflicted country as you in your judgment may think best." The paper went on to say, "Dr. Blackburn's services have been accepted by the Mayor, and he goes on duty at once."[12]

Public and the press praised Blackburn for his knowledge, compassion, and skill in controlling yellow fever epidemics for years to come. His proponents would later have this to say:

> These results [the control of the epidemics] are mainly to be attributed to the incomparable skill and efficiency of Dr. Blackburn, with whom my relations were those of unbroken harmony throughout the whole prevalence of the epidemic. In this gentleman, professional knowledge and experience were combined with sound practical judgment, a diagnostic insight into disease which seemed to be intuitive, extraordinary capability of physical endurance, and a cheerfulness and kindliness of heart, which are better than medicine to the suffering patient.[13]

Blackburn subsequently went to Shreveport to fight a yellow fever epidemic there, as well, before returning to Louisville. He continued to volunteer his services for the treatment of yellow fever. When an outbreak occurred in Memphis in 1875 he again responded. He also went to Fernandina, Florida, in 1877 for the same purpose. He was, indeed, a humanitarian when fellow Southerners were in peril.

In Louisville, Dr. Blackburn resumed his medical practice. He ventured into politics for reasons unknown, perhaps because many members of his family had served as elected officials at various levels of government. He announced his candidacy for governor of Kentucky in March 1878. On September 5, however, the mayor of Hickman, Kentucky, interrupted Blackburn's campaign for governor, asking the good doctor for help. Another outbreak of yellow fever had erupted in Hickman that month, and Blackburn willingly put his campaign for governor on hold to help treat victims of the epidemic there. He wasted no time, arriving in Hickman on September 7. Hickman sat along the Mississippi River and had a population of about 1,500.[14] There the epidemic was out of control, and nearly 30 percent of the population would become sick with the disease.

Dr. Blackburn (Figure 16) organized his usual isolation techniques and supervised the cleanup of the city, also tending to the protection of abandoned homes. He was so successful, so compassionate, and so loved that he was dubbed "the Hero of Hickman." Newspapers as far away as Los Angeles heralded Blackburn's compassion. He was described as "a stout, jolly, well-to-do and well-preserved old gentleman of nearly seventy," who "labored unceasingly." He was depicted in a "photograph representing him sitting by a hospital cot, with a sufferer's hand in his."[15] From Hickman, Blackburn went to Chattanooga, Tennessee, and then to Martin, Tennessee, to fight yet more outbreaks of yellow fever; subsequently, he returned briefly to Hickman as the yellow fever epidemic gained a brief resurgence. Ultimately, 462 Hickman residents fell victim to yellow fever, and 150 died.[16] Because of the rapidity of the devastation, many were buried in mass graves. But the epidemic was again controlled. Blackburn's reputation and fortunes rose.

The treatment for yellow fever that Blackburn recommended even as late as 1878 is interesting:

> The patient should be placed in a bed in a horizontal position; should not under any circumstances be allowed to arise from that bed; should be well covered with blankets; a foot-tub of hot water without mustard should be introduced under the blankets; the patient lying upon his back, should flex his lower limbs and place his feet in the tub; the covering should be tucked well around him, close up to his neck; he should be given hot tea, composed of balm, sage, elder blossom, boneset, corn-shock, or orange- or lemon-leaf. At the same time he should be permitted to drink ice water or to take crushed ice in sufficient quantities to allay his thirst. Free and continuous perspiration should be kept up.... The fever will continue from twenty to ninety hours. When it has passed off the blankets should be gradually withdrawn from the patient; stimulants, such as ale, porter, pure rum, and French brandy should be freely given.... Nourishment, such as rice-water, or corn-meal gruel, or chicken-water should be given cautiously and sparingly.... Should the perspiration have a glutinous, gummy touch, you may expect your patient to recover with watchful and careful nursing. But should the perspiration have a sensation like that of pure water, showing that there is no vicarious action by the skin, which gives relief to the liver and kidneys, you may know that your patient is in great danger. You will find upon an examination the tongue red and tremulous, covered with a short white fur, with great gastric fetor of the breath. It is then all-important to apply the cups [heated cups applied to the skin with the rim of the cup against the skin to form suction and removing liquid or causing blisters] or leeches to the pit of the [skin covering the] stomach in order to prevent that degree of inflammation which destroys the coat of the stomach. If neither cups, leeches, nor blisters be applied, the patient will complain of the sensation of a ball in his stomach in thirty-six hours. And in twelve hours thereafter he will throw off blood that is exuded into the stomach, known as black vomit, which has the appearance of coffee-grounds floating in an amber-colored fluid.[17]

These thoughts comprised Blackburn's qualifications for governor.

Primarily on the strength of his image as a compassionate physician, Blackburn continued to seek the office of governor of Kentucky in late 1878, running as a Democrat. His local newspaper said, "The hospitals at Hickman will make old Luke Blackburn Governor of the proud Commonwealth of Kentucky."[18] Certainly the sentiments in Hickman strongly favored Blackburn. The *Hickman Courier* said he was "a disciple of Father Matthew's total abstinence principles ... [with] a countenance which beams in every lineament with philanthropy, and wins a place in the hearts of all who come within the sphere of his influence."[19]

16. Ghoul or Governor?

The Democratic Convention was held in Louisville beginning May 1, 1879.[20] Delegates nominated Blackburn by acclamation, defeating his Democratic opponents Thomas Laurens Jones and John Cox Underwood.[21] Jones was a lawyer who had served as a United States congressman from the 6th District of Kentucky. Underwood was completing his term as the 21st lieutenant governor of Kentucky. Delegates to the convention declared Blackburn a state hero. These delegates even ignored a legal challenge to Blackburn's candidacy: he had not been a resident of the state of Kentucky for a complete seven years as required by law. His medical exploits had carried him to the governor's nomination; apparently the citizens of Kentucky thought that a relatively inexperienced politician should be made governor to reward him for his humanitarian work. Blackburn's flowery acceptance speech after becoming the Democratic nominee for governor said nothing of the controversy surrounding his service to the Confederacy during the Civil War.

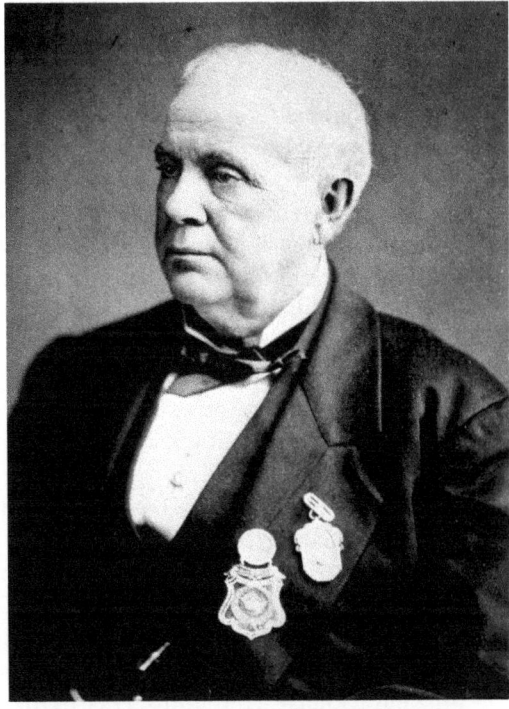

Figure 16. Dr. Luke Pryor Blackburn, exact date unspecified. The significance of the medals on his coat is unknown, but they may be the awards given to him by Queen Victoria for aiding the citizens of Bermuda during the yellow fever epidemic (National Library of Medicine, image #101410585).

But newspapers—and foes—began to suspect that the diabolical doctor who had tried to infect the North with yellow fever was one and the same as the Democratic candidate for governor. Blackburn said that he wanted "to expunge from my name that obliquy [sic] which the venal press and people of the North put upon it at a time when no friend could defend me unless at the peril of his life or liberty."[22] Accusations and denials flew from town to town, from newspaper to newspaper. But he had endeared himself to his fellow Kentuckians, even though his only real qualification for governor was his beloved status due to his tireless humanitarian efforts to treat the victims of yellow fever. His new title, "Hero of Hickman," propelled him in the standings of the candidates.

Then the election turned ugly. It was that predictable political event now called the "October Surprise." In May 1879, just after the Democratic Convention, the *Cincinnati Gazette* reported a story on the yellow fever plot, apparently never covered before in detail by newspapers in Kentucky. The editors saw the opportunity for exposing a great scandal, and the *Gazette* published a series of stories investigating the charges against Blackburn. The *Gazette* even temporarily organized a special office to run the investigation. Other newspapers, many in the North, picked up these stories, and they chastised Kentuckians for even nominating such a scoundrel for governor. Blackburn was dubbed "Dr. Black Vomit," after the cardinal symptom of yellow fever. Blackburn refused to comment on the accusations, and voters in Kentucky essentially ignored the controversy. His only statement regarding the issue was that the entire story was "too preposterous for intelligent gentlemen to believe."[23] Few Kentuckians read newspapers, particularly those publications from out of state.

Even newspapers in remote states relatively uninterested in Kentucky politics picked up the story for its controversy and its shock value. The *Weekly Kansas Chief* in Troy, Kansas, quoted the now ancient testimony from the Lincoln assassination trial, in which a Dr. Luke Blackburn was accused of attempting to spread yellow fever and smallpox among the citizens of the North. It asked in a lengthy headline, "Is He the Same? Interesting Reading for Kentuckians—A Reminiscence of the Rebellion—Is this Dr. Luke P. Blackburn the Democratic Candidate for Governor of Kentucky?" It extensively quoted the trial transcript, mostly the words of Godfrey Joseph Hyams that incriminated Blackburn. The newspaper then asked, "Is It a Case of Mistaken Identity?" While it presented the story as a question, the text supported the claims that the two Dr. Luke Blackburns were one and the same. It concluded by saying,

> We confess to some difficulty in parrying the force of these facts and circumstances. And yet we are unwilling to believe that a party which claims to contain within itself all the pride and principle, all the wealth and civilization, all the aristocracy and honor of a great State, would select for its standard bearer a man capable, under any circumstances, of participating in so base methods of warfare, methods which imperiled the health and lives alike of children and women, of the decrepit and infirm of both sexes, and which waged an indiscriminate and cruel warfare against the feeble and unprotected classes of society, at which humanity stands aghast, and which are simply an ineffaceable blot upon the character of the agents of the rebellion, and which, indeed, must truly mark their detestable and desperate character.[24]

Many newspapers were harshly critical of the plot devised by Blackburn, calling him a "fiend" or a "devil." Interest in the story was high, and Blackburn's vocal supporters were decreasing in number.

Not only did newspapers chide Blackburn for his role in "the yellow fever plot," the *Louisville Commercial* sought to discredit Blackburn for other statements accredited to him. Trying to counter the prevailing opinion that he was a humble, self-effacing servant, the newspaper quoted a statement attributed to him: "[I have] already done more for the people of Kentucky than Je...s Ch...t [*sic*] ever did."[25] This statement didn't endear Blackburn to many Christian folk from Kentucky. Blackburn, annoyed at the accusations, said, "The statements are lies, and I don't care a damn for all the Republican comment in Christendom."[26] Blackburn, of course, was running as a Democrat.

Blackburn was ill himself during the months prior to the election. A few other Democrats—Boyd Winchester, Parker Watkins Hardin, and W.C.P. Breckinridge—delivered most of the campaign speeches in his favor. His Republican opponent, Walter Evans of Hopkinsville, Kentucky, claimed that Blackburn was feigning illness. The *Hickman Courier* reported in June that Blackburn was indeed ill, as even some Democratic newspapers were taking sides with the Republicans:

> We are sorry to see some ungenerous Democratic papers re-echoing the *Radical Mountain Echoe's* insinuating that Dr. Blackburn is shamming sickness to avoid meeting Col. Evans [his opponent]. We know of our own personal knowledge that Dr. Blackburn would endanger his life by making a speech. He is very much debilitated by sickness, and can scarcely see at all out of one eye, which is still very much inflamed. Even his enemies must acknowledge that Dr. B. is incapable of such deception, and that he is afraid of neither Walter Evans nor of the head devil of Republicanism. Such insinuations are untrue, ungenerous and unmanly.[27]

By the time of the election on August 4, 1879, it was still uncertain in the eyes of most Kentuckians whether candidate Luke Pryor Blackburn was the Dr. Luke Blackburn of Bermuda infamy. Perhaps few even cared. Blackburn, the "Hero of Hickman," won handily, defeating his Republican opponent Walter Evans by 125,790 to 81,882 votes.[28] Blackburn was inaugurated on September 2, 1879, and served as governor of Kentucky from September 2, 1879, through September 5, 1883.

After Blackburn's election, however, the controversy didn't stop. Some newspapers still called the story of the yellow fever plot a fabrication, saying that it wasn't even established that Blackburn had gone to Canada during the Civil War. The *St. Clairsville (OH) Belmont Chronicle* reported, "The fact that no denial has been made leads a prominent Kentucky Democratic journal to suggest that this yellow fever Democratic hero make his denial a part of his inaugural address." The same issue of that paper reported that Blackburn "has spoken at last, but only to remark that he does not care a d—n about what the Republican newspapers care to say about him. But he did not say whether he is the same Luke P. Blackburn that attempted to infect the North with yellow fever and smallpox during the war."[29]

However, even on inauguration day, September 2, 1879, newspapers said,

"Everybody likes Blackburn, but there are few who admire him for either culture or ability. He has much personal magnetism, but is not conspicuously possessed of any of the strong traits which go to make up great men. He will succeed in looking the Governor, but as to his success in the reality, time alone can decide." The pouring rain that greeted the inaugural ceremonies that day portended the controversy that would surround his governorship. Other newspapers reported:

> Those who hoped to hear from his lips an explicit denial of charges against him in connection with yellow fever were disappointed. His only reference to the subject was the following: "Let us hope that the people of the various States will cultivate a feeling of especial amity, and that they will believe and remember that the enterprise and prosperity of a single State adds to the prosperity of all, and that the time is at hand when North, South, East, and West will turn in scorn, contempt, and loathing from those political, blatant tricksters who, for their unholy and unselfish ends, continually endeavor to excite sectional bitterness and hate."

The *New York Times*, citing the *Lexington Transcript* said,

> This serious insinuation against his character is 14 years old, but, if it be true, he cannot live long enough nor do service enough for the people to wipe out the remembrance of so diabolical a deed. Such a damnable scheme all the philanthropy of an age, could he live it, would not atone. All the deeds of a lifetime, were they all good and successful, cannot justify a people in indorsing [sic] for their highest office a man guilty of what is charged against one Luke P. Blackburn, to whom the newspapers have so often referred. In the name of all that is good, let Dr. Blackburn say something in defense of himself.[30]

The stockholders of this Cincinnati newspaper met with Ben Doering, the writer of the editorial, after it appeared and told him that he should either resign or never write again about the Blackburn yellow fever plot. Doering told the stockholders that he had supported Blackburn only on the condition that Blackburn satisfactorily answer the charges that he had tried to conduct biological warfare during the Civil War. Blackburn hadn't responded. Doering resigned.

Soon after this inauguration, more comments surfaced about the likelihood that Governor Blackburn was the same as the Dr. Blackburn of Bermuda yellow fever plot infamy. A Mr. M. McKeogh claimed to have been a hotel operator in Canada during the time Blackburn lived in Canada. McKeogh admitted his hotel was a center for Southern sympathizers, and he included Blackburn in that group. McKeogh said that the Canadian Blackburn was the same as the Governor Blackburn of Kentucky. When asked if Blackburn had tried to introduce yellow fever into the North, McKeogh replied that he was one of "the kindest-hearted men I ever knew. He wouldn't harm a flea.... He is a gentle-hearted man and a born philanthropist. I have known him to travel all night to relieve sickness and distress, when he knew he would never get a cent for it.... He gave his money, his time, and put his life in the balance, all from love and charity toward the sick and suffering."³¹ Clearly Blackburn had a charitable side as a lover of mankind, but he had allowed his politics to dictate actions he should have avoided.

Further controversy plagued Blackburn's governorship. He was accused of nepotism, appointing many of his friends and relatives to government posts. Blackburn appointed his brother-in-law, Colonel Samuel B. Churchill, to become the secretary of state of Kentucky. Not one to mince words, Blackburn answered the charges: "By God, I intend to make the appointment in spite of h-ll, and I think ... he is the most suitable man in the State for the place, and because he is my wife's brother, that is no reason why he should not be appointed."³² Blackburn's speech was inelegant; his enemies had found many reasons to criticize him.

Blackburn completed his governorship with honor, although not necessarily pleasing all of his foes. He reformed and transformed the prison system as his major accomplishment. Seeing the horrendous conditions under which the prisoners endured their sentences, he made prison life more humane. He recognized that the Kentucky prison system was grossly overcrowded—one prison had 969 prisoners and only 780 cells.³³ Other reports cite a capacity of 600 in the Frankfort Prison, with 1200–1300 prisoners housed there.³⁴ Whatever the numbers, prisons were overcrowded. Each cell was six feet wide by nine feet long by six feet high. When Blackburn realized that the government couldn't fit the prison to the convicts, he decided that he needed to fit the convicts to the prison, releasing as many as reasonable—those convicted of nonviolent crimes, those unlikely to commit violent crimes, and those needing clemency for other reasons, such as serious illnesses.³⁵ During Blackburn's governorship (Figure 17), he pardoned 850 convicted prisoners (some reports decried a

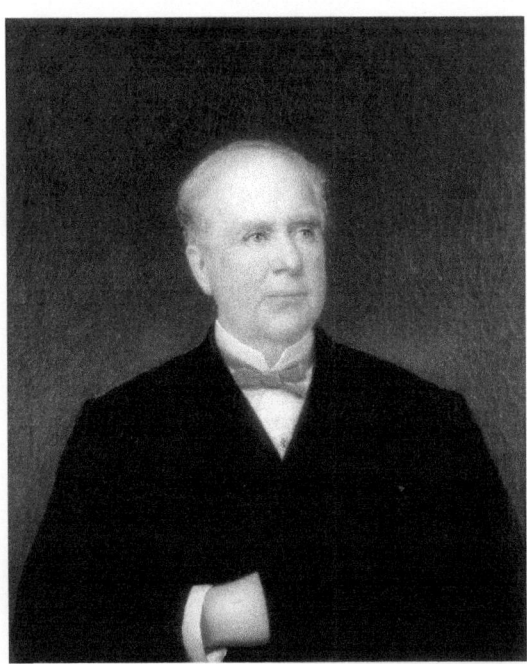

Figure 17. Oil painting of Dr. Luke Pryor Blackburn, MD, governor of Kentucky, by Nicola Marschall in 1883 at the end of Blackburn's governorship (Kentucky Historical Society, 1904.4).

total of over 1,000 pardons).[36] Because of these reforms and his frequent pardons of prisoners, his detractors called him "Lenient Luke." He pioneered the concept of parole, releasing the least dangerous offenders, especially those less likely to repeat an offence, such as those in the final stages of any illness thought to be fatal. Blackburn introduced the warden system into prison organization, and he also instituted the use of prisoners as cheap labor and improved financial aspects of Kentucky's government, even though he expended scarce dollars in his reform of the state's prisons, prompting criticism from his enemies. While his efforts at prison reform weren't necessarily popular at the time, they were later applauded by most people. Even Blackburn's wife Julia became involved, starting church classes as a Sunday school for the prisoners. Hers was one of the first prison ministries in the United States.

But Blackburn's own party was eventually displeased with him. His prison reform expenses met with widespread disapproval, and his pardons offended many even in his Democratic Party. Furthermore, Blackburn, though a Kentucky aristocrat, businessman, and physician, was rather unpolished. His detractors declared him to be crude; others called him a buffoon.

After he finished his governorship, Blackburn returned to the practice of medicine. In 1883 he heard the evangelist George Owen Barnes and experienced a Christian conversion.[37] In his early adult years, Blackburn and his wife had attended a Presbyterian congregation, but he had joined the Catholic church in 1865 during the week he was arrested in Canada. His encounter with the Reverend Barnes was rather lengthy. Barnes came from Presbyterian stock and had worked in India as a missionary for seven years. Returning to Kentucky, Barnes left the Presbyterian denomination after charges of heresy were leveled at him.[38] He preached what would earn him the title of "The Mountain Evangelist." His style and theology caused derision in some Christian circles, but his influence was unquestioned. Although he had been educated at Princeton Theological School, Barnes adopted less polished preaching techniques and was able both to identify with and to influence uneducated mountain folk. His preaching reached mostly the hill regions of Kentucky, and it's said that he was responsible for the conversion of over 26,000 souls in Kentucky (26,769 in five years and four months by Barnes' own count,[39] 20,000 of whom lived in the backwoods of the state).[40] He also preached occasionally in the cities, and Blackburn came under the spell of his charismatic messages and healing services at a three-week revival meeting in Frankfort, Kentucky, in June 1882. Barnes wrote in his memoirs about his encounter with Governor Luke Blackburn and his wife Julia:

> **June 9** ... The Governor and lady present.
> **June 11** ... At the penitentiary promptly at 9 o'clock.... After sermon three hundred and ten confessed; more whites than colored, about one third and two thirds

16. Ghoul or Governor?

the proportion. Governor Blackburn, lady, and few spectators. The most wonderful meeting of my evangelistic life. Hardly a dry eye in either [penitentiary] ward [male and female].

June 15 ... Governor and his wife there again, the dear old man seemed deeply interested. Oh, to win him.

June 21 ... An hour's talk with earnest listeners.... At night a glorious meeting. The Governor confessed.... The dear Governor made a bold confession, and was the first man to go forward.

June 26 ... The dear Governor took me aside at the hotel, and in a voice almost inarticulate with emotion, told me to always count him as a fast and loving friend.[41]

News of Blackburn's conversion rapidly made its way to newspapers, both local and afar. He returned to Protestantism and joined the Episcopal Church, where he remained faithful until his death.[42] While his conversion may have cleansed his heart, the consequence of his behavior during the Civil War— a stained reputation—would follow him to his death.

Blackburn continued his humanitarian activities. In 1884 he founded the Blackburn Sanitarium for Nervous and Mental Diseases in Louisville, though it failed to endure.[43] He maintained his medical practice in Louisville until his own health failed at age 71. As he detected his failing stamina and increasing illness, in January 1887 he returned to his beloved Frankfort, the town he had called home.

Later in 1887 Blackburn became more seriously ill and slipped into a coma about one week before he died, but he aroused three times during that week. On one occasion he said, "Oh the beauty of religion!" and then lapsed back into unconsciousness. On another of those cogent moments, five days before his death, he said, "I will only be with you five days; tell all of my relatives and friends." And indeed he died five days later, at 2:30 p.m. on September 14, 1887.[44]

At his death and thereafter, friends and supporters refused to believe that Blackburn had ever participated in any nefarious plots, though enemies would never forget his attempts to disseminate yellow fever to the North. At his burial in Frankfort, Kentucky, long and profound eulogies and life summaries from friends exuded only descriptions of his benevolence and love for mankind. One penned decades later said, he "had the brains of a man, the tenderness of a woman, the skill of a surgeon, the heart of a philanthropist, and the acumen of one born to rule."[45] Today that description would be considered politically incorrect, but when it was written in 1922 it was regarded as high praise. Another eulogy said "he was the very incarnation of the Red Cross before the Red Cross existed." Friends heaped praise upon the "Hero of Hickman," even calling him "Luke, the Beloved Physician." The Louisville newspaper reported the Bermuda yellow fever plot in his obituary only by saying, "In 1864, by the request of the Governor General of Canada, he repaired to the Bermuda Islands to look after the suffering citizens and soldiers ... and his services were afterward favorably recognized by the Queen's Court of Admiralty." Newspapers refused to mention any plot or scandal. Most people in attendance at his funeral ignored accusations against him; they wanted to believe the best about their friend and former governor. As he was put to rest, choirs sang "Safe in the Arms of Jesus," and "It Is Well with My Soul."[46] His tombstone displays a carved bas-relief depiction of the Good Samaritan, with these inscribed words:

> He earned affection which can die only with the hearts in which his memory is enshrined; and his life consecrated to duty and charity is an example of heroism and fidelity. Chief Magistrate of his native commonwealth his official record is a bright page in her illustrious history. In his great soul justice, honor, and mercy ruled together, and sordid aspirations held no sway. He rests with the blessed who have feared God and loved their fellow men.[47]

In his death his tombstone rejects the notion that he ever had "sordid aspirations."

Even over a century later, some biographers suggested that Blackburn might have been an innocent bystander, an honorable man painted as an ogre only by his political enemies.[48] Much evidence against Blackburn was circumstantial, but a lot of it was also reliable and verifiable. Some witnesses were disreputable, but many were upright and believable. Authorities found some of his trunks filled with contaminated articles in Bermuda, and these containers—tangible physical evidence—had to be buried and subsequently flooded with sulfuric acid. Blackburn was a small player in the many Canadian plots to terrorize the North, but Yankees wanted revenge. His crime was particularly odious. He had safely ensconced himself for years in Canada. By the time he returned to the United States, passions had cooled, and his soiled reputation had been largely forgotten. He was once again seen as a hero in the fight against disease. Even his political career recovered.

In a court today, Blackburn probably would be acquitted of murder, although guilty of conspiracy to commit murder. His actions had produced no victims. He transported contaminated clothing with the intent to murder and terrorize the North, but his action in fact produced no yellow fever. Transmission of yellow fever required mosquitoes—unindicted co-conspirators, so to speak. Blackburn didn't know this fact about the disease, so in practical terms his attempts were futile. His attachment to a cause overshadowed his devotion to mankind as a physician. In the recent era, physicians take an oath to bring healing to mankind. The Hippocratic Oath says, in part,

> I will follow that system of regimen which, according to my ability and judgment, I consider for the benefit of my patients, and abstain from whatever is deleterious and

mischievous. I will give no deadly medicine to any one if asked, nor suggest any such counsel.... With purity and with holiness I will pass my life and practice my art. Into whatever houses I enter, I will go into them for the benefit of the sick, and will abstain from every voluntary act of mischief and corruption....[49]

In fact, instruction in ethics was lacking in many medical schools in the 1800s, including Transylvania University. Professors thought that such instruction was trivial and unnecessary. They simply assumed that a physician's conscience and his exposure to ethics statements of various medical societies were sufficient to regulate his behavior in his medical practice.[50] They weren't.

Blackburn's life otherwise, in general, was honorable, and his achievements cannot be denied. He was physician, healer, friend, champion of prison reform, politician and statesman, tamer of epidemics, and medical observer controlling yellow fever. He ultimately rose from his proverbial ashes to return to his roots of medical compassion, to become a good politician, or at least a successful one, and to serve honorably as governor of Kentucky.

However, by targeting civilians during the Civil War instead of the opposing army, Blackburn had also violated the rules of war, as though such rules are ever likely to be followed. Indeed, all is *not* fair in love and war, as the common phrase in the affirmative would suggest. Had the technique of transporting contaminated clothing been successful, civilians would not just have been collateral damage they also would have been the primary target, the intended casualties. His victims would have been largely indiscriminate. He knew that he couldn't control the final destination of the contaminated clothing and therefore the people he would kill. It was warfare at its worst. Blackburn's goal was different from the unintended loss of civilians during the bombing of a military base. The recipients of Blackburn's tainted goods were in some cases military encampments, but others were the masses of noncombatants located in the major cities of the North.

Blackburn's devotion to the heritage and traditions of the South propelled him into a scheme that would ultimately bring him shame. He had a passion, a goal, and a method to aid the South, and to his detriment he sought valiantly to support his chosen cause. Dedicated in the extreme, he focused on an outcome to be achieved at all costs. He elevated his love of Southern society above universal love of man, giving the South a misbegotten gift of love in the form of hatred directed toward the North. His one fault emerged as his view of the injustice of the North drove him to attempt the unthinkable—germ warfare. In today's parlance, he sought to distribute a "weapon of mass destruction." He tried to send a gift of yellow fever, with misguided love, from Bermuda. His actions will forever serve as an example of indecent medical conduct. Fortunately for him, the techniques he used could never have been productive. But had he succeeded in finding clothing contaminated by smallpox, a disease transmissible by such methods, then....

Chapter Notes

Abbreviations in citations include: NARA—National Archives and Records Administration; ORA—*The War of the Rebellion: A Compilation of the Official Records of the Union and Confederate Armies. Original Records of the Civil War*; ORN—*Official Records of the Union and Confederate Navies in the War of the Rebellion. Original Records of the Civil War.*

Introduction

1. *Cincinnati Daily Gazette*, October 4, 1879.

Chapter 1

1. United States Census, Slave Schedule, Woodford County, Kentucky, 1850, pp. 31–32, https://familysearch.org; Blackburn Family Papers, 1840–1896. Louisville, Kentucky, Special Collections, Filson Historical Society.
2. United States Census, Slave Schedule, City of Natchez, Mississippi, 1850, p. 13, https://familysearch.org.
3. Webster, Noah. *Dictionary of the English Language,* Springfield, MA: G. & C. Merriam, 1865, pp. 567, 1479.
4. Filson Club Publication #20, *The History of the Medical Department of Transylvania University*, Doctor Robert Peter, ed. Johanna Peter. Louisville, KY: Filson Historical Society, John P. Morton, 1905.
5. Blackburn, Luke Prior [sic]. *An Inaugural Dissertation on Cholera Maligna Submitted to the Trustees and Medical Professors of Transylvania University for the Degree of Doctor of Medicine on the 20th of February, A.D. 1835*, Kentucky Digital Library.
6. Caldwell, Charles. *Autobiography of Charles Caldwell, M.D., with Preface, Notes, and Appendix by Harriot W. Warner.* Philadelphia: Lippincott, Grambo, 1855.
7. Blackburn, *An Inaugural Dissertation,* 4.
8. *Ibid.,* 12 and 20.
9. *Ibid.,* 2.

10. Some sources list her name as "Davidella," though her tombstone declares her to have been "Ella." Some sources spell her middle name incorrectly as "Guest." Her maiden name was "Ella Gist Boswell." Gist was her mother's maiden name.
11. Letter, Ella G. Blackburn to Lavinia L. Blackburn, October 1, 1846. M-442, frame 141: Blackburn Family Papers, 1829–1865, Lexington, University of Kentucky Special Collections Research Center, Margaret I. King Library, University of Kentucky (letter references cite beginning microfilm frame numbers for the entire letter).
12. Letter, Luke P. Blackburn to Lavinia L. Blackburn, October 10, 1846. M-442, frame 143: Blackburn Family Papers, 1829–1865, Lexington, University of Kentucky Special Collections Research Center, Margaret I. King Library, University of Kentucky; Letter, Luke P. Blackburn to Lavinia L. Blackburn, July 13, 1846. M-442, frame 107: Blackburn Family Papers, 1829–1865, Lexington, University of Kentucky Special Collections Research Center, Margaret I. King Library, University of Kentucky.
13. Letter, Ella G. Blackburn to Lavinia L. Blackburn, June 2, 1847. M-442, frame 188: Blackburn Family Papers, 1829–1865, Lexington, University of Kentucky Special Collections Research Center, Margaret I. King Library, University of Kentucky.
14. Letter, Ella G. Blackburn to Lavinia L. Blackburn, November 13, 1853. M-442, frame 345: Blackburn Family Papers, 1829–1865, Lexington, University of Kentucky Special Collections Research Center, Margaret I. King Library,

University of Kentucky; Baird, Nancy Disher. *Luke Pryor Blackburn: Physician, Governor, Reformer.* Lexington: The Kentucky Bicentennial Bookshelf, University Press of Kentucky, 1979, p. 9.

15. United States Passport of Luke Pryor Blackburn, 1857. Blackburn Family Papers, Folder 23, Filson Historical Society, Louisville, Kentucky.

16. United States Census, Slave Schedule, Woodford County Kentucky, 1850, pp. 31–32; United States Census, Slave Schedule, Desha County Arkansas, Mississippi Township, 1860, p. 19, http://interactive.ancestry.com.

17. Letter, Ella G. Blackburn to William E. Blackburn, February 24, 1849. M-442, frame 297: Blackburn Family Papers, 1829–1865, Lexington, University of Kentucky Special Collections Research Center, Margaret I. King Library, University of Kentucky.

18. Letter, Ella G. Blackburn to Lavinia L. Blackburn, February 15, 1854. M-442, frame 362: Blackburn Family Papers, 1829–1865, Lexington, University of Kentucky Special Collections Research Center, Margaret I. King Library, University of Kentucky.

19. Letter, Luke P. Blackburn to Lavinia L. Blackburn, October 10, 1846. M-442, frame 143; Letter, Ella G. Blackburn to Lavinia L. Blackburn, February 19, 1858. M-442, frame 385: Blackburn Family Papers, 1829–1865, Lexington, University of Kentucky Special Collections Research Center, Margaret I. King Library, University of Kentucky.

20. Baird, *Luke Pryor Blackburn*, 12.

21. Webster, Noah. *Dictionary of the English Language.* Springfield, MA: G. & C. Merriam, 1865, p. 41.

22. Letter, Ella G. Blackburn to Lavinia L. Blackburn, March 1, 1855. M-442, frame 371: Blackburn Family Papers, 1829–1865, Lexington, University of Kentucky Special Collections Research Center, Margaret I. King Library, University of Kentucky.

23. Letter, Ella G. Blackburn to Lavinia L. Blackburn, September 30, 1855. M-442, frame 374: Blackburn Family Papers, 1829–1865, Lexington, University of Kentucky Special Collections Research Center, Margaret I. King Library, University of Kentucky.

24. Letter, Ella G. Blackburn to Lavinia L. Blackburn, December 13, 1855. M-442, frame 376: Blackburn Family Papers, 1829–1865, Lexington, University of Kentucky Special Collections Research Center, Margaret I. King Library, University of Kentucky.

25. Letter, Ella G. Blackburn to Lavinia L. Blackburn, February 17, 1858. M-442, frame 385: Blackburn Family Papers, 1829–1865, Lexington, University of Kentucky Special Collections Research Center, Margaret I. King Library, University of Kentucky.

26. Baird, *Luke Pryor Blackburn*, 17; Find A Grave, http://www.findagrave.com.

27. Julia Churchill's family founded Churchill Downs, the Louisville racetrack that is the home to the Kentucky Derby. Opened in 1875, it was named after John and Henry Churchill.

28. Churchill Family Papers, 1735–1905. Louisville, Kentucky: Special Collections, Folder 9, LB/A/c563/9, Filson Historical Society.

Chapter 2

1. *Contagion: Historical Views of Diseases and Epidemics; The Yellow Fever Epidemic in Philadelphia, 1793.* Harvard University Library Open Collections Program, http://ocp.hul.harvard.edu; Rush, Benjamin. *Observations upon the Origin of the Malignant Bilious, or Yellow Fever in Philadelphia, and upon the Means of Preventing It: Addressed to the Citizens of Philadelphia.* Philadelphia: Budd and Bartram, 1799, http://pds.lib.harvard.edu/pds/view/6483213?n=1&printThumbnails=no.

2. Congressional Serial Set. Index to the Senate Executive Documents for the Third Session of the Forty-Second Congress of the United States of America. 1872–73. Washington: Government Printing Office, 1873. 42nd Congress, 3rd Session, Senate, Executive Document #9, *Letter from the Secretary of War Communicating, in obedience to law, information in relation to quarantine on the Southern and Gulf coasts*, pp. 1–117. Quarantine on the Southern and Gulf Coasts.

3. Woodward, Joseph Janvier. *Report on Epidemic Cholera and Yellow Fever in the Army of the United States, During the Year 1867.* Circular No. 1, War Department, Surgeon General's Office, Washington, June 10, 1868, Washington, Government Printing Office, 1868, p. xxxiv.

4. Carrigan, Jo Ann. *Yankees Versus Yellow Jack in New Orleans, 1862–1866.* Kent, Ohio: Kent State University Press, *Civil War History* 9, no. 3 (September 1963), 248–260.

5. *Ibid.,* 250.

Chapter 3

1. Harris, Thomas Maley. *Assassination of Lincoln: A History of the Great Conspiracy.* Boston: American Citizen, 1892, p. 61.

2. Boyko, John. *Blood and Daring: How Canada Fought the American Civil War and Forged a Nation.* Toronto: Knopf Canada, 2013.

3. Pitman, Benn. *The Assassination of President Lincoln and the Trial of the Conspirators*. Cincinnati: Moore, Wilstach & Baldwin, 1865, p. 379.
4. Mayers, Adam. *Dixie and the Dominion: Canada, the Confederacy, and the War for the Union*. Toronto: Dundern, 2003, p. 155.
5. Davis, Jefferson. *The Papers of Jefferson Davis, Volume 11, September 1864–May 1865*. Crist, Lynda Lasswell, Barbara J. Rozek, and Kenneth H. Williams, ed. Baton Rouge: Louisiana State University Press, 2004, p. 194.
6. Winks, Robin W. *The Civil War Years: Canada and the United States*. Montreal: McGill-Queen's University Press, 1998, pp. 140–141; *Donegana's Hotel, Montreal*. https://en.wikipedia.org/wiki/Donegana%27s_Hotel; *The Donegana Hotel, Notre Dame Street, Montreal, and Traveller's Guide to Montreal*. Montreal: Daniel Rose, 1866, pp. 1–2.
7. *New York Times*, "The Rebels in Canada; Blockade Runners from Montreal? The Trade Very Active—Secession Up North," August 17, 1863; created Aug 12, 1863.

Chapter 4

1. Deichmann, Catherine Lynch. *Rogues and Runners: Bermuda and the American Civil War*. Hamilton, Bermuda: Bermuda National Trust Collection, 2003, p. 15.
2. *Ibid.*, p. 16.
3. Officially, the name of the town is "St. George," though common usage often renders it as "St. Georges." When discussing parishes of Bermuda, the term is usually written "St. George's Parish;" for delineation of ports, the proper term is "Port of St. George" or "St. George's Port." Though the strict grammarian may object, I have arbitrarily chosen to use the designation "St. Georges" in this book for the town, not "St. George" or "St. George's."
4. Deichmann, *Rogues and Runners*, 14.
5. *Ibid.*, 42.
6. *Ibid.*, 63.
7. Measuring Worth. Exchange Rates Between the United States Dollar and Forty-One Currencies, http://measuringworth.com/datasets/exchangeglobal/result.php?year_source=1791&year_result=2007&countryE%5B%5D=United+Kingdom.
8. Deichmann, *Rogues and Runners*, p. 46.
9. *Ibid.*, 67.
10. *Ibid.*, 70.
11. *Ibid.*, 36.
12. Vandiver, Frank E. *Confederate Blockade Running Through Bermuda, 1861–1865: Letters and Cargo Manifests*. Austin: University of Texas Press, 1947, p. xxv.
13. *Bermuda Pocket Almanack, for the Year of Our Lord 1865: Calculated for Bermuda, and Containing Everything Necessary for an Almanack*. Hamilton, Bermuda: D. M'Phee Lee, Office of the Royal Gazette, 1865. Hamilton, Bermuda: Bermuda Archives, pp 35–36.
14. Vandiver, *Confederate Blockade Running*, xxi.
15. *Ibid.*, 94.
16. Stansbury Letters. Hamilton, Bermuda: Bermuda Archives.
17. Also spelled "Alexandre" in some references.
18. Vandiver, *Confederate Blockade Running*, 98.
19. Deichmann, *Rogues and Runners*, 36, 40.
20. Wiche, Glen N., ed. *Dispatches from Bermuda. The Civil War Letters of Charles Maxwell Allen, United States Consul at Bermuda, 1861–1888*. Kent, Ohio: Kent State University Press, 2008, p. 91.
21. *Papers Relating to the Treaty of Washington. Volume III—Geneva Arbitration*. Washington: Government Printing Office, 1873, p. 404.
22. Wiche, *Dispatches from Bermuda*, 23.
23. *Ibid.*, 44.
24. Deichmann, *Rogues and Runners*, 41.
25. Vandiver, *Confederate Blockade Running*, xx.
26. *Ibid.*, xxi, 64.
27. *Ibid.*, xxii–xxiii.

Chapter 5

1. Wood, Margaret. *Civil War Conscription Laws*. Library of Congress, November 15, 2012; Moore, Albert B. *Conscription and Conflict in the Confederacy*. Columbia: University of South Carolina Press, 1924.
2. Stillé, Alfred. *Therapeutics and Materia Medica: A Systematic Treatise on the Action and Uses of Medicinal Agents, Including Their Description and History*. Vols. 1 and 2. Philadelphia: Blanchard and Lea, 1860; Cunningham, H.H. *Doctors in Gray: The Confederate Medical Service*. Baton Rouge: Louisiana State University Press, 1986; Hartshorne, Henry. *Memoranda Medica; or, Note-Book of Medical Principles, Being a Concise Syllabus of Etiology, Semeiology, General Pathology, Nosology and General Therapeutics, with a Glossary for the Use of Students*. Philadelphia: Lippincott, 1860; Watson, Thomas. Revised by D. Francis Condie. *Lectures on the Principles and Practice of Physic; Delivered at King's College, London*. Philadelphia: Blanchard and Lea, 1856.
3. Tripler, Chas. S, and George C Black-

man. *Handbook for the Military Surgeon: Being A Compendium of the Duties of the Medical Officer in the Field, the Sanitary Management of the Camp, the Preparation of Food, Etc.; with Forms for the Requisitions for Supplies, Returns, Etc.; the Diagnosis and Treatment of Camp Dysentery; and All the Important Points in War Surgery: Including Gunshot Wounds, Amputation, Wounds of the Chest, Abdomen, Arteries and Head, and the Use of Chloroform.* Cincinnati: Robert Clarke & Co., 1861; Druitt, Robert. *The Principles and Practice of Modern Surgery.* Philadelphia, Blanchard and Lea, 1860.

4. Roberts, Deering J. "Organization and Personnel of the Medical Department of the Confederacy." Appendix D, pp. 349–352. In Thompson, Holland, ed. Thompson, Holland, Edward L. Munson, and Deering J. Roberts, Contributors. Volume 7. *Prisons and Hospitals.* In Miller, Francis Trevelyan, and Robert S. Lanier, ed. *The Photographic History of the Civil War in Ten Volumes.* New York: Review of Reviews, Trow, 1912.

5. Tooker, John. *Antietam: Aspects of Medicine, Nursing and the Civil War.* Trans. Am. Clin. Climatol. Assoc. 2007; 118:215–223.

6. Letterman, Jonathan. *Letterman's Report Detailing the Medical Department of the Army of the Potomac.* March 1, 1863.

7. Craven, John J. *Prison Life of Jefferson Davis: Embracing Details and Incidents in His Captivity, Particulars Concerning His Health and Habits, Together with Many Conversations on Topics of Great Public Interest.* New York: Carleton, 1866, p. 287.

8. Munson, Edward L. *The Army Surgeon and His Work.* In Thompson, Holland, ed. Thompson, Holland, Edward L. Munson, and Deering J. Roberts, Contributors, pp. 213–236. In Miller, Francis Trevelyan, and Robert S. Lanier, eds. *The Photographic History of the Civil War in Ten Volumes.* Vol. 4: *Prisons and Hospitals.* New York: Review of Reviews, Trow, 1912; Roberts, Deering J. *Confederate Medical Service,* pp. 238–250. In Thompson, Holland, ed. Thompson, Holland, Edward L. Munson, and Deering J. Roberts, Contributors. Vol. 7. *Prisons and Hospitals.* In Miller, Francis Trevelyan, and Robert S. Lanier, eds. *The Photographic History of the Civil War in Ten Volumes.* New York: Review of Reviews, Trow, 1912.

9. Paul F. Lacy Papers, Paul Christian Yates biography, written 10/5/1881 at Neosho, Missouri, Mss/C/L, pp. 23–24. Louisville, Kentucky: Special Collections, Filson Historical Society.

10. Editing, punctuation, and spacing of this narrative were added solely for clarity and readability.

11. Jones, Joseph. *The Medical History of the Confederate States Army and Navy, Comprising the Official Report of Surgeon Joseph Jones, M.D., LL.D., Surgeon-General of the United Confederate Veterans.* Southern Historical Society. Southern Historical Society Papers (1876–1905), 20:109–138, 1892.

12. No. 385. Armed Forces Personnel—Summary of Major Conflicts. Statistical Abstract of the United States, 1970, 91st Annual Edition, U.S. Department of Commerce, Bureau of Census. Washington: U.S. Government Printing Office, 1970, p. 256.

13. Civil War Facts, www.civilwar.org/education/history/faq.

14. Jacobs, Jos. *Some of the Drug Conditions During the War Between the States, 1861–1865.* Proceedings of the American Pharmaceutical Association at the Forty-Sixth Annual Meeting, Held at Baltimore, MD, August, 1898. Baltimore: American Pharmaceutical Association, 1898, pp. 192–213; Hasegawa, Guy R., and F. Terry Hambrecht. "The Confederate Medical Laboratories," *Southern Medical Journal* (2003), 96 (12), 1221–1230.

15. "Anesthetics in the Civil War." In Barnes, Joseph K., George A. Otis, and D.L. Huntington. *The Medical and Surgical History of the War of the Rebellion (1861–1865).* Part 3, Vol. 2, Ch. 13. *Anaesthetics,* pp. 887–898. Washington: Government Printing Office, 1883.

16. Civil War Battlefield Surgery. A Description of Civil War Field Surgery, http://ehistory.osu.edu/exhibitions/cwsurgeon/cwsurgeon/amputations.

17. Howey, Allan W. "Minié Ball," *Civil War Times,* October 1999. http://www.historynet.com/minie-ball.

18. Civil War Facts, www.civilwar.org/education/history/faq.

Chapter 6

1. *Report of the Adjutant General of the State of Kentucky,* vol. 2, *1861–1866.* Frankfort: Kentucky Yeoman Office, John H. Harney, 1867; Kleber, John E., ed. (chief); Clark, Thomas D., Lowell H. Harrison, and James C. Klotter, associate ed. *The Kentucky Encyclopedia.* Lexington: University Press of Kentucky, 1992, pp. 438, 513; Eubank, Damon R. *In the Shadow of the Patriarch: The John J. Crittenden Family in War and Peace.* Macon, GA: Mercer University Press, 2009, p. 44.

2. Keehn, David C. *Knights of the Golden Circle: Secret Empire, Southern Secession, Civil War.* Baton Rouge: Louisiana State University Press, 2013, pg. 1.

3. Goebel, Robert William. *Casualty of War: the Governorship of Beriah Magoffin,*

1859–1862. Louisville, KY: Electronic Theses and Dissertations, 2005. University of Louisville master's thesis, Paper 506, p. 84.
    4. *New Orleans Daily Crescent*, April 25, 1861.
    5. ORA. Correspondence, etc.—Confederate, Series 1, Volume 52 (2), chapter 64, p. 67.
    6. ORA. Correspondence, etc.—Confederate, Series 1, Volume 52 (2), chapter 64, p. 71.
    7. *Daily Nashville Patriot*, May 11, 1861.
    8. *Millersburg (OH) Holmes County Republican*, May 9, 1861.
    9. *Cincinnati Daily Press*, May 2, 1861.
    10. *Report of the Adjutant General of the State of Indiana.* Indianapolis: Alexander H. Conner, State Printer, 1869, vol. 1, p. 214.
    11. *Cincinnati Daily Press*, May 2, 1861.
    12. General Orders No. 17, 1861. Blackburn Family Papers, 1840–1896. Louisville, Kentucky: Special Collections, Miscellaneous Manuscripts Collection, MS/C/G, Filson Historical Society.
    13. ORA. Correspondence, etc.—Confederate, Series 1, Vol. 4, p. 549.
    14. NARA. Record Group 94, M 1017 and M 818, Roll 3.
    15. ORA. Correspondence, etc.—Confederate, Series 1, Volume 17, Part 2, Chapter 29, pp. 665, 676–677.
    16. Telegram, L.P. Blackburn to Maj. Genl. S. Price, August 20, 1862. Civil War Service Records, Confederate Records, www.fold3.com/image/65131016.
    17. Letter, John J. Pettus to Luke P. Blackburn, January 11, 1863 (erroneously dated 1862), citing the Legislative Act of Mississippi on January 2, 1863. Blackburn Family Papers, 1840–1896. Louisville, Kentucky: Special Collections, Filson Historical Society.
    18. Baird, *Luke Pryor Blackburn*, p. 21; Letter, Luke P. Blackburn to "Dear Sir," May 13, 1863, www.fold3.com/image/65130895.
    19. Note, Samuel Preston Moore to Luke P. Blackburn, May 20, 1863, www.fold3.com/image/65131029.
    20. Letter, Luke P. Blackburn to Major General D.H. Maury. Churchill Family Papers, 1735–1905. Louisville, Kentucky: Special Collections, A/c 563/9, Filson Historical Society; Baird, *Luke Pryor Blackburn*, 22.
    21. Wiche, Glen N., ed. *Dispatches from Bermuda: The Civil War Letters of Charles Maxwell Allen, United States Consul at Bermuda, 1861–1888.* Kent, OH: Kent State University Press, 2008, p. 44; *The War of the Rebellion: A Compilation of the Official Records of the Union and Confederate Armies*; ORA. Correspondence, etc., Series 4, Vol. 2, p. 924; Craven, John J. *Prison Life of Jefferson Davis: Embracing Details and Incidents in His Captivity, Particulars Concerning His Health and Habits, Together with Many Conversations on Topics of Great Public Interest.* New York and London: Carleton, 1866, p. 99; Steers, Edward, Jr. *Blood on the Moon: The Assassination of Abraham Lincoln.* Lexington: University Press of Kentucky, 2001, p. 47.
    22. Letter, Colonel M. Mundy to Mrs. J.L. Blackburn, July 21, 1863. Churchill Family Papers, 1735–1905. Louisville, Kentucky: Special Collections, A/c 563/9, Filson Historical Society.
    23. Letter, General J.T. Boyle to Julia Blackburn, July 24, 1863. Churchill Family Papers, 1735–1905. Louisville, Kentucky: Special Collections, A/c 563/9, Filson Historical Society.
    24. *Mitchell & Co.'s General Directory for the City of Toronto, and Gazetteer of the Counties of York and Peel for 1866.* Toronto, Ontario, Canada: Mitchell, 1866, p. 1.
    25. *City of Toronto Directory for 1867-8, Containing an Alphabetical Directory of the Citizens, a Business Directory, or Classified List of Trades and Professions.* Toronto, Ontario, Canada: James Sutherland, comp., 1867, p. 28.
    26. Pitman. *Assassination of President Lincoln*, p. 54.

Chapter 7

    1. England Census, 1851, http://interactive.ancestry.com.
    2. England and Wales, FreeBMD Marriage Index, 1837–1915, http://interactive.ancestry.com.
    3. England and Wales, Criminal Registers, 1791–1892, http://interactive.ancestry.com.
    4. New York, Passenger Lists, 1820–1957, http://interactive.ancestry.com.
    5. *Scientific American* 2, no. 7 (November 6, 1846): 54.
    6. NARA. Record Group 36, M237, Roll 172.
    7. Worley, Ted R. "Helena on the Mississippi," *Arkansas Historical Quarterly* 13 (Spring 1954): 1–15.
    8. Kohl, Rhonda M. "'This Godforsaken Town': Death and Disease at Helena, Arkansas, 1862–1863," *Civil War History* 50, no. 2 (2004): 109–144.
    9. Brent, Joseph E., and Maria Campbell Brent. *Civil War Helena: A Research Project and Interpretive Plan. Part 2: Helena and Phillips County, Arkansas, 1861–1868.* Versailles, KY: Mudpuppy and Waterdog, April 30, 2009; *Agriculture of the United States in 1860, Compiled from the Original Records of the Eighth Census.* Washington, D.C.: U.S. Government Printing Office, p. 6; *Population of the United States in 1860, Compiled from the Original*

Records of the Eighth Census. Washington, D.C.: U.S. Government Printing Office, p. 18.
10. Personal communication, Shane Williams, Helena Museum of Phillips County, November 5, 2015, Helena Arkansas.
11. Census Table 1860, Executive Office, Little Rock, Arkansas, November 14, 1860, Elias N. Conway, governor; Unreferenced Civil War display, November 5, 2015, Delta Cultural Center, Helena, Arkansas.
12. *Little Rock Arkansas True Democrat*, August 8, 1861.
13. *Memphis Daily Appeal*, September 18, 1861.
14. *Arkansas True Democrat*, October 31, 1861.
15. *Ibid.*, September 19, 1861.
16. *Memphis Daily Appeal*, August 14, 1861.
17. *Ibid.*, August 3, 1861.
18. *Little Rock Arkansas Gazette*, November 8, 1862.
19. *Helena (AR) Weekly Note-Book*, January 9, 1862. Displayed at the Helena Historical Society, Helena, November 6, 2015.
20. *New York Daily Tribune*, June 7, 1862, cited in H.L. Hanna, *The Press Covers the Invasion of Arkansas 1862*. Vol. 1, January–June, CreateSpace Independent Publishers, 2011, p. 284.
21. LeMaster, Carolyn Gray. *A Corner of the Tapestry: A History of the Jewish Experience in Arkansas, 1820s–1990s*. Fayetteville: University of Arkansas Press, 1994, p. 18; *Encyclopedia of Southern Jewish Communities—Helena, Arkansas*, http://www.isjl.org/arkansas-helena-encyclopedia.html.
22. Worley, Ted R. "Helena on the Mississippi," *Arkansas Historical Quarterly* 13 (Spring 1954), 13.
23. Eighth United States Census, 1860, NARA. Record Group 29, M 653, Roll 47; Blackburn Family Papers, 1829–1865, Lexington: University of Kentucky Special Collections Research Center, Margaret I. King Library, University of Kentucky, M-442, frame 521.
24. United States Census, Slave Schedules, Phillips County, Arkansas, Helena, St. Francis Township, 1860, http://interactive.ancestry.com.
25. United States Census, Slave Schedules, Desha County, Arkansas, Mississippi Township, 1860, p. 19, http://interactive.ancestry.com.
26. *Little Rock Arkansas Gazette*, as cited in H.L. Hanna, *The Press Covers the Invasion of Arkansas 1862*, vol. 2, July–December. CreateSpace Independent Publishers, 2012, p. 58, date of cited article not given.
27. Kohl, "This Godforsaken Town," 114.
28. Kohl, Rhonda M. "Hard Lessons of War: The Fifth Illinois Cavalry at Helena, Arkansas," *Journal of the Illinois State Historical Society* (1998–) 99, (3/4) (Fall 2006–Winter 2007): 187.
29. Dougan, Michael B. "Life in Confederate Arkansas," *Arkansas Historical Quarterly* 31, no. 1 (Spring 1972): 19–20.
30. *Ibid.*, 28–29.
31. Davenport, Edward A., ed. *History of the Ninth Regiment Illinois Cavalry Volunteers*. Chicago: Donohue & Henneberry, 1888, p. 46.
32. *ORA*. Prisoners of War and State, etc., Series 2, Volume 4, p. 316.
33. Foote, Shelby. *The Civil War: A Narrative*. Vol. 5: *Fredericksburg to Steele Bayou*. Alexandria, VA: Time-Life Books, 2000, p. 68.
34. *Little Rock Arkansas Gazette*, as cited in H.L. Hanna, *The Press Covers the Invasion of Arkansas 1862*, vol. 2, July–December. CreateSpace Independent Publishers, 2012, p. 58.
35. *Memphis Daily Appeal*, July 31, 1862, as cited in H.L. Hanna, *The Press Covers the Invasion of Arkansas, 1862*. Vol. 2: July–December. CreateSpace Independent Publishers, 2012, p. 101.
36. Kohl, "This Godforsaken Town," 117.
37. Behlendorff, Frederick. *The History of the Thirteenth Illinois Cavalry Regiment*. Grand Rapids, MI, 1888, as cited in Rhonda M. Kohl, "'This Godforsaken Town': Death and Disease at Helena, Arkansas, 1862–63." *Civil War History* 50, no. 2 (2004): 118.
38. Steiner, Paul F. *Disease in the Civil War: Natural Biological Warfare in 1861–1865*. Springfield, IL: Charles C. Thomas, 1968, p. 213; Packard Diary, October 11, 1862, as cited in Rhonda M. Kohl, "'This Godforsaken Town': Death and Disease at Helena, Arkansas, 1862–1863," *Civil War History*, 50, no. 2 (2004): 144.
39. Kohl, "This Godforsaken Town," 126.
40. *Ibid.*, 127.
41. Davis, Jefferson. *The Papers of Jefferson Davis*, vol. 8, 1862. Crist, Lynda Lasswell, Mary S. Dix, and Kenneth H. Williams, ed. Baton Rouge: Louisiana State University Press, 1995, pp. 536–537.
42. *Ibid.*, 537–538.
43. Letter, Godfrey J. Hyams to Adjutant General E.D. Townsend, December 28, 1862, https://www.fold3.com/image/300098871.
44. *Chicago Tribune*, September 3, 1879.
45. *New York Times*, May 26, 1865.
46. *Montreal Herald*, May 26, 1865.
47. *Ibid.*, May 19, 26, 27, 1865.
48. Gratiot Street Prison, http://civilwarstlouis.com/Gratiot/gratiot.htm.
49. *ORA*. Mo. Ark., Kans., Ind. T., and Dept. N.W., Series 1, Volume 22, Serial 32, Chapter 34, p. 804.

50. Speer, Lonnie R. *Portals to Hell: Military Prisons of the Civil War.* Mechanicsburg, PA: Stackpole Books, 1997, pp. 56, 88–89, 133–135, 179, 184.
51. *Montreal Herald,* May 19, 26, 27, 1865.
52. Speer, *Portals to Hell,* 211.
53. Roll of Prisoners of War, Gratiot Street Prison, 1862, p. 45, http://interactive.ancestry.com.
54. *Montreal Herald,* May 19, 26, 27, 1865.
55. *J.L. Mitchell's Toronto City Directory, 1864–1865.* J.L. Mitchell, W.C. Chewett, 1864, pp. 82, 300.
56. *Ibid.,* xviii.
57. United States Census, 1870, 1880.
58. Robinson, Rev. Stuart. "Infamous Perjuries of the 'Bureau of Military Justice' Exposed," https://ia800307.us.archive.org/17/items/cihm_63181/cihm_63181.pdf; *Montreal Herald,* May 26, 1865.
59. *Montreal Herald,* May 19, 1865.
60. *Ibid.,* May 19, 1865.
61. Baird, Nancy Disher. *Luke Pryor Blackburn: Physician, Governor, Reformer.* The Kentucky Bicentennial Bookshelf. Lexington: University Press of Kentucky, 1979, p. 29; *Chicago Tribune,* September 3, 1879.
62. *Ibid.*
63. *Montreal Herald,* May 26 and 27, 1865.

Chapter 8

1. Kline, Michael J. *The Baltimore Plot.* Yardley, PA: Westholme, 2008.
2. ORA. Correspondence, Etc.—Union and Confederate. Series 2, Vol. 8, Serial 121, p. 849.
3. *Ibid.,* 851.
4. *Ibid.,* 849.
5. Steers, *Blood on the Moon,* 42.
6. *Richmond Sentinel,* March 5, 1864; *Richmond Dispatch,* March 5, 1864; Thomas, Emory M. "The Kilpatrick-Dahlgren Raid—Part 1." *Civil War Times Illustrated* 16 (February 1978): 4–9, 46–48; "The Kilpatrick-Dahlgren Raid—Part 2." *Civil War Times Illustrated* 17 (April 1978): 26–33.
7. Steers, *Blood on the Moon,* 44–45.
8. *Richmond Examiner,* November 23, 1863, as cited in *New York Times,* November 27, 1863.
9. Letter, Maj. Gen. Benjamin J. Butler to Brig. Genl. Isaac Jones Wistar, February 4, 1864. In Butler, Benjamin F. *Private and Official Correspondence of Gen. Benjamin F. Butler During the Period of the Civil War,* vol. 3, February 1863–March 1864. Norwood, MA: Plimpton Press, 1917, pp. 373–374.
10. ORA, Correspondence, Etc.—Union and Confederate. Series 2, Vol. 8, Serial 121, p. 849.
11. *Ibid.* 848–849.
12. *Ibid.,* 853.
13. *Ibid.,* 848–849.
14. Letter, Kensey Johns Stewart to Jefferson Davis, December 12, 1864. NARA. Record Group 109, Chapter 7, Volume 24, pp. 64–65, as cited in Steers, *Blood on the Moon,* 53, 302.
15. Letter, Secretary of War James A. Seddon (CSA) to Captain T. Henry Hines, as quoted in "The Northwestern Conspiracy," in *Southern Bivouac* 2, no. 1 (June 1886): 443.
16. Mayers, Adam. *Dixie and the Dominion: Canada, the Confederacy, and the War for the Union,* Toronto: Dundern, 2003, p. 26.
17. Kinchen, Oscar A. *Confederate Operations in Canada and the North: A Little-Known Phase of the American Civil War.* North Quincy, MA: Christopher, 1970, pp. 35–36.
18. Mayers, *Dixie and the Dominion,* 23.
19. *Ibid.,* 26.
20. Bovy, Wilfrid. "Confederate Agents in Canada During the American Civil War," *Canadian Historical Review* 2, March 11, 1921: p. 47, as cited in Steers, *Blood on the Moon,* 46.
21. Mayers, *Dixie and the Dominion,* 29.
22. *Ibid.,* 27–28.
23. *Ibid.,* 40.
24. Claim, John Gordon McBain, vs. the U.S., https://www.fold3.com/image/298477971.
25. Mayers, *Dixie and the Dominion,* 28.
26. *Ibid.,* 61.
27. Kinchen, *Confederate Operations,* 37.
28. Allen, Felicity. "Jefferson Davis, Unconquerable Heart." In *Shades of Blue and Gray,* Book 1, Series edited by Herman Hattaway, Jon L. Wakelyn, and Clayton E. Jewett. Columbia: University of Missouri Press, 1999, p. 233.
29. *Ibid.,* 231–233.
30. Davis, Jefferson. *The Papers of Jefferson Davis,* vol. 6, 1856–1860. Crist, Lynda Lasswell, and Mary Seaton Dix, ed. Baton Rouge: Louisiana State University Press, 1989, p. 174.
31. Cumming, Carman. *Devil's Game: The Civil War Intrigues of Charles A. Dunham.* Urbana: University of Illinois Press, 2004, p 3.
32. Hines, Thomas H. "The Northwestern Conspiracy." *Southern Bivouac* 2, no. 1 (June 1886): 502.
33. Kinchen, *Confederate Operations,* 37–38.
34. Letter, Jacob Thompson to Secretary of State Judah P. Benjamin, December 3, 1864. ORN. The Operations of the Cruisers—Con-

federate (April 1, 1864–December 30, 1865). Series 1, Vol. 3, p. 719.

35. Bellevue, Home of James Philemon Holcombe. Application for the National Register of Historic Places, National Park Service, citing Carl Sandburg, *Abraham Lincoln: The War Years* 3:159.

36. Tidwell, William A., with James O. Hall and David Winfred Gaddy. *Come Retribution: The Confederate Secret Service and the Assassination of Lincoln.* Jackson: University Press of Mississippi, 1988, pp. 189, 197, 204, 407; Tidwell, William A. *April '65: Confederate Covert Action in the American Civil War. Eastern European Studies: 1.* Kent, Ohio, and London, England: Kent State University Press, 1995, pp. 114, 252; Cleary, William W. *Diary of William Walter Cleary, 1862–1864.* University of Kentucky, Kentucky Digital Library, image 1, p. 1. http://kdl.kyvl.org/catalog/xt7d251fkb86_1?.

37. Headley, John W. *Confederate Operations in Canada and New York.* New York and Washington: Neale, 1906. p. 214.

38. General Orders, No. 164, War Department Adjutant-General's Office, Washington, November 24, 1865, by E.D. Townsend, Assistant Adjutant-General.

39. Halmer H. Emmons Papers, Box 111, Burton Historical Collection, Detroit Public Library, Detroit, Michigan.

40. Cleary, *Diary*, 11.

41. *Ibid.*, 10.

42. *Ibid.*, 111.

43. Cleary, William W., quoted in Hines, Thomas H. "The Northwestern Conspiracy." *Southern Bivouac* 2, no. 7 (December 1886): 444.

44. *Ibid.*, 445.

45. Kinchen, *Confederate Operations*, 39.

46. Walker, Georgiana Gholson. *The Private Journal of Georgiana Gholson Walker, 1862–1865, with Selections from the Post-War Years, 1865–1876,* ed. Dwight Franklin Henderson. Tuscaloosa, AL: Confederate Publishing, Confederate Centennial Studies, Wm. Stanley Hoole, editor-in-chief, 1963, p. 67.

47. *Ibid.*, 91–93.

48. *Ibid.*, 92–93.

49. *Hamilton (Bermuda) Royal Gazette,* May 17, 1864.

50. Kinchen, *Confederate Operations*, 46.

51. *Ibid.*, 44.

52. *Ibid.*, 30.

53. Hines, Thomas H. "The Northwestern Conspiracy." *Southern Bivouac* 2, no. 8 (January 1887): 501–502.

54. Smith, Bethania Meradith. "Civil War Subversives." *Journal of the Illinois State Historical Society* 45, no. 3 (Autumn 1952): 220–240.

55. Letter, Abraham Lincoln to Horace Greeley, July 9, 1864. *Abraham Lincoln: Complete Works Comprising His Speeches, Letters, State Papers, and Miscellaneous Writings.* Ed. John G. Nicolay and John Hay. Vol. 2. New York: Century, 1894, p. 546; and Letter, Abraham Lincoln, "TO WHOM IT MAY CONCERN," July 1864, p. 550; *ORA,* Correspondence, Union Authorities. Series 3, Vol. 4, p. 501.

56. Hines, Thomas H. "The Northwestern Conspiracy." *Southern Bivouac* 2, no. 8 (January 1887), 502.

57. Kinchen, *Confederate Operations*, 41.

58. Mayers, *Dixie and the Dominion,* 81.

59. "The Plan to Rescue Johnson's Island Prisoners." *Southern Historical Society Papers* 23 (January–December 1895), 283–290, as originally reported in the *Richmond (VA) Dispatch,* December 15, 1895; Mayers, *Dixie and the Dominion,* 67, 80, 82, 86–87, 243; Downer, Edward T. "Johnson's Island." *Civil War History* 8, no. 2 (June 1962): 202–217; "Intelligence in the Civil War," Central Intelligence Agency Document, pp. 44–46, https://www.cia.gov/library/publications/intelligence-history/civil-war/Intel_in_the_CW1.pdf.

60. Sherburne, Michelle Arnosky. *The St. Albans Raid: Confederate Attack on Vermont.* Charleston, SC: History, 2014, p. 23.

61. "Intelligence in the Civil War," Central Intelligence Agency Document, p. 47.

62. Letter, Jacob Thompson to Secretary of State Judah P. Benjamin, December 3, 1864. *ORN.* The Operations of the Cruisers—Confederate (April 1, 1864–December 30, 1865). Series 1, Vol. 3, p. 718.

63. Letter, Judah P. Benjamin to Jacob Thompson, cited in Mayers, *Dixie and the Dominion,* 163.

64. Steers, *Blood on the Moon,* 52–58.

65. *Testimony of Sanford Conover, Dr. J.B. Merritt, and Richard Montgomery, Before Military Court at Washington, Respecting the Assassination of President Lincoln, and the Proofs Disproving Their Statements, and Showing Their Perjuries.* Toronto: Lovell & Gibson, 1865, p. 28.

66. *Ibid.*, 13–14; "Proceedings of Societies: American Medical Association." *Chicago Medical Examiner ("A Monthly Journal, Devoted to the Educational, Scientific and Practical Interests of the Medical Profession)* 6, no. 7 (July 1865): 415, 426. Chicago: George H. Fergus; N.S. Davis, ed.

67. *Testimony of Sanford Conover,* 25; "Proceedings of Societies," *Chicago Medical Examiner* 6, no. 7 (July 1865): 428.

68. Mayers, *Dixie and the Dominion,* 121, 125.

69. The Lost Museum Archive. "The Plot," *New York Times,* November 27, 1864.

70. Headley, *Confederate Operations*, 214–5, 278, 281, 288, 308.
71. *Ibid.*, 215.
72. *Ibid.*, 264.

Chapter 9

1. "Bermuda History—Epidemics, Yellow Fever and Biowarfare in the 1800s?" Bermuda National Library. bnl.bm/files/2011/08/Bermuda_History_Epidemics.pdf.
2. Deichmann, Catherine Lynch. *Rogues and Runners: Bermuda and the American Civil War.* Hamilton, Bermuda: Bermuda National Trust Collection, 2003, p. 72.
3. Maclean, Deputy Inspector-General. "Lecture on the Epidemic of Yellow Fever at Bermuda in 1864." *Lancet* 86 (December 16, 1865): 667–669.
4. *Ibid.*, 669.
5. Though named a "Junior," Sandy was actually the nephew of his namesake Alexander Keith, the original brewer in the family. Sandy was the son of John Keith, Alexander "Senior's" younger brother.
6. Solomon, Janet. "'Yellow Fever Fiend' Hated Abe Lincoln: A Murder Plot Hatched by Southern Agents in the Alehouses of Halifax Targeted the U.S.," http://www.care2.com/news/member/471046224/1241320.
7. Forbes, Keith Archibald. "Bermuda's History from 1800 to 1899," http://www.bermuda-online.org/history1800-1899.htm.
8. Forbes, Keith Archibald. "Bermuda's Connections with and Ties to Canada," http://www.bermuda-online.org/canada.htm.
9. *Hamilton (Bermuda) Royal Gazette*, November 18, 1809.
10. *Official Guide and Album of the Cunard Steamship Company.* Liverpool: Sutton Sharpe, 1877, p. 35.
11. *Cunard Liners: Alpha, 1863–1900*, http://www.dieselduck.info/historical/05%20documents/Cunard%20Liners.pdf; *Report of the Meteorological Committee of the Royal Society for the Year Ending 31st December 1867.* London: George E. Eyre and William Spottiswoode, 1868, pp. 40, 43, 51, 55.
12. Marquis, Greg. *In Armageddon's Shadow: The Civil War and Canada's Maritime Provinces.* Montreal: McGill-Queen's University Press, 2000, p. 94.
13. *Hamilton (Bermuda) Royal Gazette*, January 26, 1864.
14. Morgan, James Morris. *Recollections of a Rebel Reefer.* Boston and New York: Houghton Mifflin, Riverside Press Cambridge, 1917, pp. 189–190.
15. Burton, James H. "An Example of Blockade Running," http://www.csarmory.org/blockade-running.htm.
16. Gray, S. Brownlow, T.W. Barrow, Francis Cogan, Park Benjamin Tucker, J.E. Hope, D.C. Walker. "Papers Relating to the Origin and Spread of the Yellow Fever in Bermuda in 1864." Great Britain Colonial Office, Committee Appointed to Inquire into the Origin and Spread of the Yellow Fever, by Which Bermuda Was Visited in 1864. House of Commons Reports and Papers, 1866, pp. 6–7.
17. *Montreal Gazette*, May 27, 1865.
18. *Hamilton (Bermuda) Royal Gazette*, February 16, 1864.
19. Pitman, *Assassination of President Lincoln*, 30.
20. *New York Times*, May 7, 1865.
21. *Fitchburg Sentinel*, Fitchburg, MA, October 30, 1880.
22. *Hamilton (Bermuda) Royal Gazette*, April 25, 1865. Note: The proprietress of Slater's Boarding House was named Catherine Slater, though advertisements in the newspapers of the time listed her as "Catharine Slater." She was a widow with four children who would later run the Victoria Hotel, located on the site of the old Slater's Boarding House and where The Emporium now sits. I have chosen to spell Ms. Slater's name as Catharine, rather than the version that newspaper readers of the time would have seen—Author.
23. *Hamilton (Bermuda) Royal Gazette*, August 24, 1852.
24. *Hamilton (Bermuda) Royal Gazette*, July 30, 1861.
25. *Hamilton (Bermuda) Royal Gazette*, March 22, 1864.
26. Letter, Kensey Johns Stewart to Jefferson Davis, December 12, 1864. NARA. Record Group 109, Chapter 7, Volume 24, pp. 64–65, as cited in Steers, *Blood on the Moon*, 53, 302.
27. Tidwell, *April '65*, 18; Tidwell, *Come Retribution*, 323.
28. Davis, Jefferson. *The Papers of Jefferson Davis*, vol. 11, September 1864–May 1865. Crist, Lynda Lasswell, Barbara J. Rozek, and Kenneth H. Williams, ed. Baton Rouge: Louisiana State University Press, 2003, pp. 57, 93, 118, 213, 214, 254, 286, 364, 376, 426.
29. *Hamilton (Bermuda) Royal Gazette*, March 15, 1864.
30. Outwards Shipping Manifests, 21 July 1863–26 July 1864, Customs Records, Bermuda Archives, Hamilton, Bermuda.
31. *Hamilton (Bermuda) Royal Gazette*, July 26, 1865.
32. *Chicago Tribune*, October 2, 1879, quoting the Washington correspondent of the

Cincinnati Gazette from September 6, 1879, www.fold3.com/image/48479022.

33. NARA. Despatches from U.S. Consuls in Havana, 1783–1906, Record Group 59, M-899, Roll 48, June 3, 1865, to December 29, 1866; Letter, from Thomas Savage, Vice-Consul General to Havana, Cuba, to C.A. Seward, Acting Assistant Secretary of State, June 21, 1865. NARA. Despatches from U.S. consuls in Havana, 1783–1906, Record Group 59, M-899, Roll 48, June 3, 1865, to December 29, 1866; Affidavit, John D. Hopkins, undated. NARA. Despatches from U.S. Consuls in Havana, 1783–1906, Record Group 59, M-899, Roll 48, June 3, 1865, to December 29, 1866; Letter, from Thomas Savage, vice-consul general to Havana, Cuba, to W.H. Seward, secretary of state, July 8, 1865. NARA. Despatches from U.S. Consuls in Havana, 1783–1906, Record Group 59, M-899, Roll 48, June 3, 1865, to December 29, 1866; Letter, John D. Belt to John D. Hopkins, July 5, 1865; NARA Despatches from U.S. Consuls in Havana, 1783–1906, Record Group 59, M-899, Roll 48, June 3, 1865, to December 29, 1866; Affidavit, Eduardo Belot, July 24, 1865; NARA. Despatches from U.S. consuls in Havana, 1783–1906, Record Group 59, M-899, Roll 48, June 3, 1865, to December 29, 1866; Letter, from Thomas Savage, vice-consul general to Havana, Cuba, to W.H. Seward, secretary of state, August 18, 1865; NARA. Despatches from U.S. consuls in Havana, 1783–1906, Record Group 59, M-899, Roll 48, June 3, 1865, to December 29, 1866; Letter, from Thomas Savage, Vice-Consul General to Havana, Cuba, to H. N. Conger, aacting secretary of state, October 16, 1865; NARA. Despatches from U.S. consuls in Havana, 1783–1906, Record Group 59, M-899, Roll 48, June 3, 1865, to December 29, 1866; Affidavit, Edward Belot, August 11, 1865; NARA. Despatches from U.S. consuls in Havana, 1783–1906, Record Group 59, M-899, Roll 48, June 3, 1865, to December 29, 1866; Affidavit, Dr. Carlos Belot, undated; NARA. Despatches from U.S. consuls in Havana, 1783–1906, Record Group 59, M-899, Roll 48, June 3, 1865, to December 29, 1866.

34. Apparently Dr. Blackburn didn't explain to Hopkins his ulterior motive of germ warfare.

35. Published letter, Rev. Stuart Robinson to H.H. Emmons. "The Infamous Perjuries of the 'Bureau of Military Justice' Exposed," June 10, 1865, p. 5. Original publisher unknown. https://ia600307.us.archive.org/17/items/cihm_63181/cihm_63181.pdf.

36. Handwritten testimony, given by Godfrey J. Hyams to Halmer H. Emmons, at Hamilton, Ontario, April 12, 1865, pp. 3–4.

Halmer H. Emmons Papers, Box 77 (January–July, 1865), April 1865, Burton Historical Collection, Detroit Public Library, Detroit, Michigan.

37. *New York Times,* May 26, 1865.

38. Waite, P.B. *The Life and Times of Confederation, 1864–1867: Politics, Newspapers, and the Union of British North America.* Toronto: University of Toronto Press, 1962, p. 80.

39. Robinson, "Infamous Perjuries," 2. This quotation was taken from Robinson's account written in June 1865, and the date was likely incorrect. The correct date was January 15, 1865, not 1864, because a previous letter from Hyams dated February 29, 1864, spoke of his penniless pregnant wife and *child*. By January 1865 Hyams would have already had at least two children. Nevertheless, Hyams' family was impoverished for the entire time they spent in Canada, from 1863 through 1865.

40. *Detroit Advertiser,* as quoted in the *New York Times,* May 21, 1865.

41. *Montreal Herald,* May 19, 1865.

42. *Detroit Advertiser,* as quoted in the *Washington (D.C.) Evening Star,* May 22, 1865.

43. *Montreal Herald,* May 26, 1865; *Morning Chronicle,* Halifax, Nova Scotia, May 29, 1865.

44. *Montreal Herald,* May 19, 1865.

45. Handwritten testimony, given by Godfrey J. Hyams, p. 9.

46. Letter, Cordial Crane to E. M. Stanton, May 30, 1865. NARA. Investigation and Trial Papers Relating to the Assassination of President Lincoln, Record Group 153, M-599, Roll 3.

47. Tidwell, *Come Retribution,* 262.

48. Edwards, William C. *The Lincoln Assassination: The Trial Transcript.* A Transcription of NARA Microfilm File M599, Reels 8 Through 16, 2012, p. 691.

49. Pitman, *Assassination of President Lincoln,* 55–57.

50. *Ibid.,* 55.

51. Handwritten testimony, given by Godfrey J. Hyams, p. 10.

52. Spear, Donald P. "The Sutler in the Union Army," *Civil War History* 16, no. 2 (June 1970): 121–138. Sutlers traveled with the troops, setting up shop near the military camps and selling mostly nonmilitary supplies. Sutlers were the forerunners of military base commissaries. Their tents and buildings also served as the social centers for the military; men gathered there in their free time to share war stories, chat, or reminisce about home. In addition, though mostly illegal, liquor was the sutlers' most popular item for sale. His job was lucrative if he was willing to risk the danger of being close to the front lines of the war.

53. Letter, from R.C.B. (otherwise anonymous) to Secretary of War E.M. Stanton, "A" 434 (JAO) 1865, 3:215–216, May 29, 1865, as catalogued in Edwards, William C. and Edward Steers, Jr., *The Lincoln Assassination: The Evidence*. Urbana: University of Illinois Press, 2009, p. 31.
54. Handwritten testimony, given by Godfrey J. Hyams, p. 12.
55. Farnham, Thomas J., and Francis P. King. "The March of the Destroyer: The New Bern Yellow Fever Epidemic of 1864," *North Carolina Historical Review* 73, no. 4 (October 1996): 474, 481.
56. Pitman, *Assassination of President Lincoln*, 57.

Chapter 10

1. Pitman, *Assassination of President Lincoln*, 30, 34; Baird, *Luke Pryor Blackburn*, 32.
2. Cleary, W.W. *Testimony of Sandford Conover, Dr. J.B. Merritt, and Richard Montgomery, Before Military Court at Washington: Respecting the Assassination of President Lincoln, and the Proofs Disproving Their Statements, and Showing Their Perjuries*. Toronto: Lovell & Gibson, 1865; reprinted at London: Forgotten Books, 2015, p. 23. https://ia800500.us.archive.org/9/items/cihm_89111/cihm_89111.pdf.
3. Pitman, *Assassination of President Lincoln*, 30.
4. Baird, *Luke Pryor Blackburn*, 25.
5. Kennedy, Sister Jean de Chantel. *Biography of a Colonial Town: Hamilton, Bermuda, 1790–1897*. Hamilton: Bermuda Bookstore, 2nd ed., 1963, p. 313.
6. *Bermuda Pocket Almanack, for the Year of Our Lord 1865: Calculated for Bermuda, and Containing Everything Necessary for an Almanack*. Hamilton, Bermuda: D. M'Phee Lee, Office of the Royal Gazette, 1865, p. 20.
7. *Hamilton (Bermuda) Royal Gazette*, October 4, 1864.
8. *The Bermudian*, October 5, 1864.
9. Register of Burials, St. Michael's Cemetery, Toronto, entry #3010, 1865; now in the possession of Mount Hope Cemetery, Toronto. The "T.F." in the name of their second child represented initials for "Thomas Francis." Apparently the "Stonewall Jackson" part of his name was more important than the "Thomas Francis." The infant was buried in St. Michael's Cemetery, a Catholic site in Toronto. There the tombstone reads, "T.F. Stonewall Jackson Hyams" (St. Michael's Cemetery, Tombstone Inscriptions. Toronto: Ontario Genealogical Society, Toronto Branch, 1998, p. 13). The Hyams' third child, named Henry Michael Hyams, was born in Detroit on February 22, 1865, and another, named Joseph Godfrey Hyams, was born in South Carolina in about 1867. Mystery surrounds the reason that Hyams, a nominal Jew, would bury his son in a Roman Catholic cemetery. The tombstone also bears the names of the stonemasons—Mulvey and Fleming—but not the names of the parents. The designations "I.H.S." and "Requiescat In Pace," both of which are also carved on the infant's tombstone, are decidedly Catholic. "I.H.S." is commonly understood to be either the first three letters of Jesus' name—"iota eta sigma," or "Iesus Hominum Salvator," Latin for "Jesus, Saviour of men." "Requiescat In Pace" means "Rest in Peace," again in Latin as the Catholic church might choose. These certainly are not designations a typical Jewish family would use. Legend has it that the Catholic church allowed Hyams to bury his son in the St. Michael's Cemetery for a fee of only one dollar. Maybe one or both of the stonemasons, Daniel Mulvey and Alexander Fleming, were friends who donated their skills and supplies. Perhaps it was even an advertisement in return for a free headstone. One of these stonemasons' two shops was only two blocks from Godfrey Hyams and Hugh Shield's bootmaking store at 35 Queen Street West in Toronto, and Daniel Mulvey lived just one block from Hyams and Shield's business. Dates of birth for the Hyams children are inconsistent across different references, as birth records in the 1860s were irregular at best. Birth records in Ontario, Canada, weren't reliably kept until 1869. Birth records in the United States were also collected haphazardly during this era.
10. *Montreal Herald*, May 26, 1865.
11. *Hamilton (Bermuda) Royal Gazette*, April 25, 1865.
12. Personal communication, Peter Frith, Museums Manager, Confederate Museum, Globe Hotel, Bermuda National Trust Collection, St. Georges, Bermuda, July 17, 2014.
13. Nathaniel Jackson, the St. Georges nuisance inspector, rented rooms in a building on the upper floor of a building on Queen Street for the Corporation of St. Georges, and the going rate was 4–10 shillings per week (Nathaniel Jackson's Pocket Notebook, St. Georges Corporation, Miscellaneous Documents, Hamilton, Bermuda: Bermuda Archives, 1865, unpaginated).
14. Edward Cork Swan (sometimes incorrectly referred to as Edward "Coke" Swan) was born in Saint Mary, Lichfield, Stafford, England, on August 26, 1836. He emigrated to Bermuda

some time before 1860, the year he married Matilda Beresford Butterfield in St. Georges Parish on December 9 (St. Georges Parish Records, Hamilton, Bermuda: Bermuda Archives, unpaginated).

15. *Chicago Tribune*, September 3, 1879.

16. *The St. Johns Public Ledger and Newfoundland General Advertiser*, June 23, 1865.

17. Bouquet, Henry. *The Papers of Col. Henry Bouquet*, Series 21634. Stevens, Sylvester K., and Donald H. Kent, ed. Northwestern Pennsylvania Historical Series. Harrisburg: Pennsylvania Historical Commission, 1940, pp. 161 and 215.

18. *Toronto Leader*, cited in *St. John's Public Ledger and Newfoundland General Advertiser*, June 23, 1865.

19. Letter, Charles M. Allen, U.S. consul to Bermuda, April 14, 1865. In Edwards and Steers, *Lincoln Assassination: The Evidence*, 6.

20. *Washington (PA) Daily Evening Reporter*, October 28, 1880.

21. Hayward, Walter Brownell. *Bermuda Past and Present: A Descriptive and Historical Account of the Somers Islands.* New York: Dodd, 1911, p. 98.

22. *Ibid.*, 99.

23. St. Georges Corporation Minutes, Book 3, 1834–1870. Hamilton, Bermuda: Bermuda Archives, Entry for April 12, 1865, unpaginated.

24. St. Georges Corporation Minutes, Book 3, 1834–1870. Hamilton, Bermuda: Bermuda Archives: Entry for April 13, 1865, entitled, "Description of articles found in three boxes inspected on Nonsuch Island, 13th April 1865," unpaginated.

25. St. Georges Corporation Minutes, Book 3, 1834–1870. Hamilton, Bermuda: Bermuda Archives, Ledger Entry for June 3, 1865, unpaginated.

26. Letter, S. Brownlow Gray to James Thies, St. Georges Corporation Minutes, Book 3, 1834–1870. Hamilton, Bermuda: Bermuda Archives, Entry for April 17, 1865, unpaginated.

27. St. Georges Corporation, Miscellaneous Documents, 1865, Hamilton, Bermuda: Bermuda Archives

28. Letter (transcribed), Charles M. Allen, U.S. consul to Bermuda, to William H. Seward, secretary of state, April 14, 1865. In Edwards and Steers, *Lincoln Assassination: The Evidence*, 7.

29. Letter (transcribed), Charles M. Allen, U.S. consul to Bermuda, to William H. Seward, secretary of state, April 14, 1865, *Bermuda Historical Quarterly* 19, no. 1 (1962), 25–27.

30. *St. Georges Gaol Journal*, 1864–1867.

Hamilton, Bermuda: Bermuda Archives, p. 216.

31. Wiche, *Dispatches from Bermuda*, 181–182.

32. *Chicago Tribune*, September 3, 1879.

33. Frederic was also spelled "Frederick" in some reports, and Buckstaff was alternately spelled "Buxtorf" or "Buckstorf."

34. *Montreal Herald and Daily Commercial Gazette*, May 18, 1865, quoting the *Bermuda Advocate*.

35. *Ibid.*

36. *Hamilton (Bermuda) Royal Gazette*, June 13, 1865, quoting the *New York Herald*, June 6, 1865.

37. The ship was otherwise spelled *Celeste*, and also known as the *Maria Celeste* or the *Marie Celestia*. The correct version used by archaeologists today is *Mary Celestia*; the newspapers of 1864 also called it the *Mary Celestia*. This ship is not to be confused with the "ghost" ship *Mary Celeste*, a 107-foot, 282-ton brigantine sailing ship that was found abandoned off the coast of Portugal near the Azores in December 1872. The *Mary Celestia* was a fast, 225-foot, iron-hulled, side-paddle-wheel steamer weighing 207 tons used for blockade-running and owned by William and James Crenshaw from Richmond, Virginia. It had been constructed in Liverpool, England, by the William C. Miller and Sons Shipyards, launched in February 1864, and completed in May 1864 as the final boilers and engines were installed. It could achieve a speed of 15 knots, delivering war supplies to the Confederacy, most often at the port in Wilmington.

38. McNeil, Jim. *Masters of the Shoals: Tales of the Cape Fear Pilots Who Ran the Union Blockade.* Cambridge, MA: Da Capo, Perseus, 2003. p. 55–56; Delgado, James P. "Letter from Bermuda: Secrets of a Civil War Shipwreck," *Archaeology* 64, no. 6 (November/December 2011).

39. Eastman, Margaret Middleton Rivers. *Hidden History of Civil War Charleston.* Charleston, SC: History, 2012, p. 78, citing Dave Horner, *The Blockade-Runners: True Tales of Running the Yankee Blockade of the Confederate Coast.* New York: Dodd, Mead, 1968, p. 109.

40. In some reports he is incorrectly called Joseph "Headden" Rainey.

41. *St. Georges Gaol Journal*, 1864–1867. Hamilton, Bermuda: Bermuda Archives, p. 216.

42. *Hamilton (Bermuda) Royal Gazette*, May 2, 1865.

43. *St. Georges Gaol Journal*, 1864–1867. Hamilton, Bermuda: Bermuda Archives, p. 218.

44. *Ibid.*, January 1863–October 1865, p. 358.
45. *Ibid.*, pp. 349–350.
46. Bermuda Assize Records, Easter 1865 Term. Hamilton, Bermuda: Bermuda Archives.
47. *Hamilton (Bermuda) Royal Gazette,* May 9, 1865, May 30, 1865.
48. Hutchinson, William Nelson. *Standing Orders Issued to the Two Battalions, XXth Regiment, at Bermuda, in 1842.* London: W. Clowes & Sons, 1845, p. 93.
49. *Hamilton Gaol Journal,* January 1863–October 1865. Hamilton, Bermuda: Bermuda Archives, pp. 343, 352.
50. *Ibid.*, p. 270.
51. *Hamilton (Bermuda) Royal Gazette,* May 23, 1865.
52. United States Department of State. Executive Documents Printed by Order of the House of Representatives, during the First Session of the Thirty-Ninth Congress, 1865–1866. Part 2. Papers Relating to Foreign Affairs. Correspondence: Great Britain. Diplomatic Correspondence, pp. 187–189. Washington, D.C.: U.S. Government Printing Office, 1866.
53. *St. Georges Gaol Journal,* 1864–1867, p. 284.

Chapter 11

1. Wilkinson, Henry Campbell. *Bermuda from Sail to Steam: A History of the Island from 1784–1901.* London: Oxford University Press, 1973, pp. 721–723.
2. Steers, *Blood on the Moon,* 50.
3. *New York Times,* May 19, 1865.
4. Edwards and Steers, *Lincoln Assassination: The Evidence,* 468–470.
5. Letter, H.H. Emmons to Joseph Holt, April 28, 1865, in Edwards, *The Lincoln Assassination,* 468–470.
6. "The Yellow Fever Plot." Kynett, H.H., S.V. Butler, and D.G. Brinton, ed. *Medical and Surgical Reporter* 12 (35), no. 432 (June 10, 1865), 565–567. Philadelphia: Alfred Martien, 1865.
7. *New York Times,* May 24, 1865, quoting the *Toronto Globe,* May 22, 1865.
8. *New York Evening Post,* quoted in the *Hamilton (Bermuda) Royal Gazette,* May 30, 1865.
9. Kynett, "The Yellow Fever Plot," 567.
10. *New York Times,* May 26, 1865.
11. *Montreal Herald,* May 26, 1865.
12. *Ibid.*, May 27, 1865.
13. *New York Times,* May 26, 1865.
14. *Montreal Herald,* May 27, 1865.
15. Letter, James Cockburn to D. Godley, June 1, 1865. *Correspondence Relating to the Fenian Invasion: And the Rebellion of the Southern States.* Ottawa: Hunter, Rose, 1869, pp. 112–113.
16. *London Times,* June 7, 1865.
17. Letter, David Thurston to Halmer H. Emmons, May (exact date unspecified), 1865. H.H. Emmons Papers, Box 77 (January–July). Burton Historical Collection, Detroit Public Library, Detroit, Michigan.
18. Letter, Edward Cardwell to Governor Viscount Monck, July 22, 1865. *Correspondence Relating to the Fenian Invasion; And the Rebellion of the Southern States.* Ottawa: Hunter, Rose & Company, 1869, p. 112.
19. *Alton (IL) Telegraph,* September 11, 1879, citing the *Toronto Globe.*
20. *New York Times,* May 29, 1865.
21. *Philadelphia Inquirer,* August 4, 1865.
22. Letter, J. Michel to Edward Cardwell, October 27, 1865. *Correspondence Relating to the Fenian Invasion: And the Rebellion of the Southern States.* Ottawa: Hunter, Rose, 1869, p. 113.
23. Munroe, James Phinney. *Adventures of an Army Nurse in Two Wars, Edited from the Diary and Correspondence of Mary Phinney, Baroness von Olnhausen.* Boston: Little, Brown, 1904, p. 150.
24. *Hamilton (Bermuda) Royal Gazette,* June 13, 1865.
25. Pitman, *Assassination of President Lincoln,* 211; *Toronto Globe,* as quoted in the *New York Times,* May 7, 1865.
26. Earlier and later family members used the spelling "McCulloch."
27. Singer, Jane. *The Confederate Dirty War: Arson, Bombings, Assassination and Plots for Chemical and Germ Attacks on the Union.* Jefferson, NC: McFarland, 2005, pp. 98–117, 160–162.
28. Hebert, Alsace. "Civil War Terrorism, The Fiend in Gray," https://www.stormfront.org/forum/t105395/.
29. *New York Times,* April 29, 1865, quoting the *Toronto Globe,* April 27, 1865.
30. *St. John's Public Ledger and Newfoundland General Advertiser,* June 23, 1865.
31. Taylor, Thomas E. *Running the Blockade: A Personal Narrative of Adventures, Risks, and Escapes During the American Civil War.* London: John Murray, 1896, pp. 129–130.

Chapter 12

1. Pitman, *Assassination of President Lincoln,* 17.
2. *Ibid.*, 18–19.
3. *Ibid.*, 17. Note again that charging papers had Cleary's middle initial incorrect; it was "W," not "C."

4. John Surratt was tried in 1867, and the jury couldn't come to a verdict—eight jurors voted "not guilty;" four voted "guilty."
 5. Pitman, *Assassination of President Lincoln*, title page.
 6. Letter, D. Thurston, United States consul to Toronto, to W.H. Seward, secretary of state, April 7, 1865. NARA. Despatches from U.S. consuls in Toronto, 1864–1906. Record Group 59, T-491, January 15, 1864–December 29, 1866, Roll 1.
 7. Baird, *Luke Pryor Blackburn*, 34.
 8. Pitman, *Assassination of President Lincoln*, 55.
 9. Letter, Samuel Lewis to H.H. Emmons (dictated to and handwritten by John A. Posey), March 3, 1865. H.H. Emmons Papers, Box 77 (January–July). Burton Historical Collection, Detroit Public Library, Detroit, Michigan.
 10. *Toronto Directory*, J.L. Mitchell, 1866, p. 195.
 11. United States Census, 1860, http://interactive.ancestry.com.
 12. Miscellaneous papers. H.H. Emmons Papers, Box 77 (January–July), 1865. Burton Historical Collection, Detroit Public Library, Detroit, Michigan.
 13. Letter, George A. Gurnett to H.H. Emmons, March 27, 1865. H.H. Emmons Papers, Box 77 (January–July), March 1865. Burton Historical Collection, Detroit Public Library, Detroit, Michigan.
 14. Letter, Lewis to Emmons, March 3, 1865.
 15. Letter, Samuel Lewis to H.H. Emmons (dictated to, and handwritten by, John A. Posey), March 11, 1865. H.H. Emmons Papers, Box 77 (January–July), Burton Historical Collection, Detroit Public Library, Detroit Michigan.
 16. Miscellaneous Papers. H.H. Emmons Papers, Box 77 (January–July), 1865. Burton Historical Collection, Detroit Public Library, Detroit, Michigan.
 17. Letter, John A. Posey to H.H. Emmons, May 1, 1865. H.H. Emmons Papers, Box 77 (January–July). Burton Historical Collection, Detroit Public Library, Detroit, Michigan.
 18. Miscellaneous Papers. H.H. Emmons Papers, Box 77 (January–July), 1865. Burton Historical Collection, Detroit Public Library, Detroit, Michigan.
 19. Letter, Godfrey J. Hyams to H.H. Emmons, May 1, 1865. H.H. Emmons Papers, Box 77 (January–July). Burton Historical Collection, Detroit Public Library, Detroit, Michigan.
 20. Letter, John A. Posey to H.H. Emmons, June 19, 1865. H.H. Emmons Papers, Box 77 (January–July). Burton Historical Collection, Detroit Public Library, Detroit, Michigan.
 21. Letter, Samuel Lewis to H.H. Emmons, July 1, 1865. H.H. Emmons Papers, Box 77 (January–July). Burton Historical Collection, Detroit Public Library, Detroit, Michigan.
 22. Letter, John A. Posey to H.H. Emmons, January 23, 1865. H.H. Emmons Papers, Box 80 (January–June). Burton Historical Collection, Detroit Public Library, Detroit, Michigan.
 23. Letter, Dr. E.M. Clark to H.H. Emmons, April 15, 1865. H.H. Emmons Papers, Box 77 (January–July). Burton Historical Collection, Detroit Public Library, Detroit, Michigan.
 24. Mayers, *Dixie and the Dominion*, 135.
 25. Farnham, Thomas J., and Francis P. King. "The March of the Destroyer: The New Bern Yellow Fever Epidemic of 1864," *North Carolina Historical Review* 73, no. 4 (October 1996), 435–483.
 26. Handwritten testimony, given by Godfrey J. Hyams to Halmer H. Emmons, at Hamilton, Ontario, April 12, 1865, p.1. H.H. Emmons Papers, Box 77 (January–July, 1865). Burton Historical Collection, Detroit Public Library, Detroit, Michigan.
 27. Letter, Halmer H. Emmons to James Speed, April 22, 1865. H.H. Emmons Papers, Box 77 (January–July). Burton Historical Collection, Detroit Public Library, Detroit, Michigan.
 28. Letter, Alfred Russell to James Speed, April 24, 1865. NARA, catalog.archives.gov/id/6782974.
 29. Edwards and Steers, *Lincoln Assassination: The Evidence*, 1124.
 30. Telegram, Halmer H. Emmons and Alfred Russell to James Speed, May 19, 1865. H.H. Emmons Papers, Box 77 (January–July). Burton Historical Collection, Detroit Public Library, Detroit, Michigan.
 31. "Legal Services Paid by State Department and Duties of Examiner of Claims, Message from the President of the United States in Answer to A Resolution of the House of the 11th Ultimo, relative to amounts paid by the State Department since 1860 for legal services and the duties of the Examiner of Claims." 40th Congress, 2nd Session, House of Representatives, Ex. Doc. No. 221, http://www.justice.gov/jmd/ls/legislative_histories/p141-97/hdoc-221-1868.pdf.
 32. Draft of Letter and Detailed Expense Report, Halmer H. Emmons to George E. Baker, June 16, 1865. H.H. Emmons Papers, Box 77, January–July. Burton Historical Collection, Detroit Public Library, Detroit, Michigan.
 33. Letter from the secretary of state in

reply to resolution of December 20, 1867, asking for information in relation to the amounts paid for publishing United States laws and for counsel fees since March 4, 1861, pp. 1–2. In Congressional Series of United States Documents, United States Congressional Serial Set, Volume 1316, Letter from the Secretary of State, 40th Congress, 2nd Session, Senate, Ex. Doc. No. 17, p. 148.

34. Receipt from Godfrey Hyams to Halmer H. Emmons, April 13, 1865. H.H. Emmons Papers, Box 77, January–July. Burton Historical Collection, Detroit Public Library, Detroit, Michigan.

35. Telegram, James Speed to Halmer H. Emmons, April 21, 1865. H.H. Emmons Papers, Box 77 (January–July). Burton Historical Collection, Detroit Public Library, Detroit, Michigan.

36. Letter, James Speed to Halmer H. Emmons, April 21, 1865. H.H. Emmons Papers, Box 77 (January–July). Burton Historical Collection, Detroit Public Library, Detroit, Michigan.

37. Telegram, Godfrey Hyams to Halmer H. Emmons, April 21, 1865. H.H. Emmons Papers, Box 77 (January–July). Burton Historical Collection, Detroit Public Library, Detroit, Michigan.

38. Letter, Godfrey Hyams to Halmer H. Emmons, May 6, 1865. H.H. Emmons Papers, Box 77 (January–July). Burton Historical Collection, Detroit Public Library, Detroit, Michigan.

39. Note, David Thurston to Alfred Russell, May 20, 1865. H.H. Emmons Papers, Box 77 (January–July). Burton Historical Collection, Detroit Public Library, Detroit, Michigan.

40. Note, David Thurston to Alfred Russell, May 20, 1865. H.H. Emmons Papers, Box 77 (January–July). Burton Historical Collection, Detroit Public Library, Detroit, Michigan.

41. Note, Alfred Russell to Halmer H. Emmons, May 20, 1865. H.H. Emmons Papers, Box 77 (January–July). Burton Historical Collection, Detroit Public Library, Detroit, Michigan.

42. Telegram, L.C. Baker to Halmer H. Emmons, June 15, 1865. H.H. Emmons Papers, Box 77 (January–July). Burton Historical Collection, Detroit Public Library, Detroit, Michigan.

43. Draft of Letter and Detailed Expense Report, Halmer H. Emmons to George E. Baker, June 16, 1865. H.H. Emmons Papers, Box 77 (January–July). Burton Historical Collection, Detroit Public Library, Detroit, Michigan.

44. Letter, Godfrey Hyams to Halmer H. Emmons, May 30, 1865. H.H. Emmons Papers, Box 77 (January–July). Burton Historical Collection, Detroit Public Library, Detroit, Michigan.

45. "Appropriation for Secret Service, Abstract of Expenditures, Quarter Ending June 30, 1865," by John Potts, disbursing clerk for the War Department. NARA. Secret Service Account Files, Record Group 110, Records of the Provost Marshal General's Bureau (Civil War), 1861–1907, Entry #95, Accounts of Secret Service Agents, 1861–1870, National Archives Identifier 4478129, NM-65 95, Box #5, January–September 1865.

46. Payment Envelopes, War Department. NARA. Secret Service Account Files, Record Group 110, Records of the Provost Marshal General's Bureau (Civil War), 1861–1907, Entry #95, Accounts of Secret Service Agents, 1861–1870, National Archives Identifier 4478129, NM-65 95, Box #5, January–September 1865.

47. Payment Envelope for Dr. J.B. Merritt, War Department, July 7, 1865. NARA. Secret Service Account Files, Record Group 110, Records of the Provost Marshal General's Bureau (Civil War), 1861–1907, Entry #95, Accounts of Secret Service Agents, 1861–1870, National Archives Identifier 4478129, NM-65 95, Box #5, January–September 1865.

48. Entry for Letter #437 from Hyams, G.J., in Letters to Judge Advocate Col. H.L. Burnett; Register of Letters Received; Military Commission Record Book, p. 85. NARA. Investigation and Trial Papers Relating to the Assassination of President Lincoln, Record Group 153, M-599, Roll 3.

49. Letter, United States District Attorney Alfred Russell to Brig. Gen. Joseph Holt, May 11, 1865, and accompanying notarized affidavit from Godfrey J. Hyams. NARA. Investigation and Trial Papers Relating to the Assassination of President Lincoln, Record Group 153, M-599, Roll 3.

50. War Department note from C.A. Dunn (or Dana), payment envelope, and receipt from Godfrey J. Hyams. NARA. Secret Service Account Files, Record Group 110, Records of the Provost Marshal General's Bureau (Civil War), 1861–1907, Entry #95, Accounts of Secret Service Agents, 1861–1870, National Archives Identifier 4478129, NM-65 95, Box #5, January–September 1865.

51. Letter, Godfrey Hyams to Halmer H. Emmons, June 26, 1865. H.H. Emmons Papers, Box 77 (January–July). Burton Historical Collection, Detroit Public Library, Detroit, Michigan.

52. *Halifax (Nova Scotia) Morning Chronicle*, June 10, 1865; Indictment, United States District Court, Boston, Massachusetts. *The United States versus Bryan O'Brien et al.*, June

Term, June 27, 1865; *Halifax (Nova Scotia) Morning Chronicle*, June 13, 1865; *Boston Evening Transcript*, June 13, 1865; *Boston Post*, June 13, 1865; *Daily National Republican*, Washington, D.C., June 14, 1865.

53. Indictment, *U.S. versus O'Brien*.

54. *St. John's Public Ledger and Newfoundland General Advertiser*, June 23, 1865.

55. *Halifax (Nova Scotia) Morning Chronicle*, June 16, 1865; *Boston Post*, July 4, 1865. Thanks to Joe Keefe, archives specialist, NARA at Boston, for tracking down the indictment of Bryan O'Brien and for determining that the trial was never held in September or thereafter.

56. Letter, Godfrey Hyams to Halmer H. Emmons, June 26, 1865.

57. *An American Time Capsule: Three Centuries of Broadsides and Other Printed Ephemera; Wales L. Egerton & Co.'s Ladies and Gents Dining Rooms, 1866.* Library of Congress, American Memory.

58. Disturnell, John. *Disturnell's Railway and Steamship Guide.* New York: American News Company, 1865.

59. Letter, Godfrey J. Hyams to E.M. Stanton, secretary of war, July 6, 1865. NARA. Secret Service Account Files, Record Group 110, Records of the Provost Marshal General's Bureau (Civil War), 1861-1907, Entry #95, Accounts of Secret Service Agents, 1861-1870, National Archives Identifier 4478129, NM-65 95, Box #5, January-September 1865.

60. Receipts from the United States Hotel in Boston, June 30 and July 5, 1865, signed by John A. Lawyer. NARA. Secret Service Account Files, Record Group 110, Records of the Provost Marshal General's Bureau (Civil War), 1861-1907, Entry #95, Accounts of Secret Service Agents, 1861-1870, National Archives Identifier 4478129, NM-65 95, Box #5, January-September 1865.

61. Note from Judge Advocate General Joseph Holt to the Bureau of Military Justice, July 6, 1865. NARA. Secret Service Account Files, Record Group 110, Records of the Provost Marshal General's Bureau (Civil War), 1861-1907, Entry #95, Accounts of Secret Service Agents, 1861-1870, National Archives Identifier 4478129, NM-65 95, Box #5, January-September 1865.

62. Note from Edwin M. Stanton to Judge Advocate General Joseph Holt, July 8, 1865. NARA. Secret Service Account Files, Record Group 110, Records of the Provost Marshal General's Bureau (Civil War), 1861-1907, Entry #95, Accounts of Secret Service Agents, 1861-1870, National Archives Identifier 4478129, NM-65 95, Box #5, January-September 1865.

63. Note from Judge Advocate General Joseph Holt to the Bureau of Military Justice, July 8, 1865. NARA. Secret Service Account Files, Record Group 110, Records of the Provost Marshal General's Bureau (Civil War), 1861-1907, Entry #95, Accounts of Secret Service Agents, 1861-1870, National Archives Identifier 4478129, NM-65 95, Box #5, January-September 1865.

64. Payment envelope from the War Department to Godfrey J. Hyams, July 8, 1865; Appropriation documents to Godfrey J. Hyams from the "Army Contingencies"; Ledger page listing $1200 payment to Godfrey J. Hyams, approved by John Potts, Disbursing Clerk for the War Department; receipt signed by Godfrey J. Hyams for the $1200. NARA. Secret Service Account Files, Record Group 110, Records of the Provost Marshal General's Bureau (Civil War), 1861-1907, Entry #95, Accounts of Secret Service Agents, 1861-1870, National Archives Identifier 4478129, NM-65 95, Box #5, January-September 1865.

65. A payment of $1,200 in 1865 would be equivalent to $18,000-36,000 in today's money.

Chapter 13

1. Pitman, *Assassination of President Lincoln*, 45.

2. *Ibid.*, 29 and 377.

3. *Ibid.*, 38.

4. *Ibid.*, 66.

5. *Ibid.*, 39.

6. Cumming, Carman. *Devil's Game: The Civil War Intrigues of Charles A. Dunham.* Urbana: University of Illinois Press, 2004, p. 25.

7. Vanderlinden, Wolf. "On the Trail of Tumblety?," *Ripper Notes: Suspects and Witnesses*, no. 23 (July 2005). Madison, Wisconsin: Inklings, p. 39.

8. Letter, Kensey Johns Stewart to Jefferson Davis, December 12, 1864. NARA. Record Group 109, Chapter 7, Volume 24, pp. 64-65. As cited in Steers, *Blood on the Moon*, 52-54, 302.

9. Pitman, *Assassination of President Lincoln*, 375-6.

10. *Ibid.*, 47.

11. *ORA*. Series 2, Volume 8, Serial 121, p. 855.

12. Pitman, *Assassination of President Lincoln*, 380.

13. Civil War era maps refer to "Fortress" Monroe alternately as "Fort" Monroe. I have arbitrarily chosen to use the designation "Fortress" Monroe in this book. The modern-day designation is "Fort" Monroe.

14. *The Country Gentleman* 25 (January 1, 1865-July 1, 1865), 340 (May 25, 1865), Albany,

New York: Luther Tucker & Son; List of persons on board steamship *W.P. Clyde*, https://www.fold3.com/image/301568151; Letter, George E. Cooper to adjutant-general, U.S. Army, May 9, 1866. *ORA*, Correspondence, Etc.—Union and Confederate. Prisoners of War and State, Etc. Series 2, Volume 8, Serial 121, p. 908; Abbott, John Stevens Cabot. *The History of the Civil War in America: Comprising a Full and Impartial Account of the Origin and Progress of the Rebellion, of the Various Naval and Military Engagements, of the Heroic Deeds Performed by Armies and Individuals, and of Touching Scenes in the Field, the Camp, the Hospital, and the Cabin.* Springfield, MA: Gurdon Bill, 1866, vol. 2, p. 605.

15. Craven, John J. *Prison Life of Jefferson Davis, Embracing Details and Incidents in His Captivity, Particulars Concerning His Health and Habits, Together with Many Conversations on Topics of Great Public Interest.* New York and London: Carleton, 1866, p. 35.

16. *Ibid.*, 36–37.

17. Letter, Brevet Major General Nelson A. Miles to Assistant Adjutant General E.D. Townsend, July 20, 1865. NARA. Letters Received by the Office of the Adjutant General (Main Series), 1861–1870, Record Group 94, M-619B, Roll 332, 1865, File 1401 A (Part 1).

18. Craven, *Prison Life*, 183.

19. *Ibid.*, 189.

20. Letter, Secretary of War Edwin M. Stanton to Brevet Major General Nelson A. Miles, July 22, 1865. NARA. Letters Received by the Office of the Adjutant General (Main Series), 1861–1870, Record Group 94, M-619B, Roll 332, 1865, File 1401 A (Part 1).

21. Letter, George E. Cooper to the Surgeon General, January 21, 1866, https://www.fold3.com/image/301085726.

22. Letter, George E. Cooper to the Surgeon General, January 21, 1866, https://www.fold3.com/image/301085726 and https://www.fold3.com/image/301085733.

23. A traveler in the 1860s paid $2–3/day for food. The conversion factor for the value of a dollar in the 1860s, compared to now, is about 1:15 to 1:30.

24. Townsend, E.D., assistant adjutant general. Summary of the health of Jefferson Davis, May 30, 1866. NARA. Letters Received by the Office of the Adjutant General (Main Series), 1861–1870, Record Group 94, M-619B, Roll 332, 1865, File 1401 A (Part 1).

25. Telegram, Varina Davis to President Andrew Johnson, marked "Private," April 25, 1866. NARA. Letters Received by the Office of the Adjutant General (Main Series), 1861–1870, Record Group 94, M-619B, Roll 332, 1865, File 1401 A (Part 1).

26. Letter, Varina Davis to President Andrew Johnson, undated. NARA. Letters Received by the Office of the Adjutant General (Main Series), 1861–1870, Record Group 94, M-619B, Roll 332, 1865, File 1401 A (Part 1).

27. Parole of Honor, Varina Davis, May 3, 1866. NARA. Letters Received by the Office of the Adjutant General (Main Series), 1861–1870, Record Group 94, M-619B, Roll 332, 1865, File 1401 A (Part 1).

28. Townsend, Summary of the health of Jefferson Davis.

29. Letter, George E. Cooper to adjutant-general, U.S. Army, May 9, 1866. *ORA*, Correspondence, Etc.—Union and Confederate. Prisoners of War and State, Etc. Series 2, Volume 8, Serial 121, p. 908.

30. Connally, C. Ellen. "The Use of the Fourteenth Amendment by Salmon P. Chase in the Trial of Jefferson Davis." *Akron Law Review* 42 (2009), 1170–1171.

31. Not to be confused with John Cox Underwood, the 21st lieutenant governor of Kentucky and a candidate against Luke Pryor Blackburn for governor of Kentucky in 1879.

32. Connally, "Use of the Fourteenth Amendment," 1180.

33. *Ibid.*, 1177.

34. *Ibid.*

35. Thompson, James W. "The Incredible Plot of Judge Advocate General Joseph Holt." Confederate Historical Association of Belgium. Unpaginated, http://chab-belgium.com/pdf/english/Judge%20Holt.pdf.

36. Mayers, *Dixie and the Dominion*, 3.

37. Thuersam, Bernhard. "Wilmington to Canada: Blockade Runners and Secret Agents." *Cape Fear Historical Institute Papers*, Cape Fear Historical Institute, 2006, unpaginated, http://www.cfhi.net/WilmingtonsWartimeCanadianConnection.php; Herzfeld, Matt. "John Wilkes Booth Lived Here: How Montreal Fell for the Confederacy," *McGill Daily*, January 26, 2012, unpaginated, http://www.mcgilldaily.com/2012/01/john-wilkes-booth-lived-here/.

38. *Montreal Gazette*, June 29, 1968.

39. Jones, John William. *Davis Memorial Volume; or Our Dead President, Jefferson Davis, and the Tribute to His Memory.* Richmond: B.F. Johnson, 1889, p. 451.

40. Connally, "The Use of the Fourteenth Amendment," 1199.

Chapter 14

1. Boyko, *Blood and Daring*, 227.

2. Mayers, *Dixie and the Dominion*, 170, 189, 202.

3. *New York Tribune*, May 22, 1865.

4. Memorial from S.J. Gholson, John M. Simonton, and Benjamin G. Humphreys to President of the United States, https://www.fold3.com/image/22586245; https://www.fold3.com/image/22586254; https://www.fold3.com/image/22586258.

5. Letter, Jacob Thompson to Captain William Delay, August 11, 1866. In: *Letters to and from Jacob Thompson*, P.L. Rainwater, ed. *Journal of Southern History* 6, no. 1 (February 1940), 105.

6. "Jacob Thompson, Congressman, Secretary of the Interior, Pirate of the Great "Lakes," http://www.fulkerson.org/thompson.html.

7. Kinchen, *Confederate Operations*, 185.

8. Easley, Elbert L. "Clay, Clement Claiborne." *Encyclopedia of Alabama*, Alabama Humanities Foundation, 2016, unpaginated, http://www.encyclopediaofalabama.org/article/h-2951.

9. Mayers, *Dixie and the Dominion*, 201.

10. *Hamilton (Bermuda) Royal Gazette*, January 24, 1865.

11. Mayers, *Dixie and the Dominion*, 201.

12. *Ibid.*, 202.

13. Johnson, Andrew. Presidential Proclamation, May 2, 1865, https://www.fold3.com/image/301049955.

14. General Orders No. 164, by order of Andrew Johnson, president of the United States. War Department, Adjutant General's Office, November 24, 1865, declared and signed by E.D. Townsend, assistant adjutant general, https://www.fold3.com/image/301049946.

15. Note from Judge Advocate General J. Holt to Secretary of War E.M. Stanton, December 6, 1865. *ORA. Correspondence, etc.—Union and Confederate. Prisoners of War and State, Etc.* Series 2, Volume 8, Serial 121, p. 857.

16. *Ibid.*, 856.

17. Pitman, *Assassination of President Lincoln*, 45–46.

18. Note from Judge Advocate General J. Holt to Secretary of War E.M. Stanton, December 6, 1865. *ORA. Correspondence, etc.—Union and Confederate. Prisoners of War and State, etc.* Series 2, Volume 8, Serial 121, p. 860.

19. *Ibid.*, 861.

20. Letter, E.D. Townsend to N.A. Miles, April 17, 1866. In McPherson, Edward. *A Handbook of Politics for 1868*. Washington: Philp [sic] & Solomons, 1868. Volume 23, Orders and Proclamations, p. 8.

21. Beymer, Willim Gilmore. "Mrs. Greenhow," *Harper's Monthly*. New York and London: Harper & Brothers, volume 124, December 1911–May 1912, pp. 563–576.

22. Foreman, Amanda. *A World on Fire: Britain's Crucial Role in the American Civil War*. New York: Random House, 2012, pp. 684–686.

23. Letter, J. Holt to E.M. Stanton, December 29, 1865, https://www.fold3.com/image/301045917; https://www.fold3.com/image/301045935.

24. *Ibid.*, https://www.fold3.com/image/301045935.

25. *Ibid.*, https://www.fold3.com/image/301045942.

26. *Ibid.*, https://www.fold3.com/image/301045962.

27. *Ibid.*, https://www.fold3.com/image/301045965; https://www.fold3.com/image/301045968.

28. *Ibid.*, https://www.fold3.com/image/301045975; https://www.fold3.com/image/301045977.

29. Letter, James P. Holcombe to the president of the United States, Andrew Johnson, undated (covering paper dated June 28, 1865), https://www.fold3.com/image/23094457.

30. *Ibid.*, https://www.fold3.com/image/23094459.

31. *Ibid.*, https://www.fold3.com/image/23094461.

32. *Philadelphia Inquirer*, August 4, 1865.

33. Berger Stephen A., and Itzhak Shapira. "Hemorrhagic Fevers and Bioterror." *Israel Medical Association Journal* 4 (July 2002), 513–519.

Chapter 15

1. Hyams, Godfrey. Confederate Amnesty Papers, https://www.fold3.com/image/22874542; https://www.fold3.com/image/22874545; https://www.fold3.com/image/22874550; https://www.fold3.com/image/22874552; https://www.fold3.com/image/22874556; https://www.fold3.com/image/22874558.

2. Letter, Rev. Stuart Robinson to Hon. Mr. Emmons. "The Infamous Perjuries of the 'Bureau of Military Justice' Exposed," pp. 1–2.

3. Simkins, Francis Butler, and Robert Hilliard Woody. *South Carolina During Reconstruction*. Chapel Hill: University of North Carolina Press, 1932.

4. Personal communication, Nicolas Butler, PhD, historian, Charleston County Public Library, Charleston, South Carolina, October 21, 2014.

5. *Charleston City Directory*, 1867–1868. Charleston, South Carolina: Jno. Orrin Lea, p. 107.

6. Personal communication, Molly French, librarian and archivist, South Carolina Room, Charleston County Public Library, Charleston, October 22, 2014.

7. South Carolina Census, 1869, Charleston Ward 1. Charleston, South Carolina: South Carolina Room, Charleston County Public Library, p. 62.
8. Militia Enrollments of 1869, Ward 1, City of Charleston, Charleston County, S192021. Charleston, South Carolina: South Carolina Archives and History, Charleston County Public Library. vol. 5. p. 12, http://www.archives index.sc.gov.
9. Militia Enrollments, 1869, Military Department Adjutant and Inspector General. Charleston, South Carolina: South Carolina Archives Series Description, 1869, Biographical/Historical Note, http://www.archivesindex.sc.gov.
10. *Charleston (SC) Daily News*, December 1, 1866, January 4, 1867.
11. Ibid., July 18, 1867.
12. South Carolina Court Archives, Columbia, Indictment #1901, 1869. Other records are missing.
13. *Charleston City Directory*, 1869–70, 1872–1873. Charleston, South Carolina: Walker, Evans, & Cogswell.
14. South Carolina Court Archives, Columbia, Indictment #1709, L10153, 174E06, Box 20.
15. *Charleston (SC) Daily News*, July 21, 1868.
16. Letter, Godfrey Hyams to E.D. Townsend, December 26, 1862, https://www.fold3.com/image/300098761; Letter, Godfrey Hyams to Alfred Russell, January 19, 1866, https://www.fold3.com/image/22874552; Letters from Godfrey Hyams. H.H. Emmons Papers, Box 77 (January–July), 1865. Burton Historical Collection, Detroit Public Library, Detroit, Michigan.
17. *Charleston (SC) Daily News*, August 12, 1870; February 12, 1873; and February 15, 1873.
18. Ibid., June 18, 1870, and September 30, 1870.
19. King, Susan L. *History and Records of the Charleston Orphan House*, vol. 2, 1860–1899; *South Carolina Magazine of Ancestral Research (SCMAR)*, 1994, Columbia, pp. 1–5, 60, and Microfilm COH/IA/4, South Carolina Room, Charleston County Public Library, Charleston, South Carolina; Hebrew Orphan Society Papers, Folder #1057, Charleston, South Carolina: Special Collections, Addlestone Library, College of Charleston. If this Bridget Sheehan was Hyams' wife, then their first child would have been born when she was about 13 years old—unusual, but possible. During the 1860s, the age of consent in the United States varied from 10 to 16 (Saunders, April. "Age of Marriage in the U.S. in the 1800s." Demand Media, http://classroom.synonym.com/age-marriage-us-1800s-23174.html). In Missouri—the site of Godfrey Hyams' marriage to Bridget—the legal age for marriage in the 1800s was 21 for males and 18 for females. However, the legal age for consent was 15 for males and 12 for females. The law specifically stated that minor females 12 years of age or over could marry with a parent's consent (Revised Statutes of the State of Missouri, 1835. Revised Statutes of the State of Missouri, 1879, Volume 1, Section 3268. Constitutions of the United States and of the State of Missouri, Volume II, 1856, by Charles Henry Hardin). Indeed, during 1860 in some states 5 percent of males were underage, and 25.8 percent of females were minors (Report of Births, Marriages, Divorces and Deaths, Issue 8, Rhode Island Division of Vital Statistics, 1860, p 55). Overall, in the United States in 1860, in 12.4 percent of marriages the bride was under age 19 (Hacker, J. David, Libra Hilde, and James Holland Jones. "The Effect of the Civil War on Southern Marriage Patterns." *Journal of Southern History* 76, no. 1 (February 2010), pp. 39–70). So such a sequence for her marriage and childbearing is not impossible. Alternatively, her age reported at death simply may have been incorrect. Another Bridget Sheehan was reported to have immigrated through New York from Ireland in 1853 aboard the British brig *Minnet*. This Bridget was 20 years old at the time, and she could have been the Bridget who was Hyams' second wife. She would have been about 30 years old at the birth of their first child.
20. Death certificate for Bridget Hyams, http://interactive.ancestry.com.
21. Admission to the Orphan House was limited to residents of the city of Charleston, and applicants needed proof of at least three years of residency in the city to qualify for entrance. By 1870, the year when the Hyams children were accepted by the Orphan House, Godfrey and Bridget Hyams would have met that requirement.
22. Marriage Bond Book #38, Christian County, Kentucky, Series L1566, Book 9 (1870–1872 [Whites]), pp. 230–231, Christian County Public Library, Hopkinsville, Kentucky.
23. Tenth U.S. Census, 1880. NARA. Record Group 29, T 9, Roll 409.
24. *Cincinnati Commercial Tribune*, March 27, 1876.
25. *Cincinnati Daily Gazette*, October 15, 1879.
26. Christian County Tax Lists, Roll 6 (#007929), 1857–1879; Microfilm 929.3 Tax, Box #75, 5, 1848–1875, Christian County Public Library, Hopkinsville, Kentucky.
27. Collins, L., and R.H. Collins. *Collins' Historical Sketches of Kentucky: History of Ken-

tucky, vol. 1. Covington, Kentucky: Collins, 1878, p. 246.
　28. Christian County Tax Lists, District #1, Roll 8 (#008291), 1880, p. 19; Christian County Public Library, Hopkinsville, Kentucky.
　29. Christian County Tax Lists, Roll 9 (#008329), 1857–1879; Christian County Public Library, Hopkinsville, Kentucky.
　30. *Hopkinsville (KY) Semi-weekly South Kentuckian*, March 24, 1885.
　31. Twelfth Census, 1900. NARA. Record Group 29, T 623; Thirteenth Census, 1910. NARA. Record Group 29, T 624.
　32. Personal Communication. Family meeting of descendants of Godfrey Hyams: Sonny and Goldie Newcomb and Martha Gleerup, November 4, 2015, Trenton, Kentucky.
　33. *Ibid.*
　34. *Ibid.*
　35. Davis, Jefferson. *The Papers of Jefferson Davis*, vol. 14, 1880–1889. Crist, Lynda Lasswell, and Suzanne Scott Gibbs, Introduction by William C. Davis. Baton Rouge: Louisiana State University Press, 2015. Unpaginated e-book.
　36. *Ibid.*

Chapter 16

　1. *Philadelphia Inquirer*, August 4, 1865.
　2. *Nashville (TN) Daily Union and American*, December 31, 1865.
　3. Pitman, *Assassination of President Lincoln*, 373.
　4. Letter, C.C. Leathers to James Bowen, April 28, 1866, https://www.fold3.com/image/22900501; https://www.fold3.com/image/22900504.
　5. Impeachment Investigation: Testimony Taken Before the Judiciary Committee of the House of Representatives in the Investigation of the Charges Against Andrew Johnson. Second Session Thirty-Ninth Congress and First Session Fortieth Congress. Washington: Government Printing Office, 1867, p. 564.
　6. *Lewiston (ME) Evening Journal*, May 1, 1867.
　7. Letter, Luke P. Blackburn to Andrew Johnson, September 4, 1867, as cited in Bergeron, Paul H., ed. *The Papers of Andrew Johnson*, vol. 13, September 1867–March 1868. Knoxville: University of Tennessee Press, 1996, pp. 15–16.
　8. Letter, David Thurston to William H. Seward, Dispatch #223, September 17, 1867, U.S. Department of State, as cited in Bergeron, Paul H., ed. *The Papers of Andrew Johnson*, vol. 13, September 1867–March 1868. Knoxville: University of Tennessee Press, 1996, pp. 15–16.
　9. *Harrisburg (PA) Telegraph*, September 26, 1867.
　10. *Little Rock Arkansas Gazette*, July 24, 1869.
　11. U.S. IRS Tax Assessments Lists, 1862–1918, Division #2, Collection District #2, State of Arkansas, 1869, No. 97, http://interactive.ancestry.com.
　12. *Memphis Public Ledger*, September 24, 1873.
　13. Keating, J.M. *History of the Yellow Fever Epidemic of 1878 in Memphis, Tenn*. Memphis: Howard Association, 1879, p. 385.
　14. Procter, John R. "Notes on the Yellow Fever Epidemic at Hickman, KY., During the Summer and Autumn of 1878." Frankfort: Yeoman Office, E.H. Porter, 1879. Accessed at the National Library of Medicine, https://collections.nlm.nih.gov/ext/kirtasbse/9715909/PDF/9715909.pdf.
　15. *Daily Los Angeles Herald*, November 14, 1878, citing the *Louisville Courier-Journal*.
　16. Hickman City Cemetery, http://www.findagrave.com
　17. Keating, *History of the Yellow Fever Epidemic*, 56–57.
　18. *Daily Los Angeles Herald*, November 14, 1878, citing the *Louisville Courier-Journal*.
　19. *Hickman (KY) Courier*, September 5, 1879.
　20. *Cloverport (KY) Breckenridge News* (Supplement), May 14, 1879.
　21. *Hopkinsville South Kentuckian*, May 6, 1879.
　22. Letter, Luke P. Blackburn to Jefferson Davis, February 26, 1878. In Rowland, Dunbar, ed. *Jefferson Davis: Constitutionalist; His Letters, Papers and Speeches*. Volume 8. Jackson: Mississippi Department of Archives and History, 1923, pp. 118–119.
　23. Baird, Nancy D. "The Yellow Fever Plot." *Civil War Times Illustrated* 13, no. 7 (November 1974), 22.
　24. *Troy Weekly Kansas Chief*, June 26, 1879.
　25. Eberson, Frederick. "Yellow Fever and Yellow Journalism: Dr. Luke Pryor Blackburn, 1816–1887," citing the *Louisville Commercial*. In *Portraits: Kentucky Pioneers in Community Health and Medicine*, Lexington: University of Kentucky Medical Center, 1968, p. 57.
　26. *Ibid.*, 58.
　27. *Hickman (KY) Courier*, June 13, 1879, citing the *Louisville Courier-Journal*.
　28. Harrison, Lowell H., ed. *Kentucky's Governors*. Lexington: University Press of Kentucky, 2004, p. 112.
　29. *St. Clairsville (OH) Belmont Chronicle*, August 28, 1879.

30. *New York Times*, September 3, 1879.
31. *Little Rock Arkansas Gazette*, October 3, 1879.
32. Eberson, *Yellow Fever and Yellow Journalism*, 58.
33. *Appletons' American Annual Cyclopaedia and Register of Important Events of the Year 1880*. New Series, vol. 5 (Whole Series, vol. 20), D. New York: Appleton, 1881, p. 423.
34. *Rockford (IL) Daily Gazette*, April 7, 1887.
35. Duncan, Fannie Casseday. "An Appreciation of a Kentucky Physician, Surgeon, and Governor—Luke P. Blackburn." Paper read before Filson Club, May 1, 1922, Mss BI/F489b/41. Filson Historical Society, Louisville, Kentucky.
36. Ellison, T. Kyle. "Prisons." In Kleber, John E., ed., *The Kentucky Encyclopedia*. Lexington: University Press of Kentucky, 1992, pp. 742–743.
37. *Fort Wayne Daily Gazette*, July 23, 1882.
38. Deems, Charles Force. "The Mountain Evangelist," in *Frank Leslie's Sunday Magazine*. Talmage, T. De Witt, ed. New York: Frank Leslie's, volume 13, January–June 1883, pp. 7–8.
39. Price, W. T. *Without Scrip or Purse; or, "The Mountain Evangelist," George O. Barnes.* Louisville: W.T. Price, 1883, p 302.
40. Scalf, Henry P. "The Mountain Evangelist." In *Kentucky's Last Frontier*. Johnson City, TN: Overmountain Press, 1966, pp. 264–265.
41. Price, *Without Scrip or Purse*, 362.
42. *Rockford (IL) Daily Gazette*, April 7, 1887; *(KY) Big Sandy News*, September 22, 1887.
43. Blackburn, Luke Pryor. In *The Americana: A Universal Reference Library*. Beach, Frederick Converse, ed. New York: Scientific American Compiling Department, vol. 3, 1912, unpaginated.
44. John F. Jefferson Scrapbook, 1849–1887, vol. 19, pp. 83ff. Filson Historical Society, Louisville, Kentucky.
45. Duncan, "An Appreciation of a Kentucky Physician."
46. Jefferson Scrapbook.
47. Blackburn, Luke Pryor. FindAGrave.com, http://www.findagrave.com
48. Eberson, "Yellow Fever and Yellow Journalism," 52–59.
49. Hippocratic Oath, https://www.britannica.com/topic/Hippocratic-oath.
50. Wakefield, Karen June. "A Case Study of the Infusion of Bioethics into a Medical School Curriculum." Ph.D. thesis, Texas A&M University, 2014.

Bibliography

Abbott, John Stevens Cabot. *The History of the Civil War in America; Comprising a Full and Impartial Account of the Origin and Progress of the Rebellion, of the Various Naval and Military Engagements, of the Heroic Deeds Performed by Armies and Individuals, and of Touching Scenes in the Field, the Camp, the Hospital, and the Cabin.* Springfield, MA: Gurdon Bill, 1863 (vol. 1) and 1866 (vol. 2).

Appletons' American Annual Cyclopaedia and Register of Important Events of the Year 1880. New York: Appleton, 1881.

Baird, Nancy Disher. *Luke Pryor Blackburn: Physician, Governor, Reformer.* Lexington: The Kentucky Bicentennial Bookshelf, University Press of Kentucky, 1979.

Barnes, Joseph K., George A. Otis, and D.L. Huntington. *The Medical and Surgical History of the War of the Rebellion (1861–1865).* Washington: Government Printing Office, 1883.

Beach, Frederick Converse, ed. *The Americana: A Universal Reference Library.* New York: Scientific American Compiling Department, 1912.

Bermuda Pocket Almanack, for the Year of Our Lord 1865: Calculated for Bermuda, and Containing Everything Necessary for an Almanack. Hamilton, Bermuda: D. M'Phee Lee, Office of the Royal Gazette, 1865.

Bouquet, Henry. *The Papers of Col. Henry Bouquet.* Series 21634. Edited by Sylvester K. Stevens and Donald H. Kent. Northwestern Pennsylvania Historical Series. Harrisburg: Pennsylvania Historical Commission, 1940.

Boyko, John. *Blood and Daring: How Canada Fought the American Civil War and Forged a Nation.* Toronto: Alfred K. Knopf Canada, 2013.

Caldwell, Charles. *Autobiography of Charles Caldwell, M.D., with Preface, Notes, and Appendix by Harriot W. Warner.* Philadelphia: Lippincott, Grambo, 1855.

Collins, L., and R.H. Collins. *Collins' Historical Sketches of Kentucky: History of Kentucky.* Volume 1. Covington, KY: Collins, 1878.

Craven, John J. *Prison Life of Jefferson Davis, Embracing Details and Incidents in His Captivity, Particulars Concerning His Health and Habits, Together with Many Conversations on Topics of Great Public Interest.* New York: Carleton, 1866.

Cumming, Carman. *Devil's Game: The Civil War Intrigues of Charles A. Dunham.* Urbana: University of Illinois Press, 2004.

Cunningham, H.H. *Doctors in Gray: The Confederate Medical Service.* Baton Rouge: Louisiana State University Press, 1986.

Davenport, Edward A., ed. *History of the Ninth Regiment Illinois Cavalry Volunteers.* Chicago: Donohue & Henneberry, 1888.

Davis, Jefferson. *The Papers of Jefferson Davis.* Edited by Lynda Lasswell Crist, Barbara J. Rozek, and Kenneth H. Williams. Baton Rouge: Louisiana State University Press, 2003 and 2004.

_____. *The Papers of Jefferson Davis.* Lynda Lasswell Crist and Suzanne Scott Gibbs. Baton Rouge: Louisiana State University Press, 2015.

Bibliography

Deichmann, Catherine Lynch. *Rogues and Runners. Bermuda and the American Civil War.* Hamilton, Bermuda: Bermuda National Trust Collection, 2003.
Druitt, Robert. *The Principles and Practice of Modern Surgery.* Philadelphia: Blanchard and Lea, 1860.
Eastman, Margaret Middleton Rivers. *Hidden History of Civil War Charleston.* Charleston, SC: History Press, 2012.
Eberson, Frederick. *Portraits: Kentucky Pioneers in Community Health and Medicine.* Lexington: University of Kentucky Medical Center, 1968.
Edwards, William C. *The Lincoln Assassination: The Trial Transcript.* A transcription of NARA Microfilm File M599, Reels 8 Through 16, 2012. https://books.google.com/books?id=Myx3QihsH4IC&printsec=frontcover&source=gbs_ge_summary_r&cad=0#v=onepage&q&f=false.
Edwards, William C., and Steers, Edward, Jr. *The Lincoln Assassination: The Evidence.* Urbana: University of Illinois Press, 2009.
Eubank, Damon R. *In the Shadow of the Patriarch: The John J. Crittenden Family in War and Peace.* Macon, GA: Mercer University Press, 2009.
Foote, Shelby. *The Civil War: A Narrative.* Alexandria: Time-Life Books, 2000.
Foreman, Amanda. *A World on Fire: Britain's Crucial Role in the American Civil War.* New York: Random House, 2012.
Harris, Thomas Maley. *Assassination of Lincoln: A History of the Great Conspiracy.* Boston: American Citizen, 1892.
Harrison, Lowell H., ed. *Kentucky's Governors.* Lexington: University Press of Kentucky, 2004.
Hattaway, Herman, Jon L. Wakelyn, and Clayton E. Jewett. *Shades of Blue and Gray.* Columbia: University of Missouri Press, 1999.
Headley, John W. *Confederate Operations in Canada and New York.* New York: Neale, 1906.
Horner, Dave. *The Blockade-Runners: True Tales of Running the Yankee Blockade of the Confederate Coast.* New York: Dodd, Mead, 1968.
Hutchinson, William Nelson. *Standing Orders Issued to the Two Battalions, XXth Regiment, at Bermuda, in 1842.* London: W. Clowes & Sons, 1845.
Jones, John William. *Davis Memorial Volume; or Our Dead President, Jefferson Davis and the Tribute to His Memory.* Richmond: B.F. Johnson, 1889.
Keating, J.M. *History of the Yellow Fever Epidemic of 1878 in Memphis, Tenn.* Memphis, TN: Howard Association, 1879.
Keehn, David C. *Knights of the Golden Circle: Secret Empire, Southern Secession, Civil War.* Baton Rouge: Louisiana State University Press, 2013.
Kennedy, Sister Jean de Chantel. *Biography of a Colonial Town: Hamilton, Bermuda, 1790–1897.* 2nd ed. Hamilton, Bermuda: Bermuda Bookstore, 1963.
Kinchen, Oscar A. *Confederate Operations in Canada and the North: A Little-Known Phase of the American Civil War.* North Quincy, MA: Christopher, 1970.
Kleber, John E., ed. in chief; Clark, Thomas D., Lowell H. Harrison, and James C. Klotter, Associate ed. *The Kentucky Encyclopedia.* Lexington: University Press of Kentucky, 1992.
Kline, Michael J. *The Baltimore Plot.* Yardley, PA: Westholme, 2008.
LeMaster, Carolyn Gray. *A Corner of the Tapestry: A History of the Jewish Experience in Arkansas, 1820s-1990s.* Fayetteville: University of Arkansas Press, 1994.
Marquis, Greg. *In Armageddon's Shadow: The Civil War and Canada's Maritime Provinces.* Montreal: McGill-Queen's University Press, 2000.
Mayers, Adam. *Dixie and the Dominion: Canada, the Confederacy, and the War for the Union.* Toronto: Dundurn, 2003.
McNeil, Jim. *Masters of the Shoals: Tales of the Cape Fear Pilots Who Ran the Union Blockade.* Cambridge, MA: Da Capo-Perseus, 2003.
Miller, Francis Trevelyan, and Robert S. Lanier, ed. *The Photographic History of the Civil War in Ten Volumes.* New York: Review of Reviews, Trow, 1912.
Moore, Albert B. *Conscription and Conflict in the Confederacy.* Columbia: University of South Carolina Press, 1924.

Morgan, James Morris. *Recollections of a Rebel Reefer.* Boston: Houghton Mifflin, Riverside Press Cambridge, 1917.
Munroe, James Phinney. *Adventures of an Army Nurse in Two Wars, Edited from the Diary and Correspondence of Mary Phinney, Baroness von Olnhausen.* Boston: Little, Brown, 1904.
Official Guide and Album of the Cunard Steamship Company. Liverpool: Sutton Sharpe, 1877.
Official Records of the Union and Confederate Navies in the War of the Rebellion; Original Records of the Civil War [ORN] Washington: Government Printing Office, 1896.
Pitman, Benn. *The Assassination of President Lincoln and the Trial of the Conspirators.* Cincinnati: Moore, Wilstach & Baldwin, 1865.
Price, W.T. *Without Scrip or Purse; or, "The Mountain Evangelist," George O. Barnes.* Louisville, KY: W.T. Price, 1883.
Rowland, Dunbar, ed. *Jefferson Davis, Constitutionalist: His Letters, Papers and Speeches.* Volume 8. Jackson: Mississippi Department of Archives and History, 1923.
Scalf, Henry P. *Kentucky's Last Frontier.* Johnson City, TN: Overmountain Press, 1966.
Simkins, Francis Butler, and Robert Hilliard Woody. *South Carolina During Reconstruction.* Chapel Hill: University of North Carolina Press, 1932.
Singer, Jane. *The Confederate Dirty War: Arson, Bombings, Assassination and Plots for Chemical and Germ Attacks on the Union.* Jefferson, NC: McFarland, 2005.
Speer, Lonnie R. *Portals to Hell: Military Prisons of the Civil War.* Mechanicsburg, PA: Stackpole Books, 1997.
Steers, Edward, Jr. *Blood on the Moon: The Assassination of Abraham Lincoln.* Lexington: University Press of Kentucky, 2001.
Steiner, Paul F. *Disease in the Civil War: Natural Biological Warfare in 1861–1865.* Springfield, IL: Charles C. Thomas, 1968.
Stillé, Alfred. *Therapeutics and Materia Medica: A Systematic Treatise on the Action and Uses of Medicinal Agents, Including Their Description and History.* Vols. 1 and 2. Philadelphia: Blanchard and Lea, 1860.
Tidwell, William A. *April '65: Confederate Covert Action in the American Civil War.* Eastern European Studies 1. Kent: Kent State University Press, 1995.
Tidwell, William A., with James O. Hall and David Winfred Gaddy. *Come Retribution: The Confederate Secret Service and the Assassination of Lincoln.* Jackson: University Press of Mississippi, 1988.
Tripler, Chas. S., and George C. Blackman. *Handbook for the Military Surgeon: Being a Compendium of the Duties of the Medical Officer in the Field, the Sanitary Management of the Camp, the Preparation of Food, Etc.; With Forms for the Requisitions for Supplies, Returns, Etc.; the Diagnosis and Treatment of Camp Dysentery; and All the Important Points in War Surgery: Including Gunshot Wounds, Amputation, Wounds of the Chest, Abdomen, Arteries and Head, and the Use of Chloroform.* Cincinnati: Robert Clarke, 1861.
Vandiver, Frank E. *Confederate Blockade Running Through Bermuda, 1861–1865: Letters and Cargo Manifests.* Austin: University of Texas Press, 1947.
Waite, P.B. *The Life and Times of Confederation, 1864–1867: Politics, Newspapers, and the Union of British North America.* Toronto: University of Toronto Press, 1962.
Walker, Georgiana Gholson. *The Private Journal of Georgiana Gholson Walker, 1862–1865, With Selections from the Post-War Years, 1865–1876.* Edited by Dwight Henderson Franklin. Confederate Centennial Studies. Tuscaloosa: Confederate, 1963.
The War of the Rebellion: A Compilation of the Official Records of the Union and Confederate Armies; Original Records of the Civil War [ORA]. Washington: Government Printing Office, 1902.
Wiche, Glen N., ed. *Dispatches from Bermuda: The Civil War Letters of Charles Maxwell Allen, United States Consul at Bermuda, 1861–1888.* Kent: Kent State University Press, 2008.
Wilkinson, Henry Campbell. *Bermuda from Sail to Steam: A History of the Island from 1784–1901.* London: Oxford University Press, 1973.
Winks, Robin W. *The Civil War Years: Canada and the United States.* Montreal: McGill-Queen's University Press, 1998.

Index

acid, carbolic 8
Adams, Benjamin J. 47
Adelaide Street 51, 151
Aedes aegypti 20, 149, 194
Agnes Street 151
Alabama 49–50, 69, 72–74, 191, 207
alcohol 16, 42
Alexander, Gustave 34, 131, 133
Alexandria, Virginia 172
Allen, Charles Maxwell 30, 32, 35–36, 50, 96, 123–125, 127, 129–130, 133–135, 155
Alpha 77, 79, 88–91, 93–96, 103–105, 107, 110, 129
Alston, Waldeman 26, 69
Alton Prison 65, 85, 145
ambulance service 39
American Hotel 27, 114
American Museum 84
Amery, Dinah 134
Amherst, Jeffrey 123
ammunition 2, 34, 42, 47, 88, 135; *see also* munition
amnesty 168, 184, 187, 191, 193–194, 206–208
amputations 38, 43–44
antibiotics 38
antisepsis 8, 38
apoplexy 198
apprenticeship 9–10, 17, 39, 53, 199
Arkansas 15, 49, 54–64, 66, 145, 201, 208
Arnold, Samuel 154, 168
arrowroot 104
arsenic 84
arson 85, 186, 193
artist's case 202
assassin, assassinate, assassination 20, 26, 30, 68, 73, 76, 108, 117, 119, 130, 134, 143–144, 153–155, 159, 160–161, 163–165, 170–174, 179, 181–182, 186, 189–190, 192, 202, 205, 212
assault 59, 74, 197–198
assize 138–139, 147
asthma 75, 178
Astor House 113–114

Atzerodt, George A. 154, 168–169
auction, auctioneer 71, 95, 109, 114, 116, 172, 206
Augusta, Georgia 189

bacteria 8–9, 51
Bahamas 23, 32, 34, 36, 88
Baker, George E. 161–162
Baker, La Fayette C. 143, 162–164
ball, Minié or Minnie 44
ballast 104
Baltimore, Maryland 19, 78, 96, 109, 114–116, 146, 160, 164, 175
Bank of Montreal 182, 190
Barber, Samuel 89
Barclay, Curle, and Company 89
Barnes, George Owen 216
Barnum, P.T. 84–85
barque, bark 111–113, 164, 166
Barrack Hill 36, 134
Barrow, T.W. 86, 95
Bates, Louis F. 174
battery 197–198
Beall, John Yates 81
Beauregard, P.G.T. 62, 74
bedclothes 95, 134
bedding 52, 59, 67, 103, 127, 129, 131, 137, 139, 196
Belle Isle Prison 69
Bellevue, Bedford County, Virginia 192–193
Belot, Charles (Carlos) M. 105–107
Belot, Edward (Eduardo) 105–107
Belt, John B. 106–107
Benjamin, Judah P. 83, 103, 154, 189
Benton Barracks 65
Bermuda 2–5, 23, 30–37, 50, 67, 77–79, 86–91, 94–98, 100, 102–105, 107, 109, 111, 118–120, 122–125, 127, 129–130, 132, 134–142, 146, 152, 155–157, 173, 188, 191, 193–194, 205, 211, 213–214, 217–219
Bermuda Hotel 100
Beth El 57
Bethel Baptist Church 203
Bible 139, 175

245

Big #2 114, 166–117
Bingham, John A. 153–154, 174, 205
Bishop, John 65
Black, George P. 34, 122, 130–131
Black, William Anderson 89
black flag 40, 68–71, 84, 172
black ops 144, 170
Blackburn, Abby 18
Blackburn, Cary Bell 14, 17
Blackburn, Churchill H. 8, 15
Blackburn, Edward M. 7–8
Blackburn, Henrietta 57
Blackburn, James W. 57, 64, 66
Blackburn (Churchill), Julia Maria Preston Pope 17, 18, 51, 216
Blackburn, Lavinia Bell 8, 17
Blackburn Sanitarium for Nervous and Mental Diseases 217
blackmail 122, 133
Blackman, William 134
blankets 56, 95, 111, 123, 126, 132, 134, 136–138, 199, 206, 208, 210
blisters 8, 16, 210
blockade-runner 23–24, 28, 30–35, 50, 78, 81, 88, 119, 122, 135, 152, 188–189, 191
Blocking (Blockading) Squadron, West Gulf, East Gulf, North Atlantic, South Atlantic 30, 32, 36, 50, 191
Bloomer, Mr. 145
B'Nai Jeshurun 57
Booth, John Wilkes 25–26, 76, 85, 114, 144, 153–155, 163–164, 170–171, 173–174, 186–187, 190
Boston, Massachusetts 2, 19, 21, 24, 52, 85, 96, 109, 111–114, 116, 146, 161, 164–168, 175, 196
Boston Customs House 114, 146
Boswell, Ella Gist 14–17
Bouquet, Henry 123
Bourbon County, Kentucky 12
Bourne, John Tory 35
Bowen, James 206–207
Boyle, J.T. 51
brandy 26, 42, 210
Breckinridge, John C. 174
Breckinridge, W.C.P. 213
Bremier, Albert (aka Brenner) 116–117
bribes 124, 135, 146, 168
Bright's disease 194
Britain 23, 28, 32–33, 35, 88, 95
British Columbia 89
Broad Street 196–198
brogans 56–57
bronze John 19, 21
Browning, S. 27
Buchanan, James 73
Buckinghamshire, Eighth Earl of 191
Buckner, Simon Bolivar 46
Buckstaff, Frederick 130–131, 133–134, 137, 140–141

Buffalo, New York 81, 154
Bureau of Military Justice 131, 155, 167, 186–187
Burland, Benjamin 125, 127, 131–132
Burnett, H.L. 153, 163
Burns, William S. 74
Burnside, Ambrose Everett 51
Bursted, A.J. (aka Rursted) 114
Burton, James H. 90
Butler, Benjamin F. 20–22, 69, 116

Cahill, James 145
Cairo, Illinois 185
Caldwell, Charles 10–11
calomel 11, 16, 42, 120
Camden, Arkansas 57
Cameron, Frances 135–137
Cameron, John, Jr. 119
Cameron, M.C. 145, 147–148
Cameron, Simon 46
Campbell, John Archibald 69
Campbell, Robert Anson 170, 190
camphor 67, 115, 118
Canada 2, 5, 23–27, 50, 57, 63, 65–66, 70–83, 91, 93, 95–96, 106, 114–117, 125, 130–132, 142–151, 154–155, 158–164, 167–168, 170–174, 178, 181–182, 185, 188–190, 192–193, 200, 205–207, 213–214, 216–218; East 23, 24, 79, 178; Lower 23; Upper 23, 144; West 23, 24, 79, 114, 145, 205
Canadian Confederates 67, 72, 74, 77, 82, 84, 154, 160–161, 188, 203
Cape Fear 78, 135, 191
Cape Sable 112
captains 32–34, 38, 59, 63, 65, 71–72, 75, 78, 81–82, 90, 104, 111–112, 114, 135, 137, 164–166, 186, 190–191, 203
Captain Galloway's Coast Guard Company 135
Cardwell, Edward 147
Caribbean 19
carpenter 57, 157, 173, 199
Carr, Eugene A. 61
Carroll Hall 177
Carter, Jimmy 184
Carter, John C. 81
Casa de Salud 106
Castle Harbor 125
Castleman, John Breckinridge 75
Catholic 143, 216
Cawood, Charles H. 83
Champion 181
Charleston, South Carolina 2, 5, 20, 30–32, 140, 188–189, 196–200
Charleston County Militia 197
Charleston Daily News 198
Charleston Orphan House 198–199
Charlotte, North Carolina 174
Chase, Salmon Portland 180–181, 183–184
Chatham, Ontario 123, 157

Index

Chattanooga, Tennessee 209
cherries 11
Chesapeake 76
Chesapeake Affair 76, 79, 193
Chester, Samuel 171
Chestnut Street Prison 65
Chicago 24, 81–82, 84–85, 159
chickenpox 42
Childress, Eliza Miller Nichols 200
Childress, John 200
chloroform 41, 43
cholera 8–12, 15, 22, 54, 125, 150, 205
cholera maligna 10–12
Christian County, Kentucky 200–202
Christmas Day Proclamation 184, 207
Churchill, Samuel B. 215
cigars 26, 67, 115, 118
Cincinnati Commercial Tribune 200
Cincinnati Daily Gazette 201
Cincinnati Gazette 5, 105, 212
ciphers 25, 171, 173–174, 189
citizens 5, 20, 22, 32, 36, 54, 57, 59–62, 64–65, 68, 70, 106, 124, 138, 144, 148, 159, 172, 184, 191, 198, 201, 206–208, 211–212, 218
Clark, E.M. 158
Clark, Lewis 203
Clark and Jones 112
Clay, Clement 26, 72–77, 79–82, 103, 115, 117, 144, 153–154, 174–176, 178–179, 188–191, 193, 206
Cleary, William W. 70, 72, 76–80, 103, 119, 144–147, 153, 168, 171, 174, 189, 193–194
clemency 193, 215
Cleveland, Ohio 81
Clifton House 27, 77, 80, 115, 125, 131, 146
Clinton, H.V. 114
clothing 44, 52, 56, 59, 67, 71, 86, 102, 107, 110, 115–118, 124–127, 130–132, 134, 136–139, 142, 144–146, 152, 154, 156, 164, 172, 199, 208; contaminated 66–67, 103, 106–107, 111, 126, 149, 218–219
Clyde Shipyards 89, 91, 93, 175
coal 28, 32, 34, 80
coats 56, 116–117, 126, 144, 156, 210–211
coffee 9, 33, 79, 116, 210
Columbia, South Carolina 189
Columbus, Kentucky 48
Columbus, Mississippi 49
coma 9, 95, 217
Commonwealth 114
competence 83
Condor 191
Confederate Benevolence Society 67, 121
Confederate Medical Branch (Corps) 38–39, 40, 45
Confederate Ordnance Bureau 34
Confederate Secret Service 26, 71–73, 83, 147, 170, 186
Confiscation Act 61, 181
Conger, H.N. 106

Connors, C.W. 112
Conover, Sanford 108, 119, 163, 170, 206
Conrad, Thomas Nelson 83
contagion 11, 13, 19, 95, 125–126, 194, 208
contingencies, army 168
convict, convicted, conviction 2, 53, 56, 61, 82, 107, 134, 143, 148–149, 167–168, 174, 179–182, 184, 197, 215
Cooper, George E. 177–179
copperheads 79–80
Corinth, Mississippi 62, 74
Corporation of St. Georges 124, 127, 129, 132–133
cotton 32–33, 35, 42, 50, 54, 56, 61, 73–74, 123, 126, 132, 138, 207, 208
cotton gin 73
Covington, Kentucky 194
Crane, Cordial 114
Craven, Anna 178
Craven, John J. 175–178
Crenshaw, William 135
Crescent City 20
Croton Dam 84, 154
Cuba 23, 32, 50, 88, 103–109, 119
Cunard, Samuel 89
Cunard, William 89
Cunard Shipping (Cunard Lines) 88–89, 91
cupping 16
Curtis, Samuel Ryan 58–63, 145
Cynthiana, Kentucky 76, 194

Dahlgren, Ulric 69
Dahlgren Affair 69
Dalhousie Medical School 87
Dallas County, Alabama 207
dam 71, 84, 144
Dana, Charles Anderson 164, 175
Darrell, John Harvey 139
Darrell, Richard D. 130
Davenport, Robert 202
Davis, Jefferson 2, 15, 27, 36, 39, 41, 44, 49, 62, 68–72, 74–78, 80, 83, 103, 121, 147, 151, 153–155, 170–175, 177, 178–179, 181–183, 189, 192, 198–199, 202–203
Davis, Joseph Evan 75
Davis, Samuel 203
Davis, Varina 78, 178–179
death penalty 183
delirium 9, 95
Democratic National Convention 82
Denison, George T. 182
Desha County, Arkaksas 15, 55, 57
Detroit, Michigan 76, 81, 115, 143, 150, 156–160, 162, 164–165, 195–196
Detroit River 158
devil 5, 148, 212–213
Dicken, E.N. 200
disease: communicable 37, 100; infectious 4, 8–9, 12, 14, 38, 42, 45, 138; viral 19
Dixie 182

Index

Dockyard, British Royal Navy (Her Majesty's Dockyard) 30, 88
Donegana Hotel 26–27, 117
Dr. Black Vomit 212
Doctor John 202
Doering, Ben 214
Doran, John 110
Doran, Michael 110
double jeopardy 183
Douglas, H.K. 171
"Douglas Democrat" 58
Downer, Robert W. 203
Dunham, Charles A. 108, 119, 168, 170–172
Dutch courage 78
dysentery 42, 54, 60, 140
dyspepsia 177

Easter session 138
Eastern District of Michigan 159, 195
Eaton, William 173
Eccles, Henry 205
effluvia 106
Elkhorn, Tavern Battle of 58
Elliott, J.B. 28
Emmons, Halmer H. 76, 115, 143, 147, 150, 156–163, 165–166, 168
Emporium 98
England 2, 17, 33, 53, 58, 65, 88, 136, 142–143, 170, 172, 185, 198
epidemic 4–5, 8–9, 11, 13, 15–17, 19–20, 37, 51, 67, 86–87, 95–97, 102, 114, 117, 119–120, 122–124, 134, 142, 147, 149, 152, 194–195, 207–211, 219
Episcopal Church 172, 196, 217
erysipelas 177
Escorse, Michigan 158
Escorse River 158
ether 43
eulogy, eulogies 217
Europe 11, 14, 17, 28, 31–35, 84, 88, 118, 186–188, 228
Evans, Walter 4, 213
excrement 95, 102, 106, 126
execution 107, 177, 180–181, 183, 208
Exhibit Number 74 117
exile 187, 189, 206–207
explosives 151
exports 32, 86
extradition 143, 161

Fairview, Kentucky 202–203
Falmouth, England 88
false swearing 201
Fannie 119
Farmers' Hotel 110
farmworker 57
Father Matthew 210
Fay, General 163
felon, felony 191, 208
Fernandina, Florida 209

fever, gaol 19
fiend 5, 7, 144, 147, 192, 212
Finegan, Henry 171
firemen 33, 197
fomite 9, 158
Fort Caswell 135
Fort Curtis 62
Fort Delaware 175
Fort Donelson 28, 29
Fort Douglas 24, 82
Fort Fisher 78, 135, 191
Fort Lafayette 81, 85, 96
Fort McHenry 96, 175
Fort Pitt 123
Fort Warren 96, 175
Fort Washington, New York 17
Fortress Monroe 39, 175–177, 179, 189, 191
Fountain Hotel (aka Fountain Inn and Fountain House) 114–116
Four Corners of Law 196
Fourteenth Amendment 179, 182–184
Fox, John 124–125, 130, 138
Frankfort, Kentucky 14, 191, 215–217
Fraser, Trenholm and Company 185
Freemasons 66
Front Street 27, 98, 137

Gainesville, Alabama 49
Galloway, John Wesley 135–137
Galveston 30, 32, 207
gaol 19, 136, 138, 140
garments 67, 95, 102, 107, 115, 126, 134, 136, 196
Gayle, George W. 69, 207
Georgetown, South Carolina 140
Georgian 157, 167
germs 1, 8–10, 17, 33, 38, 50–51, 68, 71–74, 123, 219
Gholson, S.J. 187
Gibb's Point Lighthouse 135
Glasgow, Scotland 89
gold 32–33, 72, 83, 103, 111, 142, 146, 162, 170, 201–202, 208
Golding, William 59
Goodrich, John Zaccheus 164–165
Gorgas, Josiah 34–35
grand jury 62, 130, 151, 165, 182
Grant, Ulysses 48–49, 74, 154, 170, 207
Gratiot Street Military Prison 64, 85, 145
Gray, S. Brownlow 125, 127, 140
Greek fire 151, 159
Greeley, Horace 80, 181, 193
Green Island 112
Greenhow, Rose O'Neal 191–192
Gregor, George W. 115
grenade, hand 159
Gross, Samuel D. 17
guerrilla [guerilla] 7, 83, 190
Guernsey 126, 132
Gulf of Mexico 28

Index

Gulick, Captain 191
gunpowder 46

Habana Vieja 106
Halifax 111–113, 164–166
Halifax 24, 26–27, 32, 34–36, 50–51, 67, 77, 79, 87–89, 91, 93–96, 103–105, 107–113, 120, 122, 124, 130, 136, 143–144, 146, 148, 150, 164–166, 186, 188, 191, 193
Halifax Club 96
Halifax Hotel 87, 91, 109–111
Hall, Edwin J. 144, 146
Halleck, Henry W. 61, 176
Hallet, Henry L. 164–165
Hamilton, Bermuda 2, 30–31, 34, 96–98, 100–101, 105, 114, 117, 120, 127, 129, 134–141, 145, 159, 161, 190
Hamilton, Canada West 114, 117, 145, 159, 161, 190
Hamilton Hotel 96–98, 100–101, 120, 134–137, 140
Hamley, William George 141
Hampton Roads 175
Hand, Mr. 117
handkerchief 96, 123, 126, 132, 136–137
handwriting 3, 10, 17, 49, 157, 174
Hardin, Parker Watkins 213
Harper, George 153
Harris, J.W. 52, 67, 113–114, 116, 165, 206
Harrison, James 145
Harrison, Robert 155
Harrison County, Kentucky 76
Harrisonburg 170
Harvey, Seth 130, 133
Hastings, Sergeant Major 151
Havana, Cuba 30, 32, 50, 88, 103–106, 108–109, 123
Hawes, Richard 77
Hawthorn, George 132
Hay, John 76
Hayward, Ann 140
Hayward, Joseph M. 124, 130
Headley, John William 84–85
Helena, Arkansas 54–66, 145, 201, 208
Helena Boot and Shoe Manufactory 57
hemoglobin 9
Henderson, Kentucky 158
Herold, David 76, 154, 168–169
Hesslein's (hotel) 27
Hewett, Captain 191
Hickman, Hero of 4–5, 209, 211, 213, 217
Hickman, Kentucky 4–5, 209–211, 213, 217
Higinbothom, W.R. 127
Hill, Mr. 110
Hilton Head, South Carolina 175
Hindman, Thomas Carmichael 59–60
Hines, Thomas Henry 71, 75, 82
Hinson, Henry J. 120
Hippocratic Oath 218
Hobart-Hampton, Augustus Charles 191

Hodge, George Baird 49
Holcombe, James Philemon 72, 76–77, 79–81, 103, 108, 115, 117–118, 190–193, 206
Holt, Joseph 131, 143, 153, 155, 160, 164, 167, 174, 181, 190, 192–193
Hope, James 142
Hope, Mr. 190
Hopkins, John D. 105–107
Hopkinsville, Kentucky 2, 201, 213
hospital 14–17, 27, 39, 40, 42–43, 49–51, 60, 74, 87, 95–96, 98, 105–107, 123–124, 150, 154, 172, 175, 177–178, 199, 208–210
Hospital San Carlos 106–107
House of Representatives 140, 184
Hudson's Bay Company 23
Humphreys, Benjamin G. 187
Hunley 71
Hunter, Charles R. 114
Hunter, David 90, 104
Hunter, Frederick A.S. 140
Huntsville, Alabama 191
Hyams, Eliza 200
Hyams, Godfrey Joseph 202
Hyams, Henry Michael 121, 198–199
Hyams, Irene (Rena) 200, 202
Hyams, Jefferson Davis 121, 196, 198–199
Hyams, Joseph Godfrey 196, 198–199, 202
Hyams, Louisa 200
Hyams, Mamie 199
Hyams, Mary Jane (Mae) 196, 199, 202
Hyams, Robert Lee 200, 202
Hyams, Solomon 115
Hyams, Thomas Francis Stonewall Jackson 65, 196, 199
Hyde Park 196
Hyland, W.C.J. 130

ice 11, 16, 50, 79, 81, 210
inauguration 68, 213–214
indenture 199
indians 123
indict, indictment 61, 76, 147, 164–166, 168, 174–175, 179, 181–182, 184, 200, 218
infection, infected, infectious 4, 8–9, 12, 14, 17, 38, 42–45, 52, 67, 87, 95, 106–107, 110–111, 115, 117, 124–125, 127, 129–130, 132, 134, 137–139, 144–148, 152, 154–156, 159, 162, 164, 177, 206, 208, 211, 213
inmates 199
iodine 42
Ireland Island 88
Irwinsville, Georgia 175

Jackson, Mortimer M. 35
Jackson, Nathaniel 125, 130–132, 138
jail 53, 64, 81, 136, 138–141, 176, 194, 198
James, Edward K. 31
James, W.T. 98
jaundice 9
Jefferson County, Arkansas 54

Index

Jennings, Edward 87
Jews, Jewish 54, 57, 145, 200
Johnson, Andrew 62, 153, 166, 169–171, 174, 178, 180–182, 184, 186–187, 189, 191, 193, 206–207
Johnson, William K. 106–107, 119
Johnson's Island 24, 81, 85, 159
Jones, Thomas Laurens 211
julep 26

Kane, George Proctor 78, 95–96, 144
Keith, Alexander "Sandy" H. 87, 110
Kennedy, Robert 84–85, 186, 189–190
Kent, England 53
Kentucky 2, 4–5, 7–10, 12–15, 17–18, 38, 45, 49, 55, 66, 71–72, 75, 77, 82, 105–106, 158, 191, 194, 200–203, 207–217, 219
Kerr, Mr. 145
Key West, Florida 19
kidnap 1, 25–26, 68, 83, 144, 171–172, 203
Kilpatrick, Hugh Judson 69
Kirkwood Hotel (Kirkwood House) 164, 166
Knights of the Golden Circle 79
Koch, Robert 8

Lacey, Mr. 190
Lafarge House 85
Lafayette Square 47
Lake Ontario 181
laudanum 16
Leathers, C.C. 206
Lee, Edwin Gray 26, 83, 185–186
Lee, Robert E. 26, 28–29, 83, 156, 185
Leech, R.A. 114
leniency 180–181, 184
Lenient Luke 216
Letterman, Johnathan 39
Lewis, Samuel 156–158
Lexington, Kentucky 2, 10–12, 76, 214
Lexington, Virginia 151
Lexington Transcript 214
Libby Prison 154
limestone 54
Lincoln, Abraham 25–26, 28, 30, 36, 52, 61, 68, 70, 72, 74–76, 80, 83–84, 108, 110–111, 114, 117, 119, 130, 143–144, 148, 153–156, 159, 161, 163–166, 168, 170–171, 173–174, 179–182, 186–187, 189–190, 192–193, 196, 205–207, 212
Lincoln, William Wallace ("Willie") 75
Lister, Joseph 8, 44
Little Richmond 24
Little Rock Arkansas *Gazette* 208
Liverpool, England 88, 94, 170, 185–186
lodging house 121, 138
London, England 53, 88, 142, 196, 200
Long, Crawford Williamson 43
Long Island, New York 17
Lord of the Flies 59

Lothrop, Thornton K. 165
Louisiana 47, 207
Louisville, Kentucky 2, 38, 51, 66, 200, 208–209, 211, 213, 217
Louisville Commercial 213
Lowell, John 165–166
Luke, the Beloved Physician 217
Lusher, N.E. 98
Lusher Photographic Gallery 98
lying 87, 149, 201–203, 210

Macon, Georgia 189
Mageehan, Robert 136
Magoffin, Beriah 46–48
malaria 16, 42, 54, 59–60, 125
malevolence 11, 83
Manchester, England 53
manifests 95, 104–105
Mann, John 58
Margaret Evans 53
Marine Hospital 15–16
Marschall, Nicola 215
Martin, Hannah 53, 58, 198, 200
Martin, Robert M. 84
Martin, Tennessee 209
martyr 177, 180
Mary Celestia 135
Maryland 2, 28, 55, 116
Matamoros, Mexico 30, 32, 88
Maury, Dabney H. 50
McCulloh, Richard Sears 150–151
McDonald, William Lawrence 108, 146, 151, 167–168, 189
McGarry, Francis 143–144
McGill, John 189–190
McGregor, Captain (aka McGreggor and McGriffin) 111
McKeogh, M. 214
Meade, George G. 69
measles 42
medal 211
Medcalf, Francis Henry 145
Medical Hall of St. Georges 127
medicine 2, 8–9, 11, 14, 16, 38, 40, 42–43, 59, 205, 208–209, 211, 216, 219
Meeting Street 196
Memphis, Tennessee 54, 56, 60–61, 185, 188, 208–209
Memphis Boot, Shoe, and Leather Manufactory 56
Merritt, James B. 108, 163, 168
Meteor 63
Mexico 28, 32, 88, 189
miasma 8, 9, 11, 16, 51, 129, 150
Michigan 80–82, 85, 158–160, 165, 175, 195
Michigan 81–82, 85
Middletown, Connecticut 19
Miles, Nelson A. 176–177, 179
military commission 153–154, 167, 190
military department 153

Index

milk 11, 139, 199
Millroy's Wharf 181
ministry, prison 216
Minor, William T. 105–106, 108
misdemeanor 148
missile 151, 196
Mississippi 14–15, 45, 47, 49–50, 54–55, 57–58, 60–62, 64–65, 73–74, 84, 120, 187–188, 206, 209
Mississippi River 15, 54–55, 58, 60–61, 64–65, 209
Mississippi Township 57
Missouri 48, 55, 58, 61–62
Mobile, Alabama 20, 32, 50–51
Monck, Charles 95, 142, 147
money 14, 32, 35, 42, 72, 119, 143, 146, 158, 160–162, 164, 167–168, 170, 200, 216
Montgomery, Richard 171, 173
Montreal 2, 23–27, 67, 72, 79, 82, 108, 114–115, 117–119, 121, 142, 144, 146, 148, 150, 155, 170–171, 178, 181–182, 186, 190
Moore, Samuel Preston 49
Morgan's Raiders 71
Morton, Ellis W. 166
Morton, William T.G. 43
Mosby, John S. 83
mosquitoes 15, 20, 149–150, 194, 218
Mountain Evangelist 216
Mudd, Samuel A. 154, 168
mule 2, 55, 58–59, 63, 201
mumps 42
Munceytown 123
Mundy, Marcellus 51
munitions 32, 50, 84, 151, 159; *see also* ammunition
murder 26, 68, 70, 82, 111, 130, 144, 147, 150, 153–155, 169, 171, 179, 193, 198, 202, 218
musket 46–47
My Imprisonment and the First Year of Abolition Rule in Washington 191
Myres, G.L. (aka Myers) 116
Myrtle Street Prison 65

Nassau 30, 32, 34, 77, 88, 104–105, 119, 135, 152, 188
Natchez, Mississippi 8, 14–18, 120, 206
Natchez City Hospital 14–15
National Detective Police 143
National Hotel 116, 173
nativity 203
"Necessities and Exigencies" 73, 103
nepotism 215
neuralgia 17, 177, 179
Neuse River 149
neutrality 23, 30, 35, 41, 46–48, 71, 78, 79, 82, 143, 145, 147–148
New Bern, North Carolina 52, 109, 116–117, 124, 149–150
New Brunswick 23

New Inlet 191
New Orleans, Louisiana 5, 15, 18, 20–22, 30, 38, 46–48, 164, 207–208
New York 17, 19, 21, 24, 26–27, 34, 52–54, 57, 81, 84–85, 88, 96, 105, 114, 116, 122–123, 130, 133–134, 140, 147–148, 150, 154, 164, 181, 185–186, 188–189, 214
New York Herald 186
New York News 188
New York Times 27, 147, 214
New York Tribune 186
Newfoundland 23, 79, 111
Niagara Falls 24, 80–81, 125, 131
Niagara-on-the-Lake 182
Nichols, Jesse 200
Nichols, Kate Childress 200
Night Hawk 191
Niphon 191
noncombatants 69, 111, 148, 219
Nonsuch Island 100, 125–127, 129–132, 138
Norfolk, Virginia 52, 109, 114, 116, 124, 144
North Carolina 20, 3033, 52, 69, 73, 77, 88, 109, 117, 124, 135, 144, 149, 172, 174, 188, 191, 206
Nova Scotia 23–24, 32, 35, 76–77, 79, 87–88, 112–113, 144, 148, 150, 164
nuisance, nuisance inspector 124–125, 127, 130–132, 138–139
nurses 41, 87, 96, 134–137, 150

Oath of Allegiance 64, 191, 193, 207
Oath of Amnesty 193
O'Brien, Bryan 111–112, 164–165; *see also* John O'Brien
O'Brien, John 111, 164; *see also* Bryan O'Brien
offshore confederacy 35
Ogdensburg, New York 154
O'Laughlin, Michael 154, 168
Old Dominion 188
Old Havana 106
Oldfield's Royal Hotel Hamilton 100
Oldham, Williamson Simpson 70
Ontario 2, 23, 77, 117, 123, 155, 159, 170, 181, 190
opium 16, 42
Ord, Harry St. George 125
osteomyelitis 44
Ottawa 23, 26, 27
Ottawa Hotel 26–27
Outerbridge, R.W. 124, 130
Oxford, Mississippi 74, 188

Paine, Lewis 26
Pallen, Montrose 26, 84
pardon 117, 148, 155, 159–161, 168, 180, 184, 191–195, 203, 206–208, 215–216
Paris, France 14, 17, 188
Paris, Kentucky 9, 12
Parker House 113–114

252 Index

parole 178, 191–192, 216
passport 14
Pasteur, Louis 8
Paterson, Harrison, and Paterson 145
Paterson, James 145, 147, 162
Paterson, Robert A. 145
Patterson, William 164–165
pawn 110, 204
Payne, Lewis 26, 54
Pea Ridge, Battle of 58
Pemberton, John C. 74
penitentiary 56, 151, 216–217
Pennsylvania 116, 123
Pensacola, Florida 20, 30
perjurer, perjury 108, 156, 172, 201, 203
pestilence 2, 20, 81, 111, 119, 136, 154, 190, 193, 207–208
Pettus, John J. 49–50
phenol 8
Philadelphia, Pennsylvania 17, 19, 21, 52, 109, 114, 123, 133, 140, 144, 148, 164, 205
Philadelphia Inquirer 148, 205
Phillips County, Arkansas 54–55, 57, 63
Philo Parsons 81
photophobia 9
Pickford, Robert 89
Pickford and Black Company 89
Pine Bluff, Arkansas 54–55, 57, 208
pipe 176
Plan, Anaconda 28, 30, 88
plantation 54, 59–60, 73–74
pneumonia 42
poison 1, 8–9, 40, 44, 71–73, 84, 144, 154, 192, 204
police 34–35, 96, 124–125, 130–132, 140, 143–145, 147, 151, 197, 202
Polk, Leonidas 48
Port Royal, South Carolina 175
Porter, Richardson, and Company 56
portmanteau 126, 131–132
Posey, John Alexander 151, 157–158
Potts, John 163–164
poultice 129
pound, British 32, 127, 154
Powell, Lewis 26, 168–169
prayer book 139, 172, 175, 178
Presbyterian 15, 63, 66, 143, 216
prescriptions 14
Preston, S.S. 108, 111, 115
Price, Sterling 48–49
Prince Edward Island 23, 79
Princeton Theological School 216
Pritchard, Benjamin 175
proclamations 35, 48, 168, 181, 184, 186–187, 191, 193–194, 206–208
Proclamation of Amnesty 184, 187, 191, 193–194, 206–208
Proclamation of Neutrality 35, 48
Proclamation of Peace 181
protective custody 136

Protestantism 217
provost marshal 63–65, 143, 173
prussic acid 84
Public Enemy #1 196
Public Health Service Hospital 15
pyemia 44

quarantine 15–16, 20–22, 37, 100, 120, 125, 127, 131–132
quarantine station 37, 100, 125, 127, 131–132
Quebec 2, 23, 125, 131, 186
Queen 27, 35, 51, 65–66, 77, 121, 139, 142, 148, 162, 194, 211, 218
Queen Victoria 35, 142, 211
Queen's Court of Admiralty 218
Queen's Hotel 27, 51, 66, 77, 148, 162
quinine 16, 42

Radical Mountain Echo 213
railroads 54, 114, 149, 158
Rainey, Joseph Hayne 136, 140
Rainey, Susan 140
Raleigh 78
Rankin, G.S. 124, 130
Rattlesnake 188
reconciliation 180
reconstruction 177, 196
Red Cross 217
Redman, Francis P. 59
Reed, Walter 21
reform, prison 7, 215–216, 219
Regan, John H. 175
Regla 105–106
religion 59, 217
remedy, herbal 42, 202
repairs, shoe 108, 145, 155
repent, repentance 184
revival 216
rice 42, 79, 210
Richardson, W. 57
Richland Township, Arkansas 54
Richmond, Virginia 24, 26, 49, 68–70, 72, 77, 80, 83–84, 149–150, 154, 171–173, 181–182, 185, 192
Rise and Fall of the Confederate Government 182
Ritchie, A.J. 87
Rivals 182
Roach, Sallie 201
Roach, Sam 201
Roberts, Captain 191
Robinson, Stuart 63, 66–67, 103, 108, 110, 145–146, 195, 201, 206
rope 12, 110–111, 125, 131
Rothesay Castle 182
Royal Bermuda Yacht Club 137
Royal British Navy 142
Royal Ontario Bank 155
Rupert's Land 23
Russell, Alfred 159–163, 195

Index

sailors 14–15, 21, 33, 36–37, 95, 100, 119, 122, 125, 135, 166–167, 197
St. Albans, Vermont 24, 82, 143, 151, 154, 159, 161
St. Catharines 75, 146, 188
Saint Charles Hotel 47
St. Clairsville Belmont Chronicle 213
St. Francis Township, Arkansas 54
St. Georges 30–32, 34–36, 78, 86–88, 90, 94–95, 100, 102, 105, 120–121, 124–125, 127, 129–130, 132, 134, 136, 138–141, 194
St. John 27
St. Lawrence Hall 24–27, 82, 114, 142–144, 146, 182
St. Louis, Missouri 57, 63–65, 125, 131, 145, 164
St. Louis Hotel 125, 131
St. Michael's Episcopal Church 196
St. Paul's Episcopal Church 172
St. Thomas, Virgin Islands 32, 88–89, 91, 94, 103–105, 107, 109
salary 14, 34
saloon 89–90, 94, 148
Sanders, George 26, 76, 80–82, 119, 144, 153–154, 171, 174, 189, 193
Sandusky, Ohio 24, 81
sanitation 8, 21, 22, 42, 150
Savage, Thomas 106, 108
Savannah, Georgia 20, 30–32, 135, 175
Saverly House 27
schemes 2, 5, 24, 33, 51, 66–68, 70, 72–73, 76, 80–86, 106, 111, 115, 117–118, 130, 144, 147, 150, 155–157, 159, 161–162, 169, 173, 185, 190, 192–193, 214, 219
Schofield Barracks 65
scorched earth 58
Scotland 17, 89, 188
Scott, Winfield 28
secession 27, 32, 46, 75–76, 96, 180, 183–184
Seddon, James A. 71, 83, 103
seizures 9, 61, 63, 95
Selective Service 197
Selma (Alabama) Dispatch 207
Senate 48, 74–75, 184, 187
servant 8, 15, 96, 124, 163–164, 167, 201, 213
Seward, C.A. 106
Seward, William 27, 32, 68, 106, 130, 153–154, 156, 170, 174, 207–208
shackles 175
Sheehan, Bridget 58, 198, 200
sheets 95, 126, 132, 199
Shields, Hugh 65, 110
Shiloh, Battle of 63, 74
Shinbone Alley 36, 121, 134
shirts 52, 56, 60, 110–111, 116–117, 126, 129, 132, 137, 144, 148, 155, 165
shoe repair 108, 145, 155
shoemaker 2, 53, 55–57, 65, 71, 110, 172, 199–200, 202–203, 208
Shreveport, Louisiana 209

sickness 60, 89–90, 100, 148, 213–214
Silver Spray 146
Simonton, John M. 187
Simpson, James Young 43
Sinclair, Arthur 135
Sixth North Carolina Infantry 172
Slater, Catharine (Catherine) 97–98, 100–101, 134–137
Slater, John 87
Slaughter, H.C. 66, 108–109
slaves 8, 14–15, 26, 53, 55, 57–58, 60–62, 69, 74, 76, 140, 158, 180, 196, 201, 206
smallpox 9–10, 15, 36, 42, 51–52, 64, 86, 118, 123, 125, 154, 156, 158, 199, 212–213, 219
Smith, Andrew Jackson "Whiskey" 74
Smith, Gerritt 181
Smith, William 117
Smithfield, North Carolina 135
Snake, Scott's Great 28, 29
Sons of Israel 57
Sons of Liberty, Order of the 79–80, 82
Sons of Malta 79
South Road 135
Southern Relief Association 182
Spangler, Edward 154, 168, 173
Speed, James 158–161
Spring Station, Kentucky 7
squadrons, blockading 30, 32, 36, 50, 191
Stag 137
Stansbury, Smith 34
Stanton, Edwin M. 116, 167–168, 170, 174, 176–177, 181–182, 189, 192
Stanus, H. 155
Star 116
state borders 4, 48, 55, 72
steamboat 54–55, 63, 154
Steinacker, Henry Von 170–171
Stephens, Alexander H. 175
Stevens, Joseph Willington 136–137
Stewart, Alexander Hugh Holmes 72
Stewart, First Officer 135
Stewart, Kensey Johns 70, 103, 172–173
Stiegler and Siegel 117
Stonewall Brigade 171
"stranger's illness" 20
strychnine 84
submarines 71
sugar 42, 116
sulfuric acid 127, 132, 218
surety, sureties 130, 136, 138, 143, 147, 149
surgeons 17, 38–39, 41, 43–45, 48–49, 84, 86, 95, 132, 176–177, 217
surprise, October 4, 212
Surratt, John 26, 70, 76, 153, 168, 171–172, 174
Surratt, Mary 154, 169
sutlers 116, 206
swamp 59, 149
Swan, Christopher 140
Swan, Edward Cork 36, 121, 124, 127, 129, 131–133, 138–139, 140, 142, 155, 194

Swan, Kit 134
Swan, Matilda 132, 137, 140–141
Swayne, Noah Haynes 193
Sweet, Benjamin J. 82, 84
Swift Run Gap 170

Tappan, James Camp 63
Tappan Guards 63
Taylor, Thomas 152
Taylor, Zachary 11
Tennessee 49, 54, 62, 185, 188, 208–209
terrorism, terrorist 1, 7, 22, 68, 74, 84, 149, 150, 154
Terry, Reverend Mr. 94
Terry, William H. 173
tetanus 42, 44
Texas 28, 70, 207
Thies, James H. 124–125, 127, 130–132, 138
13th Arkansas Infantry Regiment Volunteers 63
Thistle 77–78
Thompson, Catherine 185–186, 188
Thompson, Jacob 26, 72–77, 79–84, 91, 93, 103, 115, 117–119, 143–144, 146–147, 151, 153–155, 160, 170–172, 174, 185–190, 193
Thompson, Stephen Joseph 91, 93
Thurston, David 147, 155–156, 162, 207
Tilghman, Lloyd 48
tobacco 32–33, 104, 108, 115–116, 120, 176, 203
tobacconist 115
Todd County, Kentucky 202
Toronto 23–24, 26–27, 51–53, 63, 65–67, 75, 77, 79, 103, 108, 110, 114–117, 121, 143–148, 150–151, 155–159, 162, 166, 168, 181–182, 195–196, 205, 207
Toronto Police Court 151
torpedo 151, 159
Townsend, E.D. 63, 176, 178
Tracey, Mr. 190
Train, Charles R. 165
traitor 69, 85, 152–153, 177, 187, 192, 196, 202
Transylvania University 10, 15, 76, 219
treachery 85, 203
treason 174, 179–184, 191
treatments 8–9, 11, 14–16, 35, 49, 63, 120, 134, 136–137, 176, 201, 207–210
Trent, William 123
Trenton, Kentucky 202
Trott, W.S. 124, 130
Troy, Kansas 212
trunks 44, 51, 67, 91, 95, 102–111, 113–119, 121–122, 124127, 129–134, 136–138, 140, 144, 146, 148–150, 160, 164–165, 168, 173, 190, 196, 218
Tucker, Beverly 26, 76, 120, 153–154, 171, 174, 189
Tucker, J.W. 80
Tucker, James 120
Tucker, Park B. 120

Tucker, Reverend Doctor 140
Tucker, W. Tudor 130
Tupelo, Mississippi 49, 74
Tupper, Charles 87
Tuscarora 175
typhoid 42, 54, 60
typhus 60

Uncle John 202
underclothing 126
Underwood, John Cox 211
Underwood, John Curtiss 180–184
Union Schoolhouse District 200–201
Union Secret Service 163
United States District Court 181–182
University of Mississippi 73
University of Virginia 76, 193

vaccines 10, 38
valises 110–111, 155
Vallandigham, Clement L. 80
Vancouver, British Columbia 89, 91, 93
Vancouver Island 89
Vanderbilt, Cornelius 181
Van Dorn, Earl 49, 58, 61–62
vapors 8, 43, 95, 129, 150–151
Vermont 24, 82, 159
Versailles, Kentucky 10–12, 14
vertigo 178–179
Vicksburg, Mississippi 49, 54, 62, 74
Victoria, British Columbia 89
Victoria Hotel 98, 137
Virgin, John 135–136
Virgin Islands 30, 32, 103–104, 109
Virginia 2, 28, 49, 52, 69, 72, 75–76, 109, 124, 144, 151, 171–172, 175, 179–182, 184, 189, 192–193, 200
Virginia State Penitentiary 151
viruses 9, 20, 51, 144
vitriol 127, 138
vomit, black 9, 19, 21, 87, 96, 126, 132, 150, 210, 212
vomit 8–10, 87, 95, 102, 126; *see also* black vomit
von Olnhausen, Mary Phinney 150

Wainwright, G. 124, 130
Walker, Georgiana Gholson 78, 140
Walker, James 65
Walker, L.P. 46–47
Walker, Mr. 117
Walker, Norman S. 35, 78, 122, 124, 131, 133, 138, 140
Wall, W.L. 116–117, 206
Wallace, Charlatt 201
Wallace, James 201
Wallace, James Watson 108, 119, 170
War Department 143, 162–163, 173
warden 139, 216
Ware, John 202

Index

warfare: biologic 1, 9, 156; germ 1, 10, 33, 68, 71–74, 123, 219
Washington and Lee University 151
Washington College 151
water 1, 11, 15–16, 28, 34, 54–55, 58, 60, 71–73, 78, 81, 84, 87, 94–95, 97–98, 100–101, 106, 135, 139, 144, 149, 154, 210
weapon of mass destruction 1, 84, 102, 219
Weekly Kansas *Chief* 212
Weichmann, Louis 171
Weir, Benjamin 79
Wells, Frederick B. 35
West, Absolom M. 50
West Christian County 200
Westcott, James 26
Weston, John F. 63
wetlands 149
Wheeler, Joseph 175
Whelan, Mary A. 65
White House 75, 83, 111
whooping cough 42

William P. Clyde 175
Wilmington, North Carolina 20, 30–33, 77–78, 88, 90, 135, 188, 191–192
Wilson, James H. 189
Wilson, Lieutenant 192
Winchester, Boyd 213
Winter Garden Theatre 85
witnesses 5, 54, 77, 106–108, 117, 119, 130, 132–134, 136–137, 142–146, 151, 153, 155–156, 159, 162–168, 170, 172–173, 189, 192, 195, 218
Woodford County, Kentucky 7, 9, 10, 12, 14
Woolf, Lafayette I. 197–198

Yates, Paul Christian 40
Yellow Island Lighthouse 89
yellow jack 15, 19, 21, 67
Yonge Street 27, 181
York Street 27, 157–158
Young, Bennett H. 82, 151, 159, 167–168
Young, George 153

www.ingramcontent.com/pod-product-compliance
Ingram Content Group UK Ltd.
Pitfield, Milton Keynes, MK11 3LW, UK
UKHW041935140426
5217IPUK00014B/490